The Complete Guide to Nutrition in Primary Care

Edited by

Darwin Deen, MD, MS

Professor of Clinical Family and Social Medicine
Department of Family and Social Medicine
Albert Einstein College of Medicine, New York
www.drdeen.com

Lisa Hark, PhD, RD

Director, Nutrition Education and Prevention Program
University of Pennsylvania School of Medicine
www.lisahark.com

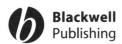

Blackwell
Publishing

© 2007 Blackwell Publishing Ltd
Blackwell Publishing, Inc., 350 Main Street, Malden, Massachusetts 02148-5020, USA
Blackwell Publishing Ltd, 9600 Garsington Road, Oxford OX4 2DQ, UK
Blackwell Science Asia Pty Ltd, 550 Swanston Street, Carlton, Victoria 3053, Australia

The right of the Author to be identified as the Author of this Work has been asserted in accordance
with the Copyright, Designs and Patents Act 1988.

First published 2007

1   2007

Library of Congress Cataloging-in-Publication Data

The complete guide to nutrition in primary care / edited by Darwin Deen, Lisa Hark.
    p. ; cm.
   Includes bibliographical references and index.
   ISBN-13: 978-1-4051-0474-6 (pbk. : alk. paper)   1. Diet therapy.   2. Nutrition.
I. Deen, Darwin.   II. Hark, Lisa.
   [DNLM: 1. Nutrition Therapy.   2. Nutrition.   3. Patient Education – methods.
4. Primary Health Care. WB 400 C7375 2007]

   RC216.C666 2007
   615.8′54 – dc22

                                                                        2006027576

ISBN 978-1-4051-0474-6

A catalogue record for this title is available from the British Library

Set in 9.5/12 Palatino by Aptara Inc., New Delhi, India
Printed and bound in Singapore by Fabulous Printers Pte Ltd

Commissioning Editor: Vicki Noyes
Editorial Assistant: Robin Harries
Development Editor: Lauren Brindley
Production Controller: Debbie Wyer

For further information on Blackwell Publishing, visit our website:
http://www.blackwellpublishing.com

The publisher's policy is to use permanent paper from mills that operate a sustainable forestry
policy, and which has been manufactured from pulp processed using acid-free and elementary
chlorine-free practices. Furthermore, the publisher ensures that the text paper and cover board
used have met acceptable environmental accreditation standards.

Contents

Editors-in-Chief

Darwin Deen, MD, MS
Professor of Clinical Family and Social
Medicine
Department of Family and Social
Medicine
Albert Einstein College of Medicine
Bronx, New York

Lisa Hark, PhD, RD
Director
Nutrition Education and Prevention
Program
University of Pennsylvania
School of Medicine
Philadelphia, Pennsylvania

Associate Editors

Jeremy Brauer, MD
Nutrition Education and Prevention
Program
University of Pennsylvania
School of Medicine
Philadelphia, Pennsylvania

Frances Burke, MS, RD
Clinical Dietitian Specialist
Cardiovascular Risk Intervention Program
University of Penn Health System *and*
Nutrition Education and Prevention
Program
University of Pennsylvania
School of Medicine
Philadelphia, Pennsylvania

Elizabeth Horvitz, BS
Nutrition Education and Prevention
Program
University of Pennsylvania
School of Medicine
Philadelphia, Pennsylvania

Randee Silverman, BSN, RN
Senior Research Coordinator
University of Pennsylvania Health System
Philadelphia, Pennsylvania

Contributors

Marianne Aloupis, MS, RD, CNSD
Clinical Dietitian Specialist
Clinical Nutrition Support Service
Hospital of the University of Pennsylvania
Philadelphia, Pennsylvania

Mary Beth Augustine, RD
Clinical Dietitian
Continuum Center for Health and Healing
Beth Israel Medical Center
New York, New York

Connie Watkins Bales, PhD, RD
Associate Director, GRECC
Durham VA Medical Center
Associate Research Professor
of Geriatric Medicine
Duke University Medical Center
Durham, North Carolina

Diane Barsky, MD
Assistant Professor of Pediatrics
University of Pennsylvania School of Medicine
Attending Physician
Division of Gastroenterology and Nutrition
Children's Hospital of Philadelphia
Philadelphia, Pennsylvania

Jeremy Brauer, MD
Nutrition Education and Prevention Program
University of Pennsylvania
School of Medicine
Philadelphia, Pennsylvania

Frances Burke, MS, RD
Clinical Dietitian Specialist
Cardiovascular Risk Intervention Program
University of Penn Health System *and*
Nutrition Education and Prevention Program
University of Pennsylvania
School of Medicine
Philadelphia, Pennsylvania

Valentine J Burroughs, MD, MBA
Chief Medical Officer
Chairman, Department of Medicine
North General Hospital
New York, New York

Katherine Chauncey, PhD, RD, FADA
Associate Professor
Department of Family and Community Medicine
Texas Tech School of Medicine
Lubbock, Texas

Charles B Eaton, MD, MS
Professor of Family Medicine
Brown University
Providence; *and*
Director, Heart Disease Prevention Clinic
Memorial Hospital of Rhode Island
Pawtucket, Rhode Island

Joel S. Edman, DSc, FACN, CNS
Director of Integrative Nutrition
Clinical Assistant Professor
Myrna Brind Center of Integrative Medicine
Thomas Jefferson University and Hospital
Philadelphia, Pennsylvania

Thomas Faust, MD
Assistant Professor of Medicine
Division of Gastroenterology
University of Pennsylvania Health System
Philadelphia. Pennsylvania

Alice Fornari, EdD, RD
Associate Professor of Family and Social Medicine
Director, Medical Education
Department of Family and Social Medicine
Albert Einstein College of Medicine
Bronx, New York

Marion J Franz, MS, RD, LD, CDE
President
Nutrition Concept by Franz, Inc.
Minneapolis, Minnesota

Kim M Gans, PhD, MPH, LDN
Associate Professor of Community Health
Deputy Directory
Institute for Community Health Promotion
Brown University
Providence, Rhode Island

Morgan B Holt, MD
Department of Family Practice
and Community Medicine
University of Pennsylvania
School of Medicine
Philadelphia, Pennsylvania

Elizabeth Horvitz, BS
Nutrition Education and Prevention Program
University of Pennsylvania
School of Medicine
Philadelphia, Pennsylvania

Arlo Kahn, MD
Professor of Family and Preventive Medicine
University of Arkansas for Medical Sciences
Little Rock, Arkansas

Benjamin Kligler, MD, MPH
Co-Director, Fellowship Programs
Continuum Center for Health and Healing
Beth Israel Medical Center *and*
Associate Professor of Family and Social Medicine
Department of Family and Social Medicine
Albert Einstein College of Medicine
Bronx, New York

Kathryn M Kolasa, PhD, RD, LDN
Professor
Nutrition Services and Patient Education
Department of Family Medicine
Brody School of Medicine at East Carolina
University; *and*
Nutrition Consultant
University Health Systems
Greenville, North Carolina

Susan Konek, MA, RD, CNSD, LDN
Inpatient Clinical Nutrition Manager
Children's Hospital of Philadelphia
Philadelphia, Pennsylvania

Katherine Margo, MD
Pre-Doctoral Director, Department of
Family Practice and Community Medicine
University of Pennsylvania
School of Medicine
Philadelphia, Pennsylvania

James M Nicholson, MD, MSCE
Assistant Professor, Department of Family
Practice and Community Medicine
University of Pennsylvania
School of Medicine
Philadelphia, Pennsylvania

Cathy A Nonas, MS, RD, CDE
Director, Diabetes and Obesity Programs
North General Hospital
New York, New York

Randee Silverman, BSN, RN
Senior Research Coordinator
University of Pennsylvania Health System
Philadelphia, Pennsylvania

Catherine Sullivan, MPH, RD, LDN, IBCLC, RLC
Affiliate Faculty, East Carolina University
State Breastfeeding Coordinator
Nutrition Services Branch
Division of Public Health
North Carolina Department of Health
and Human Services
Raleigh, North Carolina

Philippe Szapary, MD, MSCE
Cardiovascular Risk Intervention Program
University of Pennsylvania Health System
Philadelphia, Pennsylvania

Marion Vetter, MD, RD
Endocrine Fellow
Division of Endocrinology, Diabetes and
Metabolism
University of Pennsylvania
School of Medicine
Philadelphia, Pennsylvania

Richard Wender, MD
Alumni Professor and Chair
Department of Family and Community Medicine
Thomas Jefferson University
Philadelphia, Pennsylvania

Heidi K White, MD, MHSc
Associate Professor of Medicine
Duke University School of Medicine
Durham, North Carolina

Jane V White, PhD, RD, FADA, LDN
Professor, Department of Family Medicine
Graduate School of Medicine
University of Tennessee
Knoxville, Tennessee

Jennifer Williams, MS, RD, CNSD
Senior Clinical Dietitian Specialist
University of Pennsylvania Health System
Philadelphia, Pennsylvania

Preface

For the past 15 years, we have devoted our respective careers to educating medical students, physicians, and other healthcare professionals about the importance of nutrition for the prevention and management of chronic diseases. *Medical Nutrition and Disease,* Dr. Hark's first book for students is now in its 3rd edition and is one of the most widely used nutrition texts for medical, nursing, physician assistant, and dietetic training programs across the country. Frustrated by the lack of sound, common-sense nutrition resources for patients and consumers, we collaborated on *Nutrition For Life,* which is now published worldwide in 10 languages.

For years, we have been encouraged by our peers to develop a quality text for practicing professionals who have told us that their training in nutrition was inadequate. Thus, we created *The Complete Guide to Nutrition in Primary Care,* which is aimed at health professionals working in the primary care setting and registered dietitians. We believe that the primary care environment offers optimal opportunities to impact patients' diet and lifestyle behaviors on a daily basis. *The Complete Guide to Nutrition in Primary Care* was developed using a multidisciplinary approach and provides accurate, scientifically sound, and much needed, practical information for primary care clinicians to effectively counsel patients. Contributors include well-known nutrition experts who are physicians, nurses, and registered dietitians from each discipline.

The book begins with case vignettes that serve as examples of how to provide brief nutrition counseling in the office setting. Next we discuss how to change the office culture to successfully incorporate nutrition into everyday practice. With obesity and diabetes increasing morbidity and healthcare costs, we focus on various methods of weight control, including diet programs, surgery, and the latest advances in medications.

Part 2 addresses nutrition throughout the lifecycle, covering requirements and recommendations specific to children, adolescents, pregnant and lactating women, and older adults.

Part 3 reports on ways to improve diet and lifestyle behaviors when treating dyslipidemia, hypertension, metabolic syndrome, diabetes, hypoglycemia, GI disorders, urinary tract infections, kidney stones, chronic kidney disease, nutritional anemias, and patients who are HIV positive.

Part 4 includes up-to-date information about vitamins, minerals, and dietary supplements, including both evidence-based findings and opinions based on clinical experiences. We also provide some paradigm-challenging dietary protocols to be considered as part of a complimentary and alternative medicine approach.

Finally, Part 5 encompasses ways to implement all the knowledge and skills to successfully modify a patient's behavior. With the ever-growing multicultural population in the US, it is crucial to expand cultural competence by understanding and appreciating the influence of culture on diet and lifestyle behaviors. We can make an even greater impact by becoming involved in our communities to advocate for healthy behaviors in schools, resources for active neighborhoods, and reimbursement for nutrition and preventive services.

In conclusion, *The Complete Guide to Nutrition in Primary Care* provides the tools to assist you in helping your patients achieve a healthy lifestyle. Through role modeling, eating a healthy diet, leading an active lifestyle, and advocating for these behaviors in your practice and community, you can produce meaningful changes in your patient's lifestyle. Help your patients by being supportive, understanding, and above all, setting a good example. Talk to your patients about their diet, employ a registered dietitian in your office, and write exercise prescriptions every day.

For more information about us:

Darwin Deen, MD, MS (www.DrDeen.com)
Lisa Hark, PhD, RD (www.LisaHark.com)

Nutrition as preventive medicine

CHAPTER 1

Nutrition and the primary care clinician

Darwin Deen and Katherine Margo

Counseling to change a patient's diet and lifestyle has the potential to play an important role in the nation's health promotion and disease prevention efforts in the twenty-first century. *Healthy People 2010* [1] nutrition objectives for primary care clinicians focus on attaining a target of 75% of physician office visits for hyperlipidemia, cardiovascular disease, or diabetes mellitus to include nutrition counseling. Recent clinical guidelines for hypertension, hyperlipidemia, obesity, and diabetes include specific nutrition and exercise-related recommendations to be implemented by primary care clinicians [2–5].

It has been well documented that the public sees primary care clinicians as credible and acceptable sources of lifestyle advice, including dietary information [6,7]. There is no lack of enthusiasm for dietary advice among patients in primary care [8]. The literature regarding the attitude of primary care clinicians towards dietary intervention is less clear. Some studies support a positive attitude while others suggest that primary care clinicians lack the inclination to provide dietary advice. Barriers include lack of time, lack of nutrition knowledge and confidence, poor patient adherence and lack of teaching materials [9,10]. In addition, translation of nutrition recommendations into practical dietary advice may be difficult. Changes to primary care practice need to include a greater focus on diet and lifestyle if nutrition-related diseases are to managed effectively and efficiently to ultimately decrease the burden on the health care system's limited resources [11]. These changes are appropriate given the amount of trust and credibility the public has in their primary care clinicians. Our dietary advice is potentially extremely important to patient outcomes [12]. Studies such as the Lifestyle Heart Trial, DASH, and Diabetes Prevention Program all demonstrate convincingly that intensive, lifestyle-based interventions are effective at reducing disease burden and risk [3,13,14].

What is the role of the primary care clinician with regards to nutrition?

While clinical encounters need to address what patients want (with a question such as, "What can I do for you today?"), we must also consider what the patient needs. "What can I do to help you become healthier?" is the "hidden" agenda for the primary care clinician. Our role in making a patient healthier is influenced by the setting of the visit (office, home, hospital, or nursing home); by the reason for the visit (acute problem vs. chronic disease management vs. health maintenance); and by the life cycle stage of the patient. For example, when we see patients in the office, we have an opportunity to identify nutrition-related risks associated with their usual dietary intake. In the hospital, we have to ensure that their diet order promotes restoration of health while minimizing the potential for further deterioration. In the nursing home, screening for malnutrition and monitoring caloric intake are paramount. Home visits are a unique opportunity to assess how diet and lifestyle information is actually practiced.

When patients present for an acute problem we must assess the potential impact of that problem on their ability to maintain a healthy diet and monitor for problems that may be nutrition related. Patients seen for health maintenance should have a routine dietary screening and appropriate patient education. Those that have nutrition-related problems identified should have a plan generated to address that problem, part of which needs to be a follow-up visit to institute and monitor behavior change. Assessing patients' readiness to change is a critical component in this process [15,16], as discussed in detail in Chapter 15. Patients who come for chronic disease follow-up visits may benefit from significant change to their routine dietary intake and are often candidates for referral to a registered dietitian.

Reinforcement

The primary care clinician's role does not end when a referral to a nutritionist is given (just like when we refer to any specialist). We need to follow up on the nutrition consult, support the plan, and provide on-going guidance for the patient as they try to accomplish the established goals. For the infant and toddler, we need to teach parents an appropriate healthy diet to help maximize their child's growth and development while attenuating the impact of their genetic predisposition for disease. For older adults we need to screen for nutrition-related problems which affect ongoing health or a diet designed to mitigate the impact of chronic disease. For adult patients, we must help them to identify their potential disease risk and educate them about eating properly to minimize that risk or to maximize their day-to-day feeling of well being.

Giving advice

So, what is a healthy diet? What diet should primary care clinicians recommend to their patients? There is a lot of data showing that a low-fat, high fiber diet can be beneficial for long-term health promotion. On the other hand, a Mediterranean-style diet that is higher in monounsaturated fats, such as olive oil, than the typical American diet, has also been shown to be health-promoting. While it seems confusing at times, we can, in a variety of ways (as shown in the case examples) help patients to improve their diet. If weight control is an issue, a low-fat diet might be an easier way to accomplish caloric restriction or patients may choose a low carbohydrate plan to induce more rapid weight loss.

The typical American diet is too high in calories, sugar, saturated fat, and salt and limited in fruits, vegetables, and low-fat dairy foods. Fewer than 25% of Americans get five servings of fruits and vegetables daily. Even among children, calcium intake is inadequate in almost half of 3–5 year olds, and 70% of 12–19 year olds [17].

To correct these imbalances, our patients need to cut down on portion sizes (larger portions served means more calories consumed) [18]; choose healthy snacks (fruits and vegetables rather than candy bars or chips); and reduce the consumption of products made with high fructose corn syrup (soda and sweetened fruit drinks) or sugar (cakes, cookies, and pastries). Greater use of herbs and spices will flavor foods with less salt and add some health promoting antioxidants. Clinicians can recommend low-fat milk and other low-fat dairy foods, lactose-free and soy products supplemented with calcium and calcium-fortified products (like orange juice). Prescribing a calcium supplement will help address a chronic inadequate calcium intake that is prevalent in our population and may reduce the risk of osteoporosis in the elderly. (See Chapters 12, 13 and Appendices G and H).

Screening and diagnosis: what should we be looking for?

What should be expected of the busy primary care clinician? The first step for any health maintenance and prevention visit should be to include screening for a family history of risk factors, such as obesity, cardiovascular disease or diabetes. Then it is useful to get a sense of the patient's meal and exercise patterns. This can be brief, and accomplished through the use of a simple questionnaire or by routinely asking two to three questions. Body mass index (BMI) should be calculated for everyone, including children and teenagers, followed by a discussion of how the patient's weight compares to norms. Use prevention visits as an opportunity to educate patients regarding the health effects of a lack of physical activity, the problems of large portion sizes, and the hazards of excess TV time. Challenge patients to consume more fruits and vegetables and to monitor their intake on a daily basis.

Help patients who need to lose weight by identifying community resources, websites and offer help, encouragement, and referral when indicated. Suggest MyPyramid.com [20] as a resource. These general suggestions are an excellent way to start discussing healthy diets. While it is clear that our patients with hypertension, diabetes mellitus, and hyperlipidemia need our best efforts to assist them with making effective lifestyle changes, it is not enough to limit our interventions to those patients who already have medical conditions that could have been prevented had they changed their behavior earlier. To achieve primary prevention, it is important to help those patients who are not eating what they should be or those not exercising regularly to begin doing so before they develop the health problems for which these behaviors place them at risk.

US Dietary Guidelines: **Key Recommendations**

Fruits and vegetables

• Choose a variety of fruits and vegetables each day. In particular, select from all five vegetable subgroups (dark green, orange, legumes, starchy vegetables, and other vegetables) several times a week.
• Two cups of fruit and 2 ½ cups of vegetables per day are recommended for a reference 2000-calorie intake, with higher or lower amounts depending on the calorie level.

Grains

• Consume three or more one-ounce-equivalents of whole-grain products per day, with the rest of the recommended grains coming from enriched or whole-grain products. In general, at least half the grains should come from whole grains.

Carbohydrates

• Choose fiber-rich fruits, vegetables, and whole grains often.
• Choose and prepare foods and beverages with little added sugars or caloric sweeteners, such as amounts suggested by the USDA Food Guide and the DASH Eating Plan.
• Consume sugar- and starch-containing foods and beverages less frequently to reduce the incidence of dental caries.

Dairy

• Consume 3 cups/day of fat-free or low-fat milk or equivalent milk products.
• Children 2–8 years should consume 2 cups/day of fat-free or low-fat milk or equivalent milk products.
• Children 9 years of age and older should consume 3 cups/day of fat-free or low-fat milk or equivalent milk products.

Fats

• Consume less than 10% of calories from saturated fatty acids and less than 300 mg/day of cholesterol, and keep trans fatty acid consumption as low as possible.
• Keep total fat intake between 20–35% of calories, with most fats coming from polyunsaturated and monounsaturated sources, such as fish, nuts, and vegetable oils.
• When selecting and preparing meat, poultry, dry beans, and milk or milk products, make choices that are lean, low-fat, or fat-free.
• Limit intake of fats and oils high in saturated and/or trans fatty acids.

Source: [19].

For behavior change

- Set realistic goals
- Celebrate small successes
- Expect set backs
- Lavish praise
- Group visits for support
- Dietary consultation when indicated

(Also see Chapter 15)

Case examples

Case 1

A 14-year-old boy comes in for a school physical. He is 5′6″ and weighs 200 pounds. He loves junk food and hates vegetables. Mom says he watches a lot of television and when questioned, he reports playing video games for at least 3 hours every day. He is an honor roll student in school, but doesn't have many friends. You identify the following problems:

1 BMI is 32.3 (diagnostic of obesity > 95th percentile)
2 No exercise with highly sedentary activities
3 Excessive fat and sugar from junk food and sweets
4 Avoids vegetables.

Approach

This typical case can be overwhelming and it is hard to know where to start. First find out if there is any kind of exercise he likes and encourage those, such as biking, playing street hockey or tennis. Quantifying the number of hours he spends playing video games is key and then suggest that this should be limited to less than 2 hours per day, including TV time. Discuss the importance of eating less junk food, avoiding candy, cookies, and chips and emphasize healthier snacks. If Mom is around it's most helpful to include her in the discussion – and be sure to emphasize that she should stop buying junk food and offer healthier snacks and vegetables when her son is most hungry, such as after school. Often overweight children and teenagers have at least one overweight parent and the entire family's dietary choices and lifestyle need to be addressed. It's important not to expect rapid results. Lifestyle change is hard and you want it to be sustainable!

Case 2

A 21-year-old college student comes in for a Pap smear and birth control. She is 5′5″ and weighs 110 pounds. She pays a lot of attention to her looks. She exercises every day for 1–2 hours. She doesn't eat any sweets except around her period when she craves chocolate. She reports a 5 lb weight loss over the

past 6 months. She is doing well in school and has lots of friends. Her periods are normal on a birth control pill. Her identified issues are:
1 BMI is 18.8 (borderline underweight)
2 Possible eating disorder
3 Probable inadequate calcium vitamin and protein intake.

Approach
It's important to gently explore her feelings about her body and the possibility of bulimia or anorexia. You can praise her exercise, but assess if it is too much as women who have eating disorders tend to exercise more than necessary every day. Take a careful diet history to assess her caloric intake and enlist her help in improving her nutrition in a healthy and tolerable manner. If she is unable to gain any weight and continues to lose weight, she should be referred for psychological counseling.

Case 3
A 30-year-old consultant comes in for a check up. He travels a lot for work and eats most meals out. He tries to exercise regularly but says that he is too busy. He is 5′10″ and weighs 210 pounds. He played football in college and his weight has remained stable since that time. You identify the following issues:
1 BMI is 30.2 (diagnostic of obesity)
2 Eats out a lot
3 Not enough exercise.

Approach
Discussing how to eat out in restaurants in a healthy manner would be the most useful. Suggest strategies such as skipping bread, limiting wine to one glass, ordering broiled, grilled or baked fish or chicken, limiting portion sizes, especially if he orders beef, and sharing dessert when possible. In addition, brainstorm with him ways to increase exercise – using gyms at hotels, climb stairs when possible, walk instead of taxis etc.

Case 4
A 40-year-old woman is seen because of fatigue. She works full time and is a single mother. She often skips breakfast, but cooks dinner most nights for her family. She is 5′8″ and weighs 200 pounds. She used to be very thin until she had her three children. She doesn't have any time to exercise and makes very little money. You identify the following issues:
1 BMI is 30.5 (diagnostic of obesity)
2 Fatigue and probably significant stress
3 No exercise
4 Can't afford a lot of "healthy" food
5 Skips breakfast.

Approach

It is helpful to address her stress first. Moderate, regular exercise is the best form of stress relief. Fast food is often the path of least resistance for single parents. Talk about inexpensive ways to eat healthier such as using canned tuna fish, leaner cuts of ground meat, choosing poultry instead of other types of meats and avoid frying. Encourage her to buy frozen, not canned vegetables. Explain the importance of eating breakfast, as this will help regulate her appetite throughout the day. In a supportive, non-judgmental manner, emphasize that she needs to set a good example and provide a healthy diet for both herself and her children. There is so much going on in her life it would be useful to address one thing at a time, not all five concerns so as not to overwhelm her.

Case 5

A 50-year-old man comes in for a blood pressure check. He's on a diuretic and ACE inhibitor and his blood pressure (BP) is 145/90 mmHg. He works as a supervisor and his shifts are 12 hours long. He is married but he often does the cooking. He and his wife love pasta. He is 5′11″ and 200 pounds. He doesn't have any time to exercise. You identify the following issues:

1 BMI is 27.9 (diagnostic of overweight)
2 Borderline BP on medication
3 Probably ingesting too much salt
4 Not enough exercise.

Approach

Because his BP is arguably the most important health issue, it's important to discuss how to lower salt in his diet. It is helpful to discuss specific problematic foods thoroughly, such as the use of canned, processed and convenience foods, which typically contain a lot of salt. According to the Dietary Approaches to Stop Hypertension (DASH) research [ref. 3], dietary changes can significantly reduce BP. Start by asking if he uses the salt shaker during cooking or when eating. Increasing his fruit and vegetable intake can help reduce his BP. He should be questioned about his alcohol intake, as more than two drinks per day can contribute to hypertension. Suggest eating more whole grains and unsalted nuts to increase his magnesium intake. In conjunction with regular exercise, this regime can significantly impact his hypertension.

Case 6

A 63-year-old woman comes in with diabetes (HbA1C of 7.5). Her total cholesterol is 260 mg/dL and low density lipoprotein (LDL) is 170 mg/dL. She says she eats all the wrong foods and sits most of the time because of bad knees and a desk job. She is near retirement. She weighs 280 pounds and is 5′9″ tall. You identify the following issues:

1 BMI is 41.3 (diagnostic of class III obesity)
2 Type 2 diabetes
3 No exercise with arthritis
4 Life stressors of pending retirement.

Approach

This type of patient is challenging from many viewpoints. She needs a realistic approach that does not discourage her from making changes to her diet and lifestyle. She needs frequent one-on-one support and specific dietary advice that takes into account her food preferences, which may be best accomplished by referring her to a registered dietitian. A thorough exploration of her home situation is warranted to find out if she is the primary cook, and if so who else she needs to cook for. She would probably benefit from a group visit or diabetic class with group suggest.

Practice what you preach

You enhance your credibility and ability to relate by role-modeling healthy lifestyles for your patients. Become an expert on exercise options in your community, advertise fundraising walks and races in your office, join them when you can, let your patients see you out there. Participate in physical activity yourself, make sure your children are involved in local team sports, get involved in your local school district and be a voice for more physical activity and healthier cafeteria foods. Encourage your office staff to eat healthy and to exercise regularly (if we clinicians don't promote work-site health, who will?). If you maintain a library for your patients make sure that it has good nutrition information resources and send out heath promoting mailings, e-mail, etc. When your patients see how important this is to you, they will be more inclined to seek out your advice when they need help. Become a resource in your community, speak out whenever and wherever you can (block parties, town hall meetings, church suppers). Help your neighbors to identify ways to eat healthier and become more physically active. The more experience you have with these lifestyle challenges, the more of a resource you will be for your patients.

Unfortunately, the literature does not provide us with models that have been shown to be effective, so it is up to each of us to develop our own method of approach to addressing diet and activity counseling for our patients. Examples of models that have been developed are described in Chapter 2.

Barriers to adherence

Despite the fact that patients accept the old adage "You are what you eat," they do not seem able to apply that to their day-to-day dietary intake. Obesity rates have increased by 60% in the last ten years with approximately 59 million Americans adults being obese [21]. The costs associated with this epidemic of obesity and its attendant diabetes are skyrocketing (estimated at $117 billion as of 2000) [22].

The average American woman is 5'4" and weighs 140 lbs (BMI 24). The average model is 5'11" and weighs 117 pounds (BMI 18), yet our patients have trouble incorporating a diet that would yield such a body shape. In a typical primary care practice, between 26 and 40% of patients have a BMI greater than 30, while fewer than 1% have a BMI of 18 or less [23].

While most of our patients recognize how important it is to "eat right and exercise," a recent study from the Pew Research Center found that Americans see weight problems everywhere but in the mirror. According to this report, nine-in-ten American adults say most of their fellow Americans are overweight, but only seven-in-ten say this about "the people they know." And just under four-in-ten (39%) say they themselves are overweight [24].

Approximately 75% of adults are not eating enough fruits and vegetables. Our culture supports convenience, our policies favor junk food, our restaurants have huge portion sizes to increase the perception of value and even our TV habits demonstrate avoidance of exercise. Convenience foods, ever more popular, are typically not healthy choices. The primary care clinician, when attempting to counsel a patient about their diet, is faced with the barriers of time, money, taste preference, culture, family, and habit. Health is unfortunately far down on the list of factors that are considered when food choices are made.

Food is much more than nutrition for us. It represents nurturing, love, entertainment (note the popularity of the Food Network). For many Americans, a chubby baby is a healthy baby and any attempts to direct parents toward a more appropriate feeding style falls on deaf ears. The news media is not helping. Each new dietary study is trumpeted with the fanfare of a newly discovered scientific fact. So when contradictory results are found (which happens often in science), patients (and often their clinicians as well) are left confused about what to believe and what to include in a "healthy diet." Unfortunately, physicians trying to address the behaviors that lead to obesity face the same unsupportive environment that physicians faced trying to help patients quit smoking in the 1950s. Policy changes currently being considered that may help move our patients from where they are to where they need to be include: requiring fast food restaurants to include nutritional information on their packages; taxing sweetened beverages; and developing devices that monitor television viewing and video game use by our children. There is a lot more work that needs to be done and we believe that the primary care clinician can play a key role. Roll up your sleeves and get to work. *The Complete Guide to Nutrition in Primary Care* will give you the knowledge, skills and help reshape your attitudes about diet and lifestyle changes in your patient population.

References

1 *Healthy People 2010*. U.S. Department of Health and Human Services. www.Healthy People.gov
2 Klein S, Sheard NF, Pi-Sunyer X et al. Weight Management Through Lifestyle Modification for the Prevention and Management of Type 2 Diabetes: Rationale and Strategies: A statement of the American Diabetes Association, the North American Association for the Study of Obesity, and the American Society for Clinical Nutrition. *Diabetes Care* 2004;27:2067–73.

3 Appel LJ, Brands MW, Daniels SR, Karanja N, Elmer PJ, Sacks FM. Dietary approaches to prevent and treat hypertension: a scientific statement from the American Heart Association. *Hypertension*. 2006;47(2):296–308.

4 Franz MJ, Bantle JP, Beebe CA et al., American Diabetes Association. Nutrition Principles and Recommendations in Diabetes. *Diabetes Care* 2004;27:S136–46.

5 Chobanian AV, Bakris GL, Black HR et al. National Heart, Lung, and Blood Institute Joint National Committee on Prevention, Detection, Evaluation, and Treatment of High Blood Pressure; National High Blood Pressure Education Program Coordinating Committee. *JAMA*. 2003;289(19):2560–72.

6 Jackson AA. Human nutrition in medical practice: the training of doctors. *Proc Nutr Soc* 2001;60(20):257–63.

7 van Binsbergen JJ, Delaney BC, van Weel C. Nutrition in primary care: scope and relevance of output from the Cochrane Collaboration. *Am J Clin Nutr* 2003;77(4 Suppl):1083S–1088S.

8 van Weel C. Dietary advice in family medicine. *Am J Clin Nutr* 2003;77(4 Suppl):1008S–1010S.

9 Ockene JK, Ockene IS, Quirk ME et al. Physician training for patient-centered nutrition counseling in a lipid intervention trial. *Prev Med* 1995;24(6):563–70.

10 Ockene IS, Hebert JR, Ockene JK, Merriam PA, Hurley TG, Saperia GM. Effect of training and a structured office practice on physician-delivered nutrition counseling: the Worcester-Area Trial for Counseling in Hyperlipidemia (WATCH). *Am J Prev Med* 1996;12(4):252–8.

11 Ockene IS, Hebert JR, Ockene JK et al. Effect of physician-delivered nutrition counseling training and an office-support program on saturated fat intake, weight, and serum lipid measurements in a hyperlipidemic population: Worcester Area Trial for Counseling in Hyperlipidemia (WATCH). *Arch Intern Med* 1999;159(7):725–31.

12 Secker-Walker RH, Morrow AL, Kresnow M, Flynn BS, Hochheiser LI. Family physicians' attitudes about dietary advice. *Fam Pract Res J* 1991;11(2):161–70.

13 Ornish D, Scherwitz LW, Billings JH et al. Intensive lifestyle changes for reversal of coronary heart disease. *JAMA* 1998;280(23):2001–7.

14 Knowler WC, Barrett-Connor E, Fowler SE et al.; Diabetes Prevention Program Research Group. Reduction in the incidence of type 2 diabetes with lifestyle intervention or metformin. *N Engl J Med* 2002;346(6):393–403.

15 Wee CC, Davis RB, Phillips RS. Stage of readiness to control weight and adopt weight control behaviors in primary care. *J Gen Intern Med* 2005;20(5):410–5.

16 Logue E, Sutton K, Jarjoura D, Smucker W, Baughman K, Capers. Transtheoretical model-chronic disease care for obesity in primary care: a randomized trial. *Obes Res* 2005;13(5):917–27.

17 Greer FR, Krebs NF; American Academy of Pediatrics Committee on Nutrition. Optimizing bone health and calcium intakes of infants, children, and adolescents. *Pediatrics* 2006;117(2):578–85.

18 Ello-Martin JA, Ledikwe JH, Rolls BJ. The influence of food portion size and energy density on energy intake: implications for weight management. *Am J Clin Nutr* 2005;82(1 Suppl):236S–241S.

19 US Department of Health and Human Services and US Department of Agriculture. 2005 *Dietary Guidelines for Americans*. Washington, DC, US Government Printing Office, 2005. www.healthierus.gov/dietaryguidelines/

20 MyPyramid.com

21 Wyatt SB, Winters KP, Dubbert PM. Overweight and obesity: prevalence, consequences, and causes of a growing public health problem. *Am J Med Sci* 2006;331(4):166–74.

22 Tucker DM, Palmer AJ, Valentine WJ, Roze S, Ray JA. Counting the costs of overweight and obesity: modeling clinical and cost outcomes. *Curr Med Res Opin* 2006;22(3):575–86.

23 Personal Communications with Maggie Blackburn, MD. President, New York State Academy of Family Physicians, 2006.

24 Taylor P, Punk C, Craighill P, for Pew Research Center, 2006. *Americans See Weight Problems Everywhere But In the Mirror.* http://pewresearch.org/assets/social/pdf/Obesity. pdf. Report Published April 11, 2006.

CHAPTER 2

Changing the office culture to make it work

Arlo Kahn and Jane White

Introduction

Nutrition screening/assessment, diagnosis, and counseling are integral to the delivery of quality health care during the various stages of the life cycle and are a core element in the management of most of the chronic diseases that afflict Americans of all ages [1,2]. Optimal nutrition intake can reduce a patient's risk of developing chronic diseases, including coronary heart disease, diabetes, cancer and osteoporosis [3–6]. A patient's nutritional status also has an important impact on their disease onset and progression, as poor nutrition increases the morbidity and mortality irrespective of disease state [7–9]. In light of this, assessing your patients' nutritional status should be a standard part of primary care practice. Yet, without an approach to clinical practice that recognizes the impact of nutrition and incorporates the nutrition care process into daily practice, the nutritional needs of patients seen in medical settings will continue to be sporadically and incompletely addressed [10–13]. This chapter focuses on changing the office system to make nutrition screening, assessment, diagnosis, counseling and/or referral a reality, so that it benefits both patients and health care providers.

A successful systems approach

Changing the way in which individual practitioners deliver and prescribe care, particularly lifestyle interventions, is difficult. Interviews of Danish general practitioners who had taken part in a health promotion study revealed that although they believed they have an important role to play in preventing lifestyle-related illness, they are skeptical about the effectiveness of their interventions [14]. Their opinions differed widely as to whether, when, and how aggressively to provide lifestyle intervention. They were frustrated and noted that patients are chiefly interested in having their health status evaluated rather than following through on changing their behavior. Other examples of barriers to primary care physicians providing screening and intervention for behavioral change relate to the clinical setting. These include the sensitive nature of the topic, a chief complaint "perceived as unrelated" to a lifestyle trait, patient resistance, lack of available intervention tools, limited expectation of intervention effectiveness, and lack of time [15]. Historically, health care professionals have repeatedly cited poor reimbursement, limited time, and inadequate training in medical school and residency programs as barriers to providing nutrition counseling and preventive care services [16–18].

Models for brief assessment/intervention

An abundance of strong scientific evidence continues to support the fact that major causes of morbidity and mortality in the United States are related to poor diet and a sedentary lifestyle [19]. However, practice behaviors to recognize and address these problems are routinely underutilized in most health care settings. Yet, patients expect advice from primary care clinicians regarding key risk-reduction behaviors such as diet, exercise and substance abuse [11].

In order for providers to be willing to change the way they provide care or restructure the office system in which they provide care, they need to be convinced that change can be accomplished without excessive disruption, that such change will lead to improved patient health, and they can be reimbursed for the time spent providing these "nontraditional" services. Fortunately, it is possible to change the office system while satisfying all of these concerns [20]. Two principles should guide the process of an effective office system change:

1) **Keep it simple**
2) **Make it useful.**

With these principles in mind, some changes may be required in three parts of the office system (1) the appointment system; (2) the medical record; and (3) the billing and coding system. All of these will be described below.

The appointment system

The first step is for the provider to appropriately decide the frequency at which the patient's nutritional status should be evaluated. From our experience, it is reasonable that a nutrition screen or brief evaluation of nutritional status could be performed annually on the majority of patients in the primary care office setting. The appointment system, whether electronic or paper-based, should include a prompt at the time the nutrition screen is due. Patient reminders could be mailed or even emailed to the patient to ensure convenience.

Typically, primary care offices allow 15–20 minutes for most visits. With good tools, which will be described in the section on medical records, a brief evaluation of nutritional status can be accomplished in 5–7 minutes of face-to-face time. For each topic requiring physician advice, an additional 2–3 minutes of face-to-face time should suffice for brief advice and simple assistance. Further guidance can be provided by a follow-up appointment with the clinician, registered dietitian, or other health care provider.

A more in-depth annual nutrition assessment should not be attempted during a 20-minute appointment where several complicated chronic medical problems need to be addressed or where the patient's acute needs take precedence. Of course, the provider can address counseling in those areas of nutrition that relate to the chronic or acute problem for which the patient is being seen, but this would not meet the goal of an annual nutrition review. If the 20-minute visit is for a simple problem and there is additional time remaining, the assessment may be accomplished at that visit. However, time would be very limited for counseling and the patient should be rescheduled for any significant lifestyle counseling needs discussed during this assessment.

When time is insufficient, the provider should reschedule the patient to return specifically for a prevention visit, which would include a nutrition screen. The "prevention" visit, which should include an evaluation of nutrition and other lifestyle habits, relevant exposures, and past medical and family history related to preventable diseases can be scheduled for 20–30 minutes. Reimbursement is variable and will depend on policy governing the patient's health care plan/contract provisions and state/federal reimbursement policy/regulations if billing Medicaid or Medicare. Coding/coverage will be addressed in more detail below in the billing and coding section.

The key is for the provider to change the way he or she normally thinks about nutrition i.e. believing that nutrition and prevention are important enough that patients are encouraged to return within a few months for this purpose. This book provides specific examples of evidence supporting the effective use of nutrition intervention. In addition, improvement in patient satisfaction as these areas are addressed will reinforce this attitude and help providers to maintain this approach.

The medical record

Changes to the medical record should adhere to the guiding principles of simplicity and usefulness. The three essential components of the medical record to accomplish an annual nutrition evaluation are: (1) prompting mechanism; (2) assessment tools; and (3) counseling tools.

Prompt to evaluate nutrition status

This prompt should appear on the intake form where it cannot be overlooked. Assuming the physician always looks at vital signs, a prompt could be inserted in this section of the chart. An Electronic Medical Record (EMR) can be set for the prompt to appear at the desired frequency, e.g., annually, and remain until the assessment has been completed. For paper records, a section of the intake could contain the last date of completion of the assessment. In the interest of usefulness and integration, it would be best to prompt for completion of a complete risk assessment including nutrition, rather than nutrition alone. Patients can be prompted by a reminder postcard, email or phone call from the staff, which will help increase the chances of achieving this goal.

Assessment tools

Ideal screening tools for clinical settings are easily understood, brief, and easy to score/interpret. They help the clinician implement targeted interventions that are appropriate and effective. In keeping with the principles of simplicity, the evaluation tool should take approximately 5–7 minutes to complete and should be seen as a screening instrument. If indicated, more detailed dietary information can be obtained at another time and very likely by non-physician staff such as a dietitian, health educator, or nurse. A number of devices have been developed to assist clinicians in the evaluation of nutritional status throughout the lifecycle and for a variety of diseases/conditions [20]. Many of these tools are online and can be downloaded in PDF/PDA formats. Some are designed for physician/health professional administration while others can be self-administered/scored in the office reception area, exam room, or at health fairs, health clubs, or other community settings and brought to the attention of the physician if the individual is judged to be at moderate/high risk.

The AFFECTS Questionnaire (Table 2.1) addresses risky behaviors associated with alcoholic beverage use, fat, and fiber intakes, exercise, calcium/milk

Table 2.1 Diet and habit questionnaire (AFFECTS).

	Ask the patient the following questions	Potential problem*	Appropriate
A	Do you average 2 or more drinks a day (1 drink or more a day for women) of beer, wine or liquor?	Yes	No
F	Do you usually eat red meat (beef, pork or lamb) more than 3 times a week?	Yes	No
	Do you usually eat fried foods (deep fried foods, chips or French fries) more than 3 times a week?	Yes	No
	Do you usually use whole milk or milk products rather than low fat milk or low fat milk products?	Yes	No
	Do you usually use butter or margarine more than once a day?	Yes	No
F	Do you usually eat a high fiber cereal most days?	No	Yes
	Do you usually eat 2 or more pieces of whole grain bread or muffins a day?	No	Yes
	Do you take a fiber supplement regularly?	No	Yes
	Do you usually eat 5 or more servings of fruit or vegetables a day?	No	Yes
E	Do you exercise at least 30 minutes a day during most days of the week?	No	Yes
C	Do you usually have 3 or more servings of milk or milk products (including cheese or yogurt) a day?	No	Yes
	Do you take a calcium supplement every day?	No	Yes
T	Do you smoke or use tobacco in some form?	Yes	No
S	Do you usually have 2 or more sugar-containing soft drinks a day (more than 24 ounces)?	Yes	No
	Do you usually eat 2 or more servings of sweets a day (desserts, candy bars, cookies, pastries, Pop Tarts, or ice cream)?	Yes	No
	Do you take vitamins, minerals or other supplements every day?	No	Yes

*An answer in this column may suggest problem areas or need for further questioning.
Source: Arlo Kahn, MD. University of Arkansas for Medical Sciences. 2007.
Used with permission.

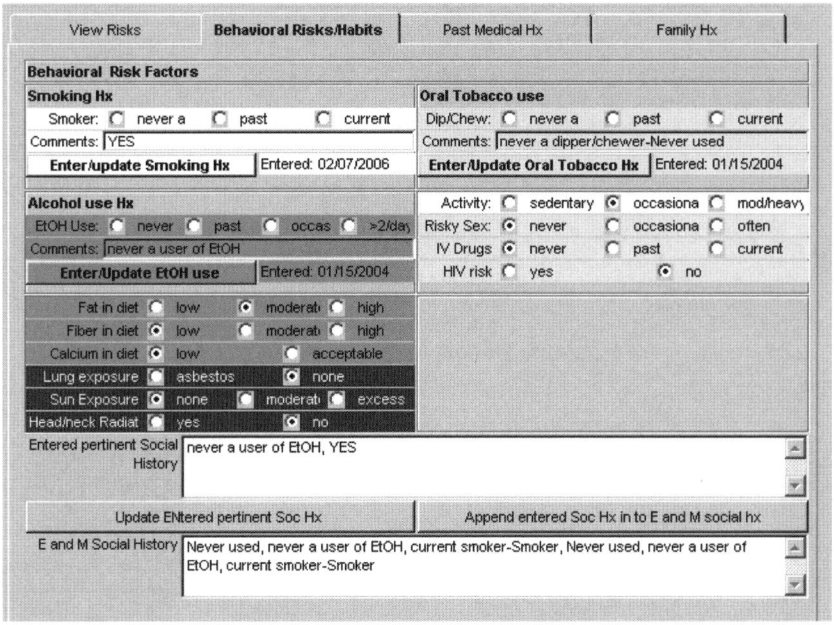

Figure 2.1 Electronic Medical Record intake form for diet and habits. Source: Arlo Kahn, MD, University of Arkansas for Medical Sciences. 2007. Used with permission.

intake, tobacco use, and sweets. It is a quick, structured way to assess the diet and lifestyle behaviors most commonly linked to chronic disease incidence in the United States [19].

To make screening more useful, it should be included as part of a diet and habit assessment that is itself a part of a risk assessment. The risk assessment should also include exposures and past medical and family history related to preventable disease. This risk assessment or "risk profile" serves as a guide to what counseling is needed. Examples of a simple EMR diet, habits, and exposures assessment form are shown in Figure 2.1.

With an EMR, items entered on the assessments can be automatically transferred to a risk profile (Figure 2.2), which should be easily accessed from the intake page with a mouse click. With a paper record, all of the risks can be displayed on a single page at the front of the chart. The EMR has the additional potential of automatically calculating BMI and alerting physicians to classes of overweight and obesity.

This assessment can also be performed by other trained office staff. However, the system is more likely to break down when there is turnover or absences. There are also tools available to allow patients to fill out the nutrition assessment. Since data will need to be reviewed for accuracy anyway, the patient-completed assessment may not really offer much advantage compared to a quick assessment by the primary care clinician. If the assessment is brief, the principle of simplicity suggests that the physician may want to do the assessment (Table 2.2).

| View Risks | Behavioral Risks/Habits | Past Medical Hx | Family Hx |

Updated (01/15/2004 8:54:2	FMC Risk Profile	Reviewed Today: ☐	SHOW
CAD Risk: Hypertension, Hx DM, Tobacco Abuse			Show CAD risks
Stroke Risk: Hypertension, Hx DM, Tobacco Abuse			Show CVA risks
Diabetes Risk: Increased risk based on race, FH T2DM (note: patient is diabetic according to problem list)			Show DM risks
Colon Ca Risk: Low fiber diet			Show Colon Ca risks
Lung Ca Risk: Smoker			Show Lung Ca risks
STD Risk: none			Show STD risks
Osteoporosis Risk: Low Ca diet, Steroid Use, Tobacco Abuse			Show bone risks
Thyroid Ca Risk: none			Show T4 risks
Oral Ca Risk: Tobacco Use			Show Oral Ca risks
Skin Ca Risk: none			Show Skin Ca risks
Breast Ca Risk: none			Show Breast Ca risks
Cervix Ca Risk: Tobacco Use			Show Cervix Ca risks
Uterus Ca Risk: none			Show Uterus Ca risks
Ovary Ca Risk: none			Show Ovary Ca risks

Figure 2.2 Electronic Medical Record risk profile form. Source: Arlo Kahn, MD, University of Arkansas for Medical Sciences. 2007. Used with permission.

Specific assessment tools have also been developed for older adults, such as the Nutrition Screening Initiative, which is described in detail in Chapter 6: Staying Healthy Later in Life.

Counseling tools

The third set of tools simplify nutrition counseling by providing structure based on strong behavioral principles. The Counseling and Behavioral Interventions Workgroup of the US Preventive Services Task Force recommends that health care professionals use the 5 A's Organizational Construct for Clinical Counseling as a frame of reference for behavior change intervention [11]. This construct defines the minimal contact interventions needed in primary care settings to facilitate behavioral change in individuals who present for care. Elements of this construct are outlined in Table 2.3 and described in detail in Chapter 15.

The first "**A**", Assessment, is accomplished with the assessment tools described above. The health care provider gives brief Advice for areas of concern as discovered in the assessment. In this case, "brief" means a few sentences. The third "**A**", Agree, will require identification of the patient's stage of readiness to change [21] (Table 2.3). The amount of Assistance from the provider depends on the stage of readiness to change and may be as simple as providing recommendations for appropriate intake of certain foods (verbally or with

Table 2.2 Role of office staff and non-physician providers in the delivery of nutrition care in primary care settings.

	Examples of role/function
Office personnel	
Receptionist	Triage
	Appointments scheduling
	Screening tools distribution/c
Nurse (RN/LPN/MA)	Screening tools distribution/collection/scoring
	Vital signs/anthropometrics/BMI
	Triage
	Supervised phone/fax/email interaction
	Basic nutrition education
Clerk	Diagnostic/procedural coding
	Billing
Non-physician providers	
Registered dietitian	Anthropometrics/vital signs
	Nutrition screening/assessment
	Nutrition-focused physical exam
	Nutrition diagnosis
	Medical Nutrition Therapy
	Nutrition education
	Food/drug interactions
	Dietary/nutrition supplement assessment/advise
	Community nutrition resources referral
Behaviorist	Cognitive/emotional assessment
	Counseling/coping skills development/stress Management
	Community services referral

Source: Jane White PhD, RD. Adapted from Reference [32]. Used with permission.
LPN, licensed practical nurse; MA, medical assistant; MNT, medical nutrition therapy; RN, registered nurse.

handouts.) Depending on the nature of the behavioral change anticipated, the provider would **A**rrange referral or follow-up to reinforce and/or modify the treatment plan.

For relatively simple topics, such as the need to increase fiber, calcium, fruits and vegetables, or to decrease saturated fat or sodium, counseling may be accomplished in a few minutes per topic. Key dietary counseling issues by age and disease are shown in Table 2.5 to accomplish this process. For more difficult areas such as weight control, hyperlipidemia, or diabetes mellitus, referral to a registered dietitian is more appropriate (see Box, below). In this case, the office may have either a registered dietitian, health educator, nurse trained in nutrition counseling, or a list of dietitians in the community to whom patients can be referred. Physicians may choose to do the intensive counseling, but in most cases will refer patients for nutritional counseling and reinforce the importance of adherence during subsequent follow-up visits, will benefit

Table 2.3 5 A's organizational construct for clinical counseling.

Assess	Ask about risky health behaviors (lifestyles) and consider factors such as age, gender, ethnicity, presence or absence of co-morbidities, literacy, etc. that would impact the choice of behavioral change goals/methods.
Advise	Provide clear, specific, individualized behavior-change advice including personalized information about the risk/benefit of lifestyle change. Advice messages from the physician can be brief (30–60 seconds), especially if provided in a team care context.
Agree	Treatment goals are mutually negotiated and selected based on the patient's interest in and readiness to change problem behaviors, and after consideration of treatment options, probable outcomes, and patient preference.
Assist	The physician, either directly, via office staff or by referral ensures that self-management skills are taught and problem-solving/coping skills development is encouraged to facilitate skills advancement, maintenance, and relapse prevention For patients not ready to commit to a specific behavioral change in the immediate future, assistance in the form of strategies that explore ambivalence can help to move patients along the change continuum.
Arrange	Regularly scheduled follow-up in person or by phone/fax/email offers continual support and allows for adjustment of the treatment plan, as the patient's condition, interest, and motivation level changes. After initial follow-up, contact is spaced based on intervention outcomes/patient need for reinforcement Referral to more intensive/specialized treatment may be indicated as co-morbidities develop or environmental/support systems change.

Source: [11].

all involved. In some cases, the referral will be more appropriately made to a behaviorist, such as when patients need help with depression, or a motivation to change a behavior, such as reducing alcohol intake.

Coding, billing, reimbursement
When coding with the expectation of reimbursement, two distinct coding sets must be used and submitted for claims processing. One to describe the chief

Table 2.4 Stages of change.

Precontemplation	No intention to change behavior in the foreseeable future
Contemplation	Aware that a problem exists and are seriously thinking about overcoming it but have not yet made a commitment to take action
Preparation	Intending to take action in the next month
Action	Modifying behavior, experiences, or environment in order to overcome their problems
Maintenance	Working to prevent relapse and consolidate the gains attained during action This stage extends from six months to an indeterminate period past the initial action

Source: [21].

Table 2.5 Dietary counseling issues by age and disease.

Infants	Fluoride, iron, calories for growth and development
Children	Fluoride, iron, calcium, calories for growth and development
Teenagers	Iron, calcium, calories for pubertal development
Pregnancy	Folate, iron, calcium, appropriate weight gain
Alcoholism	Folate, thiamin, vitamin B_{12}, calories
Anemia	Iron, vitamin B_{12}, folate
Ascites	Sodium, protein, fluid
Beriberi	Thiamin
Cancer	Adequate calories protein, vitamins, minerals and fiber
CHF	Sodium
COPD, asthma	Vitamin D, calcium, weight loss, calories
Diabetes	Carbohydrates, saturated fat, cholesterol, calories, fiber
Heart disease and hyperlipidemia	Saturated fat, monounsaturated fat, cholesterol, folate, fiber
Hypertension	Sodium, calcium, potassium, alcohol, total calories
Kidney stones	Calcium, oxalate, uric acid, protein, sodium, fluid
Liver disease	Protein, sodium, fluid
Malabsorption	Vitamins A, D, E and K, fat
Obesity	Total calories, saturated fat
Osteoporosis	Vitamin D and calcium
Pellegra	Niacin
Renal failure	Protein, sodium, potassium, phosphorous, fluid
Rickets	Vitamin D and calcium
Scurvy	Vitamin C
Vegetarian	Protein, vitamin B_{12}, iron, calcium

Source: Lisa Hark, PhD, RD. University of Pennsylvania School of Medicine. 2007.
Used with permission.
CHF, congestive heart failure; COPD, chronic obstructive pulmonary disease.

complaint (disease or condition) for which the patient presents for care [23] and the other to describe the service/procedure provided by the physician or health care professional to address the patient's reason for seeking care [24,25]. Numeric descriptors from each code set must be used and must "match", reflecting the typical patient with the disease or condition and the "accepted standard of care" used as the intervention that you provide, in order for you to be paid. For example you cannot use a CPT (Current Procedural Terminology) code for MNT (97802, MNT, initial visit, 15 minutes) and an ICD-9 (International Classification of Disease) code for otitis media (381.10) and expect to be paid. It is best to check with your practice or facility coding expert, the Centers for Medicare and Medicaid Services (CMS), or with local carriers/specific contract provisions when seeking reimbursement for nutritional care. Below are some coding alternatives that could be discussed with third party payers when seeking pre-certification or assurance of reimbursement for services delivery.

The physician who provides nutrition screening/education in the office setting might bill for these services in the context of Evaluation and Management counseling services provision (E&M CPT code) provided the exact amount of face-to-face time spent counseling is recorded and the disease/condition code (ICD-9) is compatible with the service rendered. Documentation of the

Registered Dietitians (RD) – Questions and Answers

When should I refer to a dietitian/nutritionist? When a primary care practitioner identifies a patient who needs an in-depth assessment of nutritional status or more intensive lifestyle/behavioral education and counseling than time allows in the office setting, a referral to a dietitian is necessary, especially for patients who are in the preparation, action, or relapse stage of change. RDs are health-care professionals who provide nutrition services. They have the time to individualize recommendations based on the patient's food preferences, and their unique medical, educational, cultural, and socioeconomic needs. Initial visits with the dietitian often require one hour, and follow-up visits range from 20–30 minutes depending on the diagnosis and level of health literacy.

What training is required to become a registered dietitian? Dietitians have a minimum of a bachelor's degree in foods and nutrition or similar course of study, and complete an accredited practice/training program (internship) in foods/nutrition. They are required to pass a certification exam and hold a nationally recognized credential (RD), meet state licensure requirements, and meet continuing professional education requirements. RDs use the American Dietetic Association's nationally developed MNT evidence-basssed Guides for Practice in the delivery of care for a wide range of diet-related diseases/conditions.

What should I include in the referral? When making a referral, be sure to:
• Include the diagnosis and ICD-9 code(s) for the disease/condition.
• Send recent lab data and medication list with the referral form.
• Document the medical necessity for Medical Nutrition Therapy.

Will I receive a report like other consults/specialists send? Yes. Dietitians send reports of initial and follow-up visits to the referring physician outlining their complete nutrition assessment and interpretation of the patient's diet and lifestyle. The report includes their recommendations and plans for follow-up. It is critical that the primary care provider reinforce these messages, encourage the patient to adhere to these recommendations, and monitor the patient's progress.

How do I find a dietitian? Your office staff can make an appointment with a dietitian at a local hospital outpatient clinic or the registered dietitian's private practice office. You can find a private practice dietitian by zip code at the American Dietetic Association's Web site (www.eatright.org) or call ADA's Nationwide Nutrition Network at 800/366-1655.

Source: Jane White, PhD, RD and Lisa Hark, PhD, RD., 2007. Used with permission. Adapted from [22].

length and nature of service must be placed in the patient's medical record. For example, if the physician spends 25 minutes with a patient with diabetes and hypertension, 15 minutes of which were spent counseling the patient on diet and physical activity related to managing these diseases, a 99214 E&M code may be used as long as the physician records that more than half of the visit was spent counseling the patient.

The CPT codes for preventive services for new or established patients might also be used. For example, when providing such services to children or adolescents the 99381 or 99391 codes series would be applicable. The physician might also bill using counseling and/or risk factor reduction intervention codes for individuals or groups, CPT codes such as 99420 (administration and interpretation of health risk assessment instrument) or 99429 (unlisted preventive medical service). There are also health and behavior assessment/intervention codes that apply to assessment, reassessment, and intervention for an individual or group and with family/caregiver, with/without patient that may apply. Refer to the most recent edition of the CPT coding guidelines for descriptors of these and other codes that may be used [24,25].

Coding for Nutritionist Reimbursement

CPT codes for MNT for individuals or groups are time-based codes for use by RDs or other qualified nutrition professionals (QNP) only [24]. MNT has been shown to improve patient outcomes, quality of life, and to lower healthcare costs across the continuum of care. MNT includes nutritional diagnostic, therapeutic and counseling services for the purpose of disease management. Dietitians are skilled in providing preventive services that address nutrition, physical activity and other lifestyle concerns important in maintaining and/or improving health. Dietitians also have the time to individualize recommendations based on the patient's food preferences, and their unique medical, educational, cultural, and socioeconomic needs.

Currently, Medicare reimburses for MNT for two diagnoses only: renal disease (chronic renal insufficiency and post-transplant care); and diabetes mellitus, types 1 and 2, through Medicare Part B and limits the interaction to 3–4 hours per year [22]. Dietitians cannot bill Medicare part B for MNT as "incident to" physician services but must enroll as a Medicare program provider. Services will be reimbursed for MNT delivered in an independent practice setting, hospital outpatient department or other ambulatory care setting. MNT services provided to patients during a stay in an acute care or skilled nursing facility are not reimbursable. There is also a provision for an initial nutrition/lifestyles assessment within 6 months of entry into the Medicare system [26].

Other carriers will often reimburse for MNT disease-specific care when prescribed by a physician. The military's TRICARE health program will provide inpatient and outpatient MNT, nutrition counseling and nutrition-oriented health promotion services at military medical treatment facilities [27]. Many health care plans cover MNT directly, however diabetes is the main focus [28]. Dietitian services are typically viewed as an integral component of chronic disease management/self management services. Few carriers currently reimburse for MNT, or nutrition education for weight loss counseling, or to prevent the development of co-morbidities in persons with a strong family history of chronic disease incidence. Payer attitudes toward reimbursement for prevention may change as evidence of efficacy and cost savings accumulate.

G codes, which are provisional codes that are time-based [24,25], can be used by dietitians and qualified nutrition professionals for individual and group MNT reassessment and subsequent intervention following a second referral in the same year for change in diagnosis, medical condition or treatment regimen. A physician referral is required when using these codes.

S codes are temporary non-Medicare codes that are used by some non-physician providers to document and request reimbursement from private carriers, such as S9449 – weight management and non-physician providers. Similar S-series codes for the provision of exercise classes, nutrition classes, diabetes self-management program group sessions, diabetic self-management program dietitian visits, and nutrition counseling dietitian visits are also used [24,25]. Refer to the CPT and ICD-9 publications for greater specificity regarding specific codes, coding definitions, and appropriate use [23–25].

Enhancing nutrition services delivery

Changes to the office environment and technological approaches to improve the delivery of health care to patients include the "virtual" patient care team, the EMR, group care, telemedicine, and other innovative approaches to health care services delivery. These types of innovations serve to enhance the delivery of nutritional care to patients and may improve outcomes, particularly when used to reinforce and support goals and interventions developed and implemented in the initial visit/primary consultation. Vale *et al.* [29] describe the efficacy of regular personal coaching involving telephone conversations and mailings to achieve reductions in coronary risk factors including reductions in total and saturated fat intake and increases in dietary fiber intake. Robinson *et al.* [30] described a telephone-based dietitian managed computerized tracking system to streamline the management of lipid lowering drug therapy. The dietitian called patients to review laboratory results and reinforce issues such as weight, diet, and exercise. Mean lipid values improved significantly during the study period with 61% of patients achieving the National Cholesterol Education Program target LDL (low density lipoprotein cholesterol) level. A lower program dropout rate was observed than with patients receiving usual care. Stock *et al.* [31] describe a model for geriatric care that includes site-based care coordination, longer appointment times, utilization of an EMR, interdisciplinary team management and a wellness/prevention focus. The goal of this model is to improve access to care, including nutrition care, health outcomes and quality of life, by addressing the interrelatedness of senior health care delivery [31].

Continuous quality improvement

The final step to changing the office system is to evaluate the effectiveness of the system revisions on an ongoing basis. Providers should meet with staff regularly to modify systems that are not working effectively. Reports can be generated to provide feedback as to whether assessments have been completed, whether counseling has been provided, and whether providers have used appropriate coding and billing procedures. The use of an EMR can greatly simplify the generation of these reports. Surveys addressing patient satisfaction with the provision of nutrition services can guide further changes in the office system. As Pay for Performance measures are put into place in 2007 in institutional settings and move to office settings over the next 3–5 years, provision and documentation of nutritional care will become even more important.

Summary

The repeated assessment of nutrition status and interventions to prevent or treat diseases or conditions associated with poor nutrition are essential to the delivery of quality health care. Patients expect their physician to recognize and address nutritional concerns. The physician can provide this care directly or can refer when the provision of nutrition intervention is highly complex, likely to be time/labor intensive, involves individuals with altered cognitive or emotional states that are likely to impede compliance, or is outside the physician's level of comfort or expertise. The important thing is to recognize nutrition's importance to health, well-being and recovery, and to adopt a routine, systematic approach to problem identification and intervention for every individual that presents for care.

Resource 2.1 Body mass index

Overweight and obesity are now defined using body mass index (BMI) which can be calculated using the following equation:

$$BMI = \frac{weight\ (kg)}{height\ (m^2)}$$

Classification of obesity according to BMI

According to the NHLBI (National Heart, Lung, and Blood Institute) Clinical Guidelines, BMI provides a more accurate measure of total body fat than body weight alone. BMI should therefore be used, along with waist circumference and other risk factors, to assess an individual's risk of overweight. The guidelines define overweight individuals as those with a BMI of 25–29.9 kg/m² and obese individuals as those with a BMI of 30 kg/m² and above.

Source: [21].

Resource 2.2 Key diet history questions for brief intervention

Questions for all patients
- How many meals and snacks do you eat everyday?
- How often do you eat out? What kinds of restaurants?
- What do you like to drink during the day, including alcohol? How many glasses?
- How often do you eat fruits and vegetables?
- How often do you eat dairy products? Low fat or regular type?
- Do you usually finish what is on your plate or leave food?
- How often do you exercise, including walking?

In addition to the questions above

Questions for patients with dyslipidemia (See Chapter 7)
- How often do you eat fatty meats? (hot dogs, bacon, sausage, salami, pastrami, corned beef)
- How often do you eat fish? How is it prepared?
- What do you spread on your bread?
- What types of fats do you use in cooking?
- What type of snacks and desserts do you eat?

Questions for patients with high blood pressure (See Chapter 7)
- Do you use a salt shaker at the table or in cooking?
- Do you read food labels for sodium content? (<400 mg/serving permitted)
- How often do you eat canned, smoked, frozen, and processed foods?

Questions for patients with diabetes mellitus levels (See Chapter 8)
- What time do you take your diabetes medication (including insulin)?
- What time do you eat your meals and snacks?
- Do you ever skip meals during the day?
- How many servings of starchy foods such as breads, cereals, pastas, corn, peas, or beans do you eat during a typical day?

Source: Lisa Hark, PhD, RD, University of Pennsylvania School of Medicine. 2007.
Used with permission.

References

1 Truswell AS, Hiddink GJ, Blom J. Nutrition guidance by family doctors in a changing world: problems, opportunities, and future possibilities. *Am J Clin Nutr* 2003;77 (suppl):1089S–1092S.

2 Truswell AS. Family physicians and patients: is effective nutrition interaction possible? *Am J Clin Nutr* 2000;71:6–12.

3 Lagiou P, Olsen J, Trichopoulos D. Consumption of vegetables and fruits and risk of breast cancer. *JAMA* 2005;293(18):2209.

4 Nieves JW. Osteoporosis: the role of micronutrients. *Am J Clin Nutr* 2005;81(5):1232S–9S.

5 Ford ES, Kohl HW 3rd, Mokdad AH, Ajani UA. Sedentary behavior, physical activity, and the metabolic syndrome among U.S. adults. *Obes Res* 2005;13(3):608–14.

6 The Diabetes Prevention Program (DPP): description of lifestyle intervention. Diabetes Care. 2002;25:2165–71.

7 Committee on Nutrition Services for Medicare Beneficiaries, Food and Nutrition Board, Institute of Medicine. The Role of Nutrition in Maintaining Health in the Nation's Elderly: evaluating coverage of nutrition services for the medicare population. Washington, DC. national academies press, 2000.

8 Stratton RJ, Elia M. Depriciation linked to malnutrition risk and mortality in hospital. *Brit J Nutr* 2006;96:870–6.

9 Vecchiarino P, Bohannon RW, Ferullo J, Maljanian R. Short-term outcomes and their predictions for patients hospitalized with community acquired pneumonia. *Heart Lung* 2004;33(5):301–7.

10 Hakel-Smith N, Lewis NM. A standardized nutrition care process and language are essential components of a conceptual model to guide and document nutrition care and patient outcomes. *J Am Diet Assoc* 2004;104:1878–84.

11 Whitlock EP, Orleans CT, Pender N, Allan J. Evaluating primary care behavioral counseling interventions: an evidence based approach. *Am J Prev Med* 2002;22:267–84. www.preventiveservices.ahrq.gov (Accessed 07/07/06).

12 Mihalynuk TV, Knopp RH. Scott CS, Coombs JB. Physician informational needs in providing nutritional guidance to patients. *Fam Med* 2004;36:722–6.

13 Solberg LI, Kottke TE, Conn SA, Brekke ML, Calomeni CA, Conboy KS. Delivering clinical preventive services is a systems problem. *Ann Behav Med* 1997; 19(3):271–27.

14 Jacobsen ET, Rasmussen SR, Christensen M, Engberg M, Lauritzen T. Perspectives on lifestyle intervention: the views of general practitioners who have taken part in a health promotion study. *Scand J Public Health* 2005;33:4–10.

15 Aria M, Kauhanen L, Larivaara P, Rautio P. Factors influencing inquiry about patients' alcohol consumption by primary health care physicians: qualitative semi-structured interview study. *Fam Pract* 2003;20:270–5.

16 Glanz K, Tziraki C, Albright CL, Fernandes J. Nutrition assessment and counseling practices: attitudes and interests of primary care physicians. *J Gen Intern Med* 1995;10: 89–92.

17 Levine BS, Wigren MM, Chapman DS, Kerner JF, Bergman RL, Rivlin RS. A national survey of attitudes and practices of primary-care physicians relating to nutrition: strategies for enhancing the use of clinical nutrition in medical practice. *Am J Clin Nutr* 1993;57: 115–19.

18 Bruer RA, Schmidt RE, Davis H. Nutrition counseling–should physicians guide their patients? *Am J Prev Med* 1994;10:308–11.

19 US Department of Health and Human Services and US Department of Agriculture. 2005 *Dietary Guidelines for Americans*. Washington, DC, US Government Printing Office, 2005. www.healthierus.gov/dietaryguidelines/

20 AAFP Physicians Panel on Obesity. Practical advice for family physicians to help overweight patients. *Ann American Family Physician Monograph*. 2003.

21 Prochaska JO, DiClemente CC. Transtheoretical therapy toward a more integrative model of change. *Psychotherapy: Theory, Research and Practice* 1982;19(3):276–87.

22 American Dietetic Association. Referring your patients for Medicare Medical Nutrition Therapy Services . . . As Easy As 1, 2, 3. ADA Fact Sheet, 2001. www.eatright.org

23 ICD-9 Code Set, *International Classification of Disease-9th revision Clinical Modification*. Volumes 1 and 2, American Medical Association, Chicago, IL, 2006.

24 American Medical Association. Current Procedural Terminology. Professional Editor. CPT 2007. Chicago, AMA press, 2006.

25 American Medical Association. Healthcare Common Procedure Coding System. Medicare's National level II Codes. NCPCS 2007. Chicago. AMA press, 2006.

26 Infante M, Michael P. Medicare part B coverage and billing for medical nutrition therapy. *J Am Diet Assoc* 2002;102:32.

27 Hutson V. Military's TRICARE health care program provides benefits to millions, nutrition services to some. *J Am Diet Assoc* 2004;104:1541–4.

28 Fitzner K, Myers E, Caputo N, Michael P. Are health plans changing their views on nutrition service coverage? *J Am Diet Assoc* 2003;103:157–61.

29 Vale MJ, Jelinek MV, Grigg LE, Newman RW. Coaching patients on achieving cardiovascular health (COACH). A multiicenter randomized trial in patients with coronary heart disease. *Arch Intern Med* 2003;163:2775–83.

30 Robinson JG, Conroy C, Wickemeyer WJ. A novel telephone-based system for management of secondary prevention to a low-density lipoprotein cholesterol<=100 mg/dl. *Am J Cardiol* 2000;85:305–8.

31 Stock RD, Reee D, Cesario L. Developing a comprehensive interdisciplinary senior health care practice. *J Am Geriatr Soc* 2004;52:2128–33.

32 White JV, Blackburn GL. Nutrition Screening and Intervention Extended Care Facilities: A Practical, Systematic Approach. *J Med Direct* 1993;3:33–37.

Further reading

Geboers H, Mokkink H, Van Montfort P, Van Den Hoogen H, van den Bosch W, Grol R. Continuous quality improvement in small general medical practices: the attitudes of general practitioners and other practice staff. *Int J Qual Health Care* 2001;13:391–7.

Goldsmith G, Ward K, Howard J. Office-based management of diabetes: two-year trial of primary care quality improvement. *J Ark Med Soc* 2004 Mar;100(9):300–5.

Lapidos S, Rothschild SK. Interdisciplinary management of chronic disease in primary practice. *Manag Care Interface* 2004 17(7):50–3.

Nicholas LG, Pond CD, Roberts DC. Dietitian-general practitioner interface: a pilot study on what influences the provision of effective nutrition management. *Am J Clin Nutr* 2003;77 (4 suppl):1039S–1042S.

Porta M, Trento M. ROMEO Writing Committee. ROMEO: rethink organization to improve education and outcomes. *Diabet Med* 2004;21(6):644–5.

CHAPTER 3

Methods of weight control

Cathy Nonas, Jennifer Williams and Valentine J Burroughs

In a country where 65% of the adults are either overweight or obese (and the number is increasing), it is imperative that good clinical practice include weight management.

However, there are both real and presumed difficulties that make primary care clinicians reticent to treat patients who are overweight or obese. The predominant difficulty is reimbursement; obesity is seldom a reimbursable diagnosis. In a survey of 1,103 primary care physicians, lack of adequate reimbursement was identified as a barrier to treating obesity [1]. In most cases, physicians bill for associated co-morbidities not for obesity itself. Another perceived barrier is lack of time: if the primary care clinician is monitoring a patient during weight loss, but not acting as the primary source for weight management, then follow-up visits can be brief. Other identified barriers include lack of knowledge and low physician confidence [1]. This is not surprising given the inadequacy of nutrition education in medical school [2] and the constant influx of new diets; within the last decade alone there have been more than 1,200 diet books published [3].

This chapter will provide primary care clinicians with a description of the current popular diets and simple ways to evaluate a patient's monitoring needs within the parameters with in the primary care office practice.

First rule of thumb: address the issue

Although clinicians admit that weight management is on the top of their patients' list of nutrition topics [4] and the U.S. Preventive Services Task Force recommends that clinicians should counsel all obese patients on lifestyle behaviors (diet and physical activity), there is overwhelming evidence that most do not address the issue [5]. In a study of more than 12,000 overweight and obese adult patients, 58% said that their weight was never discussed with their primary care clinician. This finding is particularly disappointing given the evidence that clinicians who provided weight loss counseling increased threefold the odds that their patients would actually attempt weight loss [6].

Part of the problem may be a lack of understanding of what is deemed to be "acceptable" or "successful" weight loss. In a study by Foster *et al.* [7], 620 primary care clinicians were asked what percentage of weight loss would be considered acceptable, successful, and ideal for their patients. Responses were: 14% weight loss would be acceptable, 25% would be considered successful and 31% would be ideal [7]. Existing evidence proves otherwise: 5–10% weight loss statistically improves a patients' health profile – a fact that 75% of these same physicians readily acknowledged. In fact, in the Diabetes Prevention Program, a randomized trial of over 3,000 people conducted by the National Institutes of Health, the prevalence of metabolic syndrome was significantly reduced and diabetes prevented in people who lost just 5–7% of their weight [8]. Losing 30% of one's bodyweight is considered a success after bariatric surgery [9], but not realistic with dietary therapy.

The patient who initiates a weight loss diet may not need treatment by the primary care clinicians office, but it is incumbent upon the clinician to investigate the diet thoroughly enough to assess the patient's risks and any need for further monitoring and follow-up.

Assessment

For those weight loss diets that can be divided into categories by their macronutrient ratios, clinical monitoring can also be categorized by diet-type.

Before any weight loss treatment can be recommended, a baseline physical is warrented to assess the effects of their weight on disease risk as well as any additional risks that may occur during the weight loss phase. In order to help, The National Heart, Lung, and Blood Institute created a guide for primary care clinicians to determine which patients need weight reduction and guidelines for intervention [10] (See Table 3.1).

Anthropometrics as vital signs

Every progress note should prompt the clinician for a weight, body mass index (BMI) (Table 3.2), blood pressure and pulse measurement. In order to assure accurate blood pressure readings, the office should have adult, large adult and thigh cuffs; the scale should be able to weigh patients over 350 pounds, and waiting room and office chairs should be armless to accommodate large girth. Although BMI is a standard guideline for risk, as well as potential insurance reimbursement, many clinicians are not using it. In a survey of internal medicine

Table 3.1 Treatment protocols by body mass index.

BMI	Diet	Exercise	Behavior	Pharm	Surgery
25–30	×	×	×		
27–30 w/risk factors	×	×	×	×	
30–40	×	×	×	×	
35–40 w/risk factors	×	×	×	×	×
≥40	×	×	×	×	×

Source: Adapted from [10].

Table 3.2 Body mass index valves and classification.

Column groupings — Normal: BMI 19–24; Overweight: BMI 25–29; Obesity Class I: BMI 30–34; Obesity Class II: BMI 35–39; Obesity Class III: BMI 40–54. Body weight given in pounds.

Height (inches)	19	20	21	22	23	24	25	26	27	28	29	30	31	32	33	34	35	36	37	38	39	40	41	42	43	44	45	46	47	48	49	50	51	52	53	54
58	91	96	100	105	110	115	119	124	129	134	138	143	148	153	158	162	167	172	177	181	186	191	196	201	205	210	215	220	224	229	234	239	244	248	253	258
59	94	99	104	109	114	119	124	128	133	138	143	148	153	158	163	168	173	178	183	188	193	198	203	208	212	217	222	227	232	237	242	247	252	257	262	267
60	97	102	107	112	118	123	128	133	138	143	148	153	158	163	168	174	179	184	189	194	199	204	209	215	220	225	230	235	240	245	250	255	261	266	271	276
61	100	106	111	116	122	127	132	137	143	148	153	158	164	169	174	180	185	190	195	201	206	211	217	222	227	232	238	243	248	254	259	264	269	275	280	285
62	104	109	115	120	126	131	136	142	147	153	158	164	169	175	180	186	191	196	202	207	213	218	224	229	235	240	246	251	256	262	267	273	278	284	289	295
63	107	113	118	124	130	135	141	146	152	158	163	169	175	180	186	192	197	203	208	214	220	225	231	237	242	248	254	259	265	270	278	282	287	293	299	304
64	110	116	122	128	134	140	145	151	157	163	169	174	180	186	192	197	204	209	215	221	227	232	238	244	250	256	262	267	273	279	285	291	296	302	308	314
65	114	120	126	132	138	144	150	156	162	168	174	180	186	192	198	204	210	216	222	228	234	240	246	252	258	264	270	276	282	288	294	300	306	312	318	324
66	118	124	130	136	142	148	155	161	167	173	179	186	192	198	204	210	216	223	229	235	241	247	253	260	266	272	278	284	291	297	303	309	315	322	328	334
67	121	127	134	140	146	153	159	166	172	178	185	191	198	204	211	217	223	230	236	242	249	255	261	268	274	280	287	293	299	306	312	319	325	331	338	344
68	125	131	138	144	151	158	164	171	177	184	190	197	203	210	216	223	230	236	243	249	256	262	269	276	282	289	295	302	308	315	322	328	335	341	348	354
69	128	135	142	149	155	162	169	176	182	189	196	203	209	216	223	230	236	243	250	257	263	270	277	284	291	297	304	311	318	324	331	338	345	351	358	365
70	132	139	146	153	160	167	174	181	188	195	202	209	216	222	229	236	243	250	257	264	271	278	285	292	299	306	313	320	327	334	341	348	355	362	369	376
71	136	143	150	157	165	172	179	186	193	200	208	215	222	229	236	243	250	257	265	272	279	286	293	301	308	315	322	329	338	343	351	358	365	372	379	386
72	140	147	154	162	169	177	184	191	199	206	213	221	228	235	242	250	258	265	272	279	287	294	302	309	316	324	331	338	346	353	358	368	375	383	390	397
73	144	151	159	166	174	182	189	197	204	212	219	227	235	242	250	257	265	272	280	288	295	302	310	318	325	333	340	348	355	363	368	378	386	393	401	408
74	148	155	163	171	179	186	194	202	210	218	225	233	241	249	256	264	272	280	287	295	303	311	319	326	334	342	350	358	365	373	378	389	396	404	412	420
75	152	160	168	176	184	192	200	208	216	224	232	240	248	256	264	272	279	287	295	303	311	319	327	335	343	351	359	367	375	383	391	399	407	415	423	431
76	156	164	172	180	189	197	205	213	221	230	238	246	254	263	271	279	287	295	304	312	320	328	336	344	353	361	369	377	385	394	402	410	418	426	435	443

Source: Adapted from [10].

Table 3.3 Classification of overweight and obesity by body mass index (BMI), waist circumference, and associated disease risks.

| | BMI (kg/m²) | Obesity class | Disease risk* relative to normal weight and waist circumference† | |
			Men 102 cm (40 in) or less Women 88 cm (35 in) or less	Men >102 cm (40 in) Women >88 cm (35 in)
Underweight	<18.5		–	–
Normal	18.5–24.9		–	–
Overweight	25.0–29.9		Increased	High
Obesity	30.0–34.9	I	High	Very high
Extreme	35–39.9	II	Very high	Very high
Obesity	40.0+	III	Extremely high	Extremely high

*Disease risk for type 2 diabetes, hypertension, and CVD.
†Increased waist circumference can also be a marker for increased risk even in persons of normal weight.
Source: [10].

residents in urban university-based residency programs to assess the prevalence of BMI use, 60% did not know the minimum BMI for diagnosing obesity [11]. Classifications of overweight and obesity by BMI are listed in Table 3.3.

Quick tip

Post BMI tables in every examining room and as icons on computers (see Table 3.2) or request the result on the electronic medical record.

Past medical history

• The patient should be assessed for metabolic syndrome and impaired glucose tolerance. These syndromes increase the risk for cardiovascular disease and are associated with other disorders such as polycystic ovary syndrome and non-alcoholic fatty liver disease. Metabolic syndrome is characterized by at least three of the following five risk factors: low-HDL, elevated blood pressure, insulin resistance, elevated triglycerides and elevated waist circumference. The most clinically sensitive test for impaired glucose is a 2-hour oral glucose tolerance test. Diet, weight loss and increased physical activity will improve risk factors associated with metabolic syndrome (see Chapter 7.)
• Although the benefits of weight loss in patients with diabetes has been well-documented, before starting a weight loss diet, it is important to assess any complications from type 2 diabetes that may be exacerbated by changes in diet and weight. Patients with type 2 diabetes often have undiagnosed vascular disease. Therefore, an EKG is important to rule out any potential heart damage (such as myocardial infarction). Other basic assessments such as HbA1c,

tests for creatinine and microalbumin should be considered, as well as exams for neuropathy and retinopathy if they have not been done within the past year.

Biochemical data

Every patient should have baseline, fasting labs that include a complete blood count (CBC), comprehensive metabolic panel, liver function tests, lipid profile, uric acid and if the patient has type 2 diabetes, glycosylated hemoglobin (HbA1c). It is well documented that obese patients, particularly those with fat distribution in the upper body, are susceptible to non-alcoholic fatty liver disease (NASH). Serum lipid levels will give the clinician an indication of whether diet alone may resolve the abnormalities or whether pharmacotherapy (such as a statin), would also be indicated. The uric acid level, which is no longer part of many lab panels, is important, particularly in patients with metabolic syndrome or when a patient is following a low-carbohydrate diet. Serum potassium levels should be measured and evaluated in follow-up visits, particularly after significant or rapid weight loss or if the patient is using diuretics. One of the most underdiagnosed syndromes associated with obesity is sleep apnea. Indications of sleep apnea include neck >16 cm in circumference; the presence of snoring loudly or if the patient complains of feeling tired during the day.

A baseline electrocardiogram (EKG) can be helpful as well as a TSH screening. Obesity is often times associated with left ventricular hypertrophy to compensate for the increased cardiac work. Weight loss can also bring an extra stressor to the heart [12].

Medication use

Patients should be questioned about their medication use, as anxiety, depression, seizures, arrhythmias, allergies, diabetes and asthma medications may cause significant weight gain by increasing the patient's appetite. It is helpful to take a careful history of weight gain and time of initiation of medication, and to consider alternate medications that do not affect appetite. Buproprion, for example, is a weight-neutral serotonin reuptake inhibitor (SSRI) and exenatide for type 2 diabetes can result in weight loss.

Dieting risks

From a theoretical perspective, the healthiest weight loss diet would have three features: 1) it would be something to which a dieter could adhere for a lifetime; 2) it would result in slow, steady weight loss and long-term weight maintenance, and 3) it would be adequate in all nutrients. In reality, weight loss diets are usually followed for a short period of time, recidivism is extremely high, rate of weight loss is variable, and the diet regimen is usually incomplete in some vitamins or minerals.

Tips to Improve Effectiveness

1 Have Consumer Questions flyers from the Partnership for Health Weight Management (www.consumer.gov), which are free of charge, in your waiting room. It gives the patient questions to ask before starting any diet program.

2 Upon each visit, the physician should ask patients if they have made any dietary changes or started a new diet since the last visit. The response will lead to a conversation on weight loss. (See chapter 15)

3 Schedule more frequent visits. Have an overweight patient with a high risk profile or an obese patient return for follow-up appointments at shorter intervals: this can be an effective way of monitoring the patient's progress, getting them to be more familiar with the support that you can provide, and still remain billable visits.

4 Use other medical management protocols as the paradigm for the overweight or obese patient. For example, if a mildly hypertensive patient does not want blood pressure medication, the clinician typically suggests a follow-up visit within 1–3 months in order to evaluate the blood pressure another time. When a hypertensive patient is prescribed a new medication, the clinician would schedule a follow-up visit within the month to evaluate the medication's effects. The same holds true for overweight and obesity: if the patient is beginning a new diet regimen, schedule a follow-up appointment within the month to evaluate the effects; if the patient is not interested in beginning a diet, schedule a visit in three months to ensure that the patient has maintained a stable weight. If the patient has gained weight, revisit their readiness to change. (See chapter 2)

Thus far research is clear: successful weight loss is about calories consumed versus calories expended. Although low-carbohydrate diets seem to confer some advantage in the short-term when compared to low-fat diets, in the long-term there is no difference between diets [13–16]. Attrition rate in these studies is high. What matters in terms of weight loss success seems to be that the dieter is willing to adhere to the diet [17,18]. What matters to the practitioner is safety and improved clinical parameters.

There may be a myriad of diets, but they all manipulate three of the four calorie-producing macronutrients: fat, carbohydrate, and protein (the only other macronutrient is alcohol which is a source of "empty calories" and should be reduced or eliminated as part of any weight loss program). Protein: except for the Rice Diet and some gimmicks, almost all diets for weight loss are high in protein. Protein preserves lean tissue when calories are reduced. Since the 1970's when 58 people died while using a liquid formula diet with inadequate protein, formulas for weight loss contain protein of good biological value: somewhere between 18–30% of total calories. In an analysis of menus based on popular diet books, daily protein ranged from 67–83 g/day for all diets but Atkins (higher), Ornish (lower) and the first phase of South Beach (higher) [19]. Likewise, there is little controversy about types of fat: except for old versions of the Atkins diet, most diets today restrict saturated fat and promote controlled amounts of monounsaturated fat. Quantity of fat varies from 10–40% of total calories.

The real controversy surrounds carbohydrates. Carbohydrates are contained in vegetables, fruit, starch, milk, and foods with added sugar. Although the Atkins diet goes to the extreme by cutting out all of these food categories (except for a small amount of certain vegetables), most "low-carbohydrate" diets restrict the amount and type of carbohydrates, with particular emphasis on those from the starch category. Therefore, except for gimmick diets, most can be categorized into three major categories: low carbohydrate, moderate carbohydrate and high carbohydrate.

Is one diet more harmful than another? Recent research seems to indicate that diets for weight loss are generally safer than we once thought. This may be due to the fact that weight loss itself tends to improve a patients' health profile.

Monitoring the patient during weight loss

Monitor rate of weight loss in order to protect lean tissue loss and avoid any complications due to rapid weight loss. National guidelines suggest weight loss of no more than 1–2 pounds/week. Blackburn and others have also used the guideline of 1% weight loss per week [20], irrespective of the diet-type. See Table 3.4 for medical monitoring during weight loss.

Table 3.4 Medical monitoring.

Medical parameter	Low carbohydrate <20% kcal/day	Moderate carbohydrate 40–60% kcal/day	High carbohdyrate >60% kcal/day	Gimmicks
General				
Weight	★	★	★	★
Blood				
Creatinine	★			★
Glucose	★	★	★	★
HDL-cholesterol			★	★
LDL-cholesterol	★			★
Potassium	★	★	★	★
Triglyceride			★	★
Uric acid	★			★
Urine				
Glomerular filtration rate	★			
Ketones	★			★
Protein	★			★

Source: Cathy Nonas, RD, North General Hospital, New York. 2007. Used with permission.

Dietary effects on lipids

Abnormally high triglycerides (200–500 mg/dL) Dieters who follow a low-carbohydrate diet show a statistically greater improvement in serum triglycerides compared to those who follow a high-carbohydrate diet [13]. Conversely, those who follow a high-carbohydrate diet and who have abnormally high serum triglycerides, may have to be monitored more frequently to ensure that the triglycerides do not continue to rise.

Abnormal LDL-cholesterol (>130 mg/dL) Although the average change in LDL has not been significant, there is some concern about increases in LDL in patients following low-carbohydrate diets [21]. In one study, three subjects following the low-carbohydrate diet regimen had LDL levels that increased 40–100 mL/dL in 12 weeks. Thirty percent of the patients experienced a 10% increase in LDL levels [22].

Abnormally low HDL Some studies show an increase in HDL levels in patients following the low-carbohydrate diet [13]. Diets high in carbohydrate tend to reduce HDL levels in the short-term [13].

Dietary effects on kidney function

The mechanisms by which obesity causes kidney dysfunction is not well understood, but obesity-related glomerulopathy has increased tenfold over the last 15 years. Excess weight increases renal sodium resorption, thereby increasing both the renin angiotensin system (RAS) and the sympathetic nervous system, causing a rise in the systemic arterial pressure. These compensatory changes may increase the stress on the glomerular capillary cell wall, resulting in cell proliferation and glomerular sclerosis.

Although proteinuria and glomerulosclerosis usually decrease with weight loss, in women with pre-established abnormal glomerular filtration rates (GFR), weight loss on a diet that contains higher than normal protein intake may worsen renal function. In a study of 1,624 women enrolled in the Nurses' Health Study, protein intake was not correlated with a change in renal indices in those with normal GFR (defined as ≥ 80 mL/min per 1.73 m^2), but was correlated with a worsening of renal indices in those women with even mild renal insufficiency [23]. In this study, the highest quintile of total protein intake was a median of 93 g/day (86.5–163.7 g/day). Furthermore, consumption of animal protein was correlated with the greatest decline in estimated GFR. Therefore, all patients following a diet of >85 g protein/day may need a baseline evaluation of kidney function, and acute and chronic monitoring of creatinine and proteinuria if GFR is abnormal.

Dietary effects on uric acid

There is a greater risk of hyperuricemia in patients following a high protein, very low-carbohydrate diets than those on moderate- or high-carbohydrate diets. This is because the ketone bodies, products of fat oxidation, compete with urate for tubular reabsorption. Ketones are preferentially excreted to maintain acid–base balance so uric acid levels tend to increase. A baseline uric acid level, as well as a family or personal history of gout [23] can be helpful in monitoring the patient more closely during the first six weeks of any diet, particularly a low-carbohydrate one [24]. It is often the case that the uric acid level increases significantly at first, but then drops over time.

Obesity and weight loss effects on the gallbladder

Cholelithiasis is associated with obesity. Cholesterol production is linearly related to the amount of body fat. There is approximately 20 mg of additional cholesterol produced for each kilogram of extra body fat causing an increased flow of cholesterol into bile, leading to supersaturation. The bile acids do not increase in response, and so precipitation of cholesterol gallstones in the gallbladder is common among obese patients. Gallbladder disease is also prevalent in patients who lose weight, but particularly high with rapid weight loss. The flow of cholesterol continues to increase without bile acid compensation. Furthermore, the gallbladder is stagnant when the diet is low in fat, causing greater risk. The risk of gallbladder disease in high-fat, low-carbohydrate diets is currently under investigation, but no data has yet been published. Studies indicate that ≥10 g of fat in one meal/day triggers gallbladder contraction, emptying cholesterol, and reducing the risk of disease [18]. Very low-fat diets, very low-calorie diets and rapid weight loss confer the greatest risk of gallbladder disease symptoms.

Dietary effects on glycemic control

Obesity and type 2 diabetes are increasing at parallel rates. Obesity is the promoter of type 2 diabetes, and therefore, weight loss is often the best treatment. A 5–10% weight loss will significantly improve blood glucose, total cholesterol, triglycerides and blood pressure [25]. However, depending upon the severity of caloric and/or carbohydrate restriction, blood glucose may drop precipitously and warrant short-term, continuous adjustment of medication.

For example, a morning dose of a sulfonylurea has a peak action in mid-afternoon. If the only change in the diet is a liquid meal replacement at lunch (a significantly reduced calorie amount from usual), hypoglycemia may occur in mid-afternoon, particularly if the glucose had been well-controlled. In studies of people with diabetes who are prescribed very-low-calorie diets, 30–50% of the change in glucose can be seen in the first 5–10 days [26]. From a clinical perspective, in the short-term, it is better to keep the blood glucose slightly elevated during the weight loss phase rather than risk hypoglycemia. At the very least, hypoglycemia will cause the patient to overeat to compensate (conversely, it is inappropriate to suggest food as a safety net for a high dose of hypoglycemic mediation.) In the meal replacement case, for example, the most appropriate advice for a patient in glycemic control would be to halve the morning sulfonylurea dose.

To avoid complications from hypoglycemia:
• Establish a glucose threshold above which weight loss alone should not be used as a first-line treatment (in our clinical practice, we use 250 mg/dL) because many medications increase weight and may increase hypoglycemia after weight loss or when calories are very restricted.
• If blood glucose is ≤250 mg/dL, adjust the hypoglycemic medication downward to avoid hypoglycemia, particularly if the diet is very low in calories or very low in carbohydrates.
• If your patient does not monitor his/her glucose, and is on hypoglycemic medication, have them start monitoring before beginning any diet.
• If your patient monitors his/her glucose, have them call in the results on a daily or every-other-day basis and adjust the medication dosage accordingly. Otherwise, give that patient a sliding scale to make his/her own adjustments as the blood glucose falls.

The diets

The diets described below have been chosen because of their current popularity. They are organized by topic. Many of the diets have been categorized by carbohydrate level: high carbohydrate (>60% carbohydrate); moderate carbohydrate (40–60% carbohydrate); and low carbohydrate (<20% carbohydrate). Other diets have been categorized by similarities such as liquid formulas (both very-low-calorie and meal replacement), non-medical programs and gimmicks. (see Table 3.5) Few actual diets have any supportive peer-reviewed

Table 3.5 Categorization of the major diets.

High carbohydrate	Moderate carbohydrate	Low carbohydrate	Gimmicks/Fad diets
>60% carbohydrate 15–20% protein 10–19% fat	40–60% carbohydrate 15–30% protein 20–30% fat	<20% carbohydrate 25–35% protein 55–65% fat	Varies
Eat More, Weight Less	Glucose Revolution	Carbohydrate Addicts	Cabbage Soup
Eat to Live	SlimFast	Dr Atkins	Eat Right for Your Type
Pritikin	South Beach	Protein Power	Fit for Life
	Sugar Busters		Fat Flush
	Volumetrics		French Women Don't Get Fat
	Weight Watchers		Grapefruit
	Zone		pH Miracle for Weight Loss
	Whole Grain Diet Miracle		Somersizing
			The Ultimate Weight Solution: The 7 Keys to Weight Loss Freedom

Source: Lisa Hark, PhD, RD, University of Pennsylvania School of Medicine. 2007.
Used with permission.

published data, and even fewer have data from randomized control studies; SlimFast has published the most, followed by Atkins and Weight Watchers.

High carbohydrate/very low fat

Originally developed for treatment of heart disease, high carbohydrate (>60% carbohydrate), very-low-fat diets were popular in the 1990s and continue to have supporters today. The diets are high in complex carbohydrates from fruits, vegetables and whole grains that are also naturally high in fiber and low in energy density. These diets advocate little-to-no animal protein or added fat. Overweight individuals who are used to consuming a high fat diet often lose weight on this type of diet [27].

Eat More, Weigh Less, Revised and Updated: Dr. Dean Ornish's Life Choice Program for Losing Weight Safely While Eating Abundantly
Claim
Limiting energy intake from fat ($\leq$10%) allows for consumption of larger volumes of low-fat, low-calorie foods resulting in weight loss. Data from the Ornish Multicenter Lifestyle Demonstration Project show that mean weight decreased from baseline to 3 months (4.2 kg), 1 year (4. kg), 2 years (4.9 kg), and 3 years (3.3 kg) [28–29].

Regimen
Three meals/day plus one-or-two snacks, unlimited in beans, legumes, fruits, grains, and vegetables. Non-fat dairy products, non-fat or very low-fat commercially available products are allowed in moderation. Foods to avoid include meats, oils, avocados, olives, nuts and seeds, high-fat or low-fat dairy products, sugar and simple sugar derivatives. Approximately 74% carbohydrate, 18% protein, 7% fat, 2% saturated fat [30].

Others
Other popular high carbohydrate diets include: *Pritikin* (www.pritikin.com) and *Eat to Live* (www.drfuhrman.com).

Moderate carbohydrate/moderate fat

These diets are moderate for two reasons: the percentage of macronutrients is not extreme and they do not restrict any category of food. Monounsaturated fats are emphasized as well as high fiber food choices, while added sugars and saturated fats are limited. These diets have the potential to meet the *US Dietary Guidelines* and the Dietary Reference Intakes (DRIs) for vitamins and minerals. Moderate carbohydrate diets have resulted in weight losses of 6% [31]. The current evidence suggests that hypocaloric weight-loss diets should be moderate in carbohydrate (35–50% of energy), moderate in fat (25–35% of energy), and moderate in protein (25–30% of energy) [32].

These diets often refer to the glycemic index (GI) which uses a numerical ranking system for carbohydrates to indicate the degree to which different foods raise blood sugar immediately after consumption as compared with the rise generated by eating white bread or glucose. Proponents claim that a food with a low GI (<50) is more desirable because the slower release of glucose into the bloodstream reduces surges of insulin and flattening of the insulin curve increases satiety, thereby reducing energy intake.

Studies suggest that low-GI diets lower the insulin response to certain carbohydrates, but the results are inconclusive regarding whether these diets decrease hunger or promote weight loss. In a randomized crossover study comparing isocaloric high- vs. low-GI diets, there was no observed benefit of the low-GI diet on insulin sensitivity [33]. The effects of low-GI diets have more to do with increments in dietary fiber than differences in available carbohydrates [34].

Regarding insulin, diet books have tried to distinguish themselves by promoting some "magical" weight loss property. The following are some that emphasize their effects on insulin but fall into the moderate category.

Sugar Busters
Claim
Refined carbohydrate intake results in an overproduction of insulin and suppression of glucagon, promoting fat storage and inhibiting fat loss. By balancing the carbohydrate : protein ratio, glucagon levels will rise and stimulate the release of glucose into the bloodstream, enhancing weight loss.

Regimen
Three meals/day plus snacks of unrefined grains, lean meats, and high fiber vegetables with a low GI. This diet tends to be 40% carbohydrate, 28% protein, 32% fat, 9% saturated fat [30]. Exercise is emphasized to lower insulin levels and enhance insulin sensitivity.

The Zone Diet
Claim
Eating the proper ratio of carbohydrates, fat, and protein keeps the body's insulin production within a therapeutic zone, making it possible to burn excess body fat and lose weight. Weight, TG (triglycerides), insulin and waist circumference levels all decrease on the Zone Diet [17,27].

Regimen
The diet is 40% carbohydrate, 30% protein, and 30% fat. Meals and snacks are distributed with the same percent ratio of carbohydrate : protein : fat (40 : 30 : 30). The diet focuses on lean meats, small amounts of high-fiber grain products, vegetables, and some fruits.

The South Beach Diet

Claim
Limiting consumption of refined carbohydrates resolves the insulin resistance. There are no peer-reviewed studies to support the claims of the *South Beach* diet.

Regimen
Phase I (two weeks): carbohydrates are eliminated – this is a low-carbohydrate diet initially. Phase II: low GI carbohydrates reintroduced at 45% of total calories until target weight is achieved. Phase III: all carbohydrates are allowed in defined portions. Monounsaturated fats are recommended throughout all three phases along with high protein between-meal snacks.

Volumetrics

Claim
Eating large volumes of low-calorie foods and small volumes of calorically dense foods leads to satiety, which indirectly limits calorie consumption. A growing body of laboratory-based, clinical, and epidemiological data suggests that less-energy-dense diets are associated with lower energy intakes and body weight [35,36].

Regimen
Three meals/day plus snacks. Weight loss phase: calorie deficit of 500–1000 calories/day [55% carbohydrate (as whole grains, fruits, and vegetables), 15% protein (low fat fish, skinless poultry, and lean meats), and 30% fat]. Foods less than one calorie per gram are considered to be low in energy density.

Others

Other popular moderate carbohydrate diets include: *The Glucose Revolution*.

Low carbohydrate

Low carbohydrate diets are generally <20% carbohydrate (<100g/day), 25–30% protein, and 55–65% fat [3]. Supporters believe that carbohydrate consumption leads to hyperinsulinemia, which increases fat storage while decreasing intracellular shifts of free fatty acids (FFA) for oxidation. They also suggest that higher glucagon levels inactivate lipoprotein lipase, which is responsible for cleavage of fatty acids from glycerol with resultant increase of FFA into the adipocyte, while activating hormone-sensitive lipase, which results in release of FFA from the adipocyte.

The facts: only when energy consumption exceeds energy expenditure are excess glucose and TG stored in adipocytes. There is no evidence to support a long-term metabolic advantage from low-carbohydrate diets. However, evidence from outcomes of uncontrolled trials, non-randomized trials, and observational studies shows that free-living overweight individuals who self-select high-fat, low-carbohydrate diets consume fewer calories and lose weight [3]. It is speculated that the protein content promotes increased satiety and short-term weight loss secondary to enhanced compliance with hypocaloric diets [32]. Compared with a low-fat diet, low-carbohydrate diet programs have been shown to have better short-term (24 weeks) participant retention and weight loss (mean change −12.9%). In a 6 month study, subjects on a very-low-carbohydrate diet lost more weight than those on the low-fat diet (5.8 vs. 1.9 kg) [14]. Other studies have corroborated this finding [13,15].

Dr. Atkins' New Diet Revolution
Claim
Intake of refined carbohydrates over-stimulates insulin and results in uncontrolled hunger and eating. Carbohydrate restriction leads to ketosis, resulting in the utilization of fat for energy. Weight loss results from carbohydrate restriction rather than calorie restriction so individuals can eat as much as they want and still lose weight.

Regimen
Four phases defined by the amount of carbohydrates allowed: induction (20 g/day); weight loss (30–60 g/day); pre-maintenance and maintenance (10 g/day increments until weight loss slows and is maintained).

Protein Power
Claim
Calories are self-regulating when eaten in the right metabolic balance. Optimizing intake of effective carbohydrates (total carbohydrate content minus grams of fiber) helps maintain metabolic balance, based on the theory that fiber does not raise insulin levels.

Regimen
Three meals/day plus between-meal snacks. The diet provides 0.75 g protein/kg ideal body weight/day. Three phases: phase I (≤30 g carbohydrate/day), phase II (≤55 g carbohydrate/day), and phase III (progressive increase in "effective carbohydrate" intake until weight stabilizes). Advocates emphasize high fat food choices, but permit limited amounts of fruits and vegetables.

Medically supervised very low calorie programs
Medically supervised programs include Health Management Resources (HMR), Optifast, and Medifast. Each one includes behavior modification modules that are mandatory in conjunction with the very-low-calorie formulas. These programs are only franchised for physician-supervised offices or hospitals, and require close medical supervision. Monitoring by the primary care doctor may not be necessary due to the intensive medical monitoring usually associated with the program itself.

Very low calorie diets provide ≤800 kcal/day, and a high protein intake (70–100 g/day) to preserve lean body mass.

HMR and Optifast have published safety and efficacy studies. Mean weight loss is ≥1.4 kg weekly for the first few months [37]. One randomized trial and several case series of medically supervised low calorie diet programs found that patients who complete treatment lose up to 25% of initial weight compared with 16% for persons who drop out [37]. Reports have shown low attrition rates (≤2.5%) at twelve weeks, but attrition rates of 45% to 56% at the end of 26 weeks [36]. At one- and four-year follow-up, participants maintained a loss of 9% and 4.7%. Serious complications, including death, have been reported in obese persons who consumed very-low-calorie diets without medical supervision. An expert panel convened by the National Heart, Lung, and Blood Institute does not recommend the use of very-low-calorie diets after reviewing randomized trials that showed no long-term (≥1 year) advantage of very-low-calorie diets over conventional diets providing 1200–1500 kcal/day [10].

Claim
High quality, complete nutrition in pre-portioned and calorie-controlled servings can result in quick, safe weight loss because no food choices are made.

Regimen
Three meals are replaced by the company's products (liquid, bars, or self-contained frozen or vacuum-packed) for ≤800 kcal/day. There is a transition phase after approximately 16 weeks (part formula and part food) until weight maintenance is reached, followed by a maintenance phase. Behavior modification group classes cover physical activity, stress management, and social support.

Programmatic diets

These are diets that are developed nationally but run locally, without medical monitoring. The sessions are often taught by a non-clinician, and someone who has successfully followed the program. Most of these programs include information about behavior modification and physical activity as well as offering a low calorie diet. The most well-known of these is *Weight Watchers: Turnaround Program*.

Weight Watchers
Claim
Individualization of the diet via a POINTS® program, counseling, group support, and exercise results in weight loss and enables life-long maintenance of a healthy diet. Of three randomized controlled trials of Weight Watchers, the largest reported a loss of 3.2% of initial weight at two years. Two randomized trials found that persons who regularly attended Weight Watchers lost

approximately 5% of initial weight over 3–6 months [37]. Weight loss at one year was 3 kg [17].

Regimen
Foods are assigned a POINTS® value based on the calorie, fat, and fiber content. Healthier food choices are assigned the lowest points, encouraging healthy lifestyle changes. A daily multiple vitamin–mineral supplement is suggested. Support includes weekly group sessions.

Others
Other programmatic diets include: Jenny Craig, LA Weight Loss and Take Off Pounds Sensibly (TOPS).

Low-calorie meal replacement
Low-calorie meal replacements come in the form of shakes, bars, or self-contained meals and are vitamin/mineral fortified. A systematic evaluation of six randomized controlled trials utilizing a partial meal replacement plan suggests that these types of interventions can safely and effectively produce significant sustainable weight loss (~7–8% body weight at 1 year compared with ~3–7% for those on a reduced calorie diet) [38]. Thus far, the only randomized clinical trial data comes from SlimFast.

The SlimFast diet
Claim
Replacing one-to-two meals/day with a standardized, portion-controlled, nutritious and inexpensive formula can reduce energy intake and result in weight loss. Dietary compliance and convenience are viewed more favorably by participants who consume meal replacements than by those in a conventional weight loss program [39].

Regimen
Two daily SlimFast products plus one balanced, portion-controlled regular food meal, and fruit, vegetables, or a SlimFast snack bar for between meal snacks provides 1200–1500 kcal/day.

Gimmicks
Food-combining
The science for food combining is unfounded. Most foods contain all three macronutrients together. The concept of daily cycles is based on normal hormonal changes in the body, but there is no evidence to support the claim that these fluctuations influence nutritional requirements or when individuals should eat specific foods.

Somersizing
Claim
Eating certain macronutrients and proteins together cancels out certain enzymes resulting in weight gain. By providing a constant source of energy with frequent small meals and plenty of fresh fruit and vegetables, the body can be reprogrammed to burn fat.

Regimen
Carbohydrates should not be eaten with fat and other carbohydrate-rich foods. Proteins and fats can be eaten together with vegetables. Fruits should be eaten alone or on an empty stomach.

Fit for Life
Claim
The body operates in cycles: appropriation (noon–8 pm), assimilation (8 pm–4 am), and elimination (4am–noon). Combining food in certain ways and eating them at certain times improves digestive processes and leads to successful weight loss. Calories are only bad if they come from highly processed or ill-combined foods.

Regimen
The diet is high in fruits and vegetables and limited in dairy products and meats. Breakfast: only fruit. When fruit is eaten throughout the day, it should not be eaten with other foods. Lunch: raw vegetables with whole grain bread or vegetable soup. Dinner: salad with grain and meat. No processed or cooked foods.

Detox
Hundreds of detoxification diets are available. They have been described as cell cleansing, immunity rejuvenating, skin revitalizing, body flushing, colon decontaminating, and liver purging. Detox approaches are contrary to scientific consensus and medical evidence [40].

Fat Flush Diet
Claim
The author claims to melt fat away by attacking the five weight gain factors: an over-worked liver, water clogged tissues, fear of eating fat, hyperinsulinemia, and stress. Liver toxicity is responsible for weight gain. Inefficient bile production can slow weight loss.

Regimen
Fat-flush supplements and a mixture of unsweetened cranberry juice and water four times/day. Phase I: 1100–1200 kcal/day. Phase II: 1200–1500 kcal/day. Phase III ≥1500 kcal/day. Foods claimed to have detox capacities are red meat

(l-carnitine), eggs (taurine, cysteine, and methionine), cruciferous vegetables, garlic, onions, and some herbs.

Effects of certain diets with medication for weight loss

Weight loss medication can and should be offered to patients when diet and exercise alone have failed to result in a 5–10% weight loss. These medications can improve weight loss effects of diet and exercise when diet and exercise alone are not sufficient. The FDA approves weight loss drugs if studies show that by using the drug along with intensive diet therapy, more subjects can safely reach and maintain a 5–10% weight loss than with intensive diet therapy and placebo [41].

As the maintenance of weight loss becomes integral to treatment paradigms, long-term effects of medications become important criteria for success [41]. Therefore, any FDA-approved medications for long-term weight loss, the 'gold' standard for all new weight loss medications, must show safety and efficacy for two years or more [41]. Currently there are only two drugs approved for long-term use: sibutramine (Meridia) and orlistat (Xenical), but others are in phase III trials now [42–44]. Rimonabant is classified as an endocannabinoid receptor antagonist, has an approval letter from the FDA and should be available by 2007 [43].

Sibutramine (Abbott) is the only long-term FDA-approved weight loss medication that is a reuptake inhibitor of norepinephrine, serotonin and dopamine, with norepinephrine occurring in greatest amounts [44]. Available since 1997, it has been proven to be safe and effective. Originally designed as an antidepressant, it was found to reduce appetite rather than depression. There is normal physiologic release of neurotransmitters, but it acts as a reuptake inhibitor. The use of sibutramine is associated with small but clinically insignificant increases of less than 1 to 3 mm Hg for diastolic blood pressure, as well as an average increase in heart rate of approximately 4 to 5 beats per minute. In a small group of patients, blood pressure and heart rate show greater increases, but the weight loss associated with sibutramine may also attenuate those blood pressure effects. However, sibutramine should not be prescribed for patients with high blood pressure. Sibutramine is prescribed in 5, 10 and 15 mg/day doses. It is prescribed once per day, usually in the morning to avoid insomnia. There are no dietary restrictions with this medication, but behavior modification and lifestyle changes are important adjuncts to success. In a recent one year study, it was found that combining Sibutramine with lifestyle counseling yielded a larger weight loss than medication or lifestyle counseling alone [45]. An even higher weight loss resulted when food intake records were added on a frequent basis [45].

Unlike other FDA-approved weight-loss medications, orlistat (Xenical by Hoffman-LaRoche) is the first non-systemic weight-loss medication, acting entirely on the gut, not the brain. Weight loss occurs because of reduced absorption of fat calories. Approximately 30% of dietary fat is eliminated in the stool. Orlistat is prescribed in 120 mg doses to be taken three times per day, at meals [44]. Since its mechanism of action is influenced by the amount of fat in the meal, when someone is following a low-fat diet, side effects are few; however, when someone consumes a high fat meal, side effects can be significant, including flatulence, oily stools, severe diarrhea, and abdominal cramping.

Orlistat, at 60 mg (half the dose of Xenical), has recently been approved by the FDA for over-the-counter (OTC) use [46]. The product will be called Alli and it is the first weight loss medication to be approved by the FDA for OTC use. It will be sold in stores to people who are over 18 years of age and will most likely be available for the spring of 2007. The introductory package will include education materials such as a glossary of fat grams in foods, how to modify recipes to reduce fat, how to make healthy choices in restaurants, how to increase physical activity and record food intake [46].

Rimonabant (FDA approval pending) represents a new class of drugs that are endocannabinoid receptor antagonists or selective CB1 blockers [43]. Cannabinoid receptors are found in two areas of the body: CB1 receptors are primarily in the brain and limbic system, and CB2 receptors are found primarily in the immune system. CB1 receptors influence appetite. In the Rimonabant in Obesity (RIO)-Lipids study, a multi-center randomized, placebo-controlled study of 1,036 obese patients with dyslipidemia, results showed significant weight loss as well as improvement in HDL-cholesterol, triglycerides, and in the higher doses, LDL particle size. Specifically, Rimonabant induces weight loss greater than 5% in 30–40% of patients and greater than 10% weight loss in 10–20% of patients, above both a dietary run-in and long-term hypo-caloric management over a 2-year period [47]. All groups reported a low level of drug-related side effects. Rimonabant therapy is associated with an extra 8–10% increase in HDL-cholesterol and a 10–30% reduction in triglycerides, as well as improvements in insulin resistance, glycemic control in patients with diabetes, and C-reactive protein (CRT) levels over the hypo-caloric diet therapy group [47].

The FDA has also approved Exenatide (Lilly and Amylin) as adjunctive therapy to improve blood sugar control in patients with type 2 diabetes who have not achieved adequate control on metformin and/or a sulfonylurea. Exenatide is the first in a new class of medicines known as incretin mimetics. Exenatide is a synthetic protein (from the Gila monster) that mimics the activity of the naturally occurring hormone glucagons-like peptide-1 (GLP-1) [48]. GLP-1 binds to pancreatic beta-cell receptors to stimulate the release of insulin. In response to food intake GLP-1 will stimulate the release of insulin by binding to the pancreatic beta-cell receptors [49].

In clinical trials, Exenatide has been shown to improve blood sugar control by lowering both post-meal and fasting glucose levels, leading to better long-term control as measured by hemoglobin A1C. Weight loss appears to be an added benefit [50]. Exenatide has been shown to do this through several actions, including the stimulation of insulin secretion only when blood sugar is high and by restoring the first-phase insulin response, an activity of the insulin-producing cells in the pancreas that is lost in patients who have type 2 diabetes. The major side effects appear to be nausea.

Medications for weight loss have had a dubious history, because of inappropriate practices, severe side effects and transitory effects [44]. However, currently prescribed medications for short-term use have been shown to be safe and effective when used appropriately. FDA-approved medications for long-term use (orlistat and sibutramine) have been on the market for almost a decade, and their safety profiles remain good. There are two things that stand in the way of weight loss medications becoming more popular- their high cost, which is usually not reimbursable by insurance, and the high expectations of the public. Clinicians may also expect that a weight loss medication will do more than result in modest weight loss. But it's important to remember that medications may help a patient reach that critical 5–10% weight loss better than with diet and exercise alone. And after all, modest can make a big improvement in the patient's health profile.

Bariatric Surgery

In the last decade, the number of obesity-related surgeries has increased 644%, making bariatric surgery the fastest growing field in all of medicine [51]. The operative mortality ranges from 0.3–1.6%. Perioperative complications (ex. thromboembolic events, gastrointestinal leak, and hemorrhage) occur in ~10% of patients. Long-term complications include malnutrition, dehydration, weight loss failure, dumping syndrome, anemia, and vitamin and mineral deficiencies [51,51]. Adherence to diet and vitamin/mineral prescriptions significantly ameliorates these risks. The most commonly deficient vitamins and minerals following weight loss surgery include protein, iron, vitamin B_{12}, thiamin, folate, calcium, the fat-soluble vitamins (A, D, E, K), and other micronutrients [52]. The deficiencies appear to be more substantial following malabsorptive procedures such as bilio-pancreatic diversion (BPD), but occur with restrictive procedures as well [52].

Bariatric surgery should be reserved for individuals with a BMI $\geq 40\,\mathrm{kg/m^2}$ or a BMI of 35–39.9 kg/m^2 with co-morbidities such as diabetes or hypertension [53]. With appropriate patient selection, education, and post-surgical care, 75–80% of patients lose >50% of their excess weight or 30% of total weight. After 15 years of follow-up, gastric bypass patients have maintained a mean excess weight loss of over 49% [51]. Even for those who satisfy the weight requirement, non-surgical weight loss, including diet, exercise, and pharmacotherapy should be considered first [52–55].

Procedures are designed either to cause nutrient malabsorption, restrict food intake, or a combination of both. Currently, there is no universally accepted "best" procedure [54,55]. Restrictive procedures with some degree of malabsorption (roux-en-Y gastric bypass) are the most common in the US. The pouch is small, with a capacity (15–30 mL) which causes early satiety. Sugar and fat intake must be decreased to avoid dumping syndrome and fat intake secondary to poor tolerance. Daily caloric intake during the first year after surgery is estimated to be <900 kcal/day [51].

Post-operatively, follow-up visits should include documentation about weight loss, any vomiting, dumping syndrome, food intolerances, and adherence to prescribed daily multivitamins, calcium, and any other supplementation [52,56,57]. Lab work should include CBC, ionized magnesium, comprehensive metabolic panel, ferritin, iron, TIBC at 1 month, 3 months and 6 months post surgery, plus serum vitamin D (25,OH Vit D), intact PTH every 6 months and bone density test annually [52,56,57].

References

1 Kushner RF. Barriers to providing nutrition counseling by physicians: a survey of primary care practitioners. *Prev Med* 1995;24(6):546–52.

2 Pearson TA, Stone EJ, Grundy SM, McBride PE, Van Horn L, Tobin WB. Translation of nutritional sciences into medical education: the Nutrition Academic Award Program. *AJCN* 2001;74(2):164-70

3 Freedman MR, King J, Kennedy E. Popular diets: A scientific review. *Obes Res* 2001;9 (suppl 1):1–40S.

4 Mihalynuk TV, Knopp RH, Scott CS, Coombs JB. Physician informational needs in providing nutrition guidance to patients. *Fam Med* 2004;36(10):722–6.

5 Snow V, Barry P, Fitterman N, Qaseem A, Weiss K. Pharmacologic and Surgical Management of Obesity in Primary Care: A Clinical Practice Guideline from the American College of Physicians. *Ann Int Med* 2005;142:525–31.

6 Galuska DA, Will JC, Serdula MK, Ford ES. Are health care professionals advising obese patients to lose weight? *JAMA* 1999;282(16):1581–2.

7 Foster GD, Wadden TA, Makris AP *et al*. Primary care physicians' attitudes about obesity and treatment. *Obes Res* 2003;11:1168–77.

8 Orchard TJ, Temprosa M, Goldberg R *et al*. The effect of metformin and intensive lifestyle intervention on the metabolic syndrome: The Diabetes Prevention Program Randomized Trial. *Ann Intern Med* 2005;142:611–19.

9 Choban P. Surgical Treatment, Overview. In: Foster GD, Nonas CA (eds). *Managing Obesity: A clinical guide*. American Dietetic Association; Chicago, IL, 2004;175–84.

10 National Institute of Health, National Heart, Lung, and Blood Institute, North American Assocation for the Study of Obesity. *The Practical Guide: Identification, Evaluation, and Treatment of Overweight and Obesity in Adults*. NIH Publication Number 00-4084, October 2000.

11 Block JP, DeSalvo KB, Fisher WP. Are physicians equipped to address the obesity epidemic? Knowledge and attitudes of internal medicine residents. *Prev Med* 2003;36(6):669–75.

12 Nonas CA. Clinical Monitoring. In: Foster GD, Nonas CA (eds). *Managing Obesity: A clinical guide*. American Dietetic Association; Chicago, IL, 2004.

13 Foster GD, Wyatt HR, Hill JO *et al*. A randomized trial of a low-carbohydrate diet for obesity. *NEJM* 2003;348(21):2082–90.

14 Samaha FF, Iqbal N, Seshadri P, Chicano KL, Daily DA, McGory J, Williams T, Williams M, Gracely EJ, Stern L. A low-carbohydrate as compared with a low-fat diet in severe obesity. *NEJM* 2003;348(21):2074–81.

15 Brehm BJ, Seeley RJ, Daniels SR, D'Alessio DA *et al.* A randomized trial comparing a very low carbohydrate diet and a calorie-restricted low fat diet on body weight and cardiovascular risk factors in healthy women. *J Clin Endo Metab* 2003;88(4):1617–23.

16 Stern L, Iqbal N, Seshadri P *et al.* The effects of low-carbohydrate versus conventional weight loss diets in severely obese adults: one-year follow-up of a randomized trial. *Ann Int Med* 2004;140:778–85.

17 Dansinger ML, Gleason JA, Griffith JL, Selker HP, Schaefer EJ. Comparison of the Atkins, Ornish, Weight Watchers, and Zone Diets for weight loss and heart disease risk reduction: A randomized trial. *JAMA* 2005;293(1):43–53.

18 Wing RR, Phelan S. Long term weight maintenance. *Am J Clin Nutr* 2005;82 (suppl 1): 222–5.

19 Nonas CA, Foster GD. Popular diets in the management of obesity. In: Carson JS, Burke FM, Hark LA (eds). Cardiovascular Nutrition. American Dietetic Association, 2005.

20 Blackburn GL. Comparison of medically supervised and unsupervised approaches to weight loss and control. *Ann Int Med* 1993;199:714–18.

21 Seshadri P, Iqbal N, Stern L *et al.* A randomized study comparing the effects of a low-carbohydrate diet and a conventional diet on lipoprotein subfractions and C-reactive protein levels in patients with severe obesity. *Am J Med* 2004;117(6):398–405.

22 Yancy WS, Olsen MK, Guyton JR, Bakst RP, Westman EC. A low-carbohydrate, ketogenic diet versus a low-fat diet to treat obesity and hyperlipidemia: a randomized control trial. *Ann Int Med* 2004;140:769–77.

23 Knight EL, Stamfer MJ, Hankinson SE, Spiegelman D, Curhan GC. The Impact of protein intake on renal function decline in women with normal renal function or mild renal insufficiency. *Ann Intern Med* 2003;138:460–7.

24 Nonas C, Pi-Sunyer FX, Foster GD. Obese women with metabolic syndrome. In: *Medical Nutrition and Disease: A Case-Based Approach.* 3rd edition. Malden, Mass: Blackwell Publishing. 2003:25–38.

25 Klein S, Burke LE, Bray GA, Blair S, Allison D, Pi-Sunyer FX, Hong Y, and Eckel RH Clinical Implications of Obesity With Specific Focus on Cardiovascular Disease: A Statement for Professionals From the American Heart Association Council on Nutrition, Physical Activity, and Metabolism: Endorsed by the American College of Cardiology Foundation *Circulation* 2004;110:2952–2967.

26 Wing RR. Weight loss in the management of type 2 diabetes. In: Gerstein H and Haynes B (eds). *Evidence-Based Diabetes Care.* BC Decker, Ontario. 2000, Chapter 14.

27 McAuley KA, Hopkins CM, Smith KJ *et al.* Comparison of high-fat and high-protein diets with a high-carbohydrate diet in insulin-resistant obese women. *Diabetologia* 2005;48(1):8–16.

28 Ornish D. *Eat More, Weigh Less, Revised & Updated: Dr. Dean Ornish's Life Program for Losing Weight Safely While Eating Abundantly.* New York, NY: Harper Collins Publishers, Inc; 2001.

29 Ornish D, Brown SE, Scherwitz LW *et al.* Can lifestyle changes reverse coronary heart disease? The Lifestly Heart Trial. *Lancet* 1990;336:129–33.

30 Anderson JW, Konz EC, Jenkins DJA. Health advantages and disadvantages of weight-reducing diets: A computer analysis and critical review. *J Am Coll Nutr* 2000;19(5):578–90.

31 Johnston CS, Tjonn SL, Swan PD. High-protein, low-fat diets are effective for weight loss and favorably alter biomarkers in healthy adults. *J Nutr* 2004;134:586–91.

32 Schoeller DA, Buchholz AC. Energetics of obesity and weight control: Does diet composition matter? *J Am Dietet Assoc* 2005;105:S24–S28.

33 Kiens B, Richter EA. Types of carbohydrate in an ordinary diet affect insulin action and muscle substrates in humans. *Am J Clin Nutr* 1996;63:47–53.

34 Hu FB, van Dam RM, Liu S. Diet and risk of type II diabetes: the role of types of fat and carbohydrate. *Diabetologia* 2001;44:805–17.

35 Kral TVE, Roe, LS, Rolls BJ. Combined effects of energy density and portion size on energy intake in women. *Am J Clin Nutr* 2004;79:962–8.

36 Rolls BJ, Drewnowski A. Ledikwe JH. Changing the energy density of the diet as a strategy for weight management. *J Am Dietet Assoc* 2005;105:S98–S103.

37 Tsai AG, Wadden TA. Systematic review: An evaluation of major commercial weight loss programs in the United States. *Ann Int Med* 2005;142:56–66.

38 Heymsfield SB, van Mierlo CAJ, van der Knapp HCM, Heo M, and Frier HI. Weight management using a meal replacement strategy: meta and pooling analysis from six studies. *Int J Obesity* 2003;27:537–49.

39 Noakes M, Foster PR, Keogh JB, Clifton PM. Meal replacements are as effective as structured weight-loss diets for treating obesity in adults with features of metabolic syndrome. *J Nutr* 2004;134:1894–9.

40 Clemens R, Pressman P. Detox diets provide empty promises. *Food Tech* 2005;59(5):18.

41 Department of Health and Human Services. Food and Drug Administration. *Guidance on the Clinical Evaluation of Weight Control Drugs.* FDA, 2004. www.fda.gov.

42 Hofbauer KG, Nicholson JR. Pharmacotherapy of obesity. *Exp Clin Endocrinol Diabetes* 2006;114(9):475–84.

43 Cooke D, Bloom S. The obesity pipeline: current strategies in the development of anti-obesity drugs. *Nat Rev Drug Discov* 2006;5(11):919–31.

44 Kushner RF, Manzano H. Obesity pharmacology: past, present and future. *Curr Opin Gastroenterol* 2002;18(2):213–20.

45 Wadden, TA, Berkowitz, RI, Womble, LG et al. Randomized trial of lifestyle modification and pharmocotherapy for obesity. *N Engl J Med* 2005;353(20):2111–20.

46 Food and Drug Administration. Orlistat approved for over-the-counter use by FDA. January 2006. www.fda.gov.

47 Scheen AJ, Van-Gaal LG, Despres JP, Pi-Sunyer X, Golay A, Honotin C. Rimonabant improves cardiometabolic risk factor profile in obese or overweight subjects: overview of RIO studies. *Rev Med Suisse (French)* 2006; 23(76):1916–23.

48 Triplitt C, Chiquette, E. Exenatide: from the Gila monster to the pharmacy. *J Am Pharm Assoc* 2006; 46(1):44–52.

49 Barnett, AH. Exantide. *Drugs Today* 2005;41(9); 563–78.

50 Heine, RJ, Van Gaal, LF, Johns, D. Exenatide versus insulin Glargine in patients with suboptimally conrolled type 2 diabetes. *Ann Intern Med* 2005;143:559–569.

51 Shikora SA. Severe obesity: A growing health concern ASPEN should not ignore. *JPEN* 2005;29(4):288–297.

52 Bloomberg RD, Fleishman A, Nalle JE, Herron DM, Kinni S. Nutritional deficiencies following bariatric surgery: what have we learned. *Obes Surg* 2005;15(2):145–154.

53 Choban P. Surgical Treatment, Overview. In: Foster GD, Nonas CA (eds). *Managing Obesity: A Clinical Guide.* American Dietetic Association. Chicago, IL. 2004.

54 Friedrich MJ. Better strategies sought against obesity. *JAMA* 2006;296(13):1577–9.

55 Wadden TA, Tsai AG. Bariatric surgery: crossing a body mass index threshold. *Ann Intern Med* 2006;144(9):689–91.

56 Fujioka K. Follow-up of nutritional and metabolic problems after bariatric surgery. *Diabetes Care* 2005;28:481–484.

57 Malinowski SS. Nutritional and metabolic complications of bariatric surgery. *Am J Med Sci* 2006;331(4):219–25.

Further reading

Boden G, Sargrad K, Homko C, Mozzoli M, Stein TP. Effect of a low-carbohydrate diet on appetite, blood glucose levels, and insulin resistance in obese patients with type 2 diabetes. *Ann Int Med* 2005;142(6):403–11.

Brehm BJ, Spang SE, Lattin BL, Seeley RJ, Daniels SR, D'Alessio DA. The role of energy expenditure in the differential weight loss in obese women on low-fat and low-carbohydrate diets. *J Clin Endocrinol Metab* 2005;90(3):1475–82.

Fukagawa NK, Anderson JW, Young VR, Minaker KL. High-carbohydrate, high-fiber diets increase peripheral insulin sensitivity in healthy young and old adults. *Am J Clin Nutr* 1990;52:524–8.

Gleason JA, Griffith JL, Selker HP, Schaefer EJ. Comparison of the Atkins, Ornish, Weight Watchers and Zone Diets for weight loss and heart disease risk reduction. *JAMA* 2005:293:43–53.

Klauer J. How the Rich Get Thin: Park Avenue's Top Diet Doctor Reveals the Secrets to Losing Weight and Feeling Great. St. Martin's Press, 2006.

Lara-Castro C, Garvey T. Diet insulin resistance, and obesity: Zoning in on data for Atkins dieters living in South Beach. *J Clin Endocrinol Metab*. 2004;4197–205.

LaRosa JC, Fry AG, Muesing R, Rosing DR. Effects of high-protein, low-carbohydrate dieting on plasma lipoproteins and body weight. *J Am Diet Assoc* 1980;77:264–70.

Ornish D. Avoiding revascularization with lifestyle changes: the Multicenter Lifestyle Demonstration project. *Am J Cardiol* 1998;82:72T–76T.

Freedman MR, Ornish D, Scherwitz LW, Bilings JH *et al.* Intensive lifestyle changes for reversal of coronary heart diseas. *JAMA* 1998;280:2001–7.

Wadden, TA, Berkowitz, RI, Womble, LG. Randomized Trial of Lifestyle Modification and Pharmocotherapy for Obesity. *N Engl J Med* 2005 Nov 17;353(20):211–20.

Wright JD, Kennedy-Stephanson J, Wang CY, McDowell MA, Johnson CI. Trends in intake of energy and macronutrients – United States, 1971–2000. *MMWR Morb Mortal Wkly Rep.* 2004;53:80–82.

Nutrition through the life-cycle

CHAPTER 4

Growing up healthy

Susan Konek and Diane Barsky

Adequate and appropriate nutrition from infancy through adolescence is critical for the developing human being. Proper nutrition supplies the immediate energy needs for physical activity, the protein to develop and grow, and the micronutrients that support these processes. Dietary intake and genetic predisposition set the stage for adult health. The incidence of overweight and obesity in all sectors of the population has increased at an alarming rate in recent years. Health care providers need to identify those families at risk and provide age appropriate anticipatory guidance for prevention of chronic diseases.

Growth

Evaluation of growth is the cornerstone of pediatric nutrition assessment [1]. Inadequate nutritional intake impacts growth and ultimately may interfere with the child achieving their developmental potential. Children undergo two rapid periods of growth: the first during infancy and early childhood, the second in adolescence. Between these, slow, steady growth is seen. Growth is documented by serial measurements of weight and length from birth to 18 years, and head circumference from birth to 36 months, plotted on growth curves derived from observations of large numbers of normal, healthy children. These curves, first developed by the National Center for Health Statistics (NCHS) in 1977, have been revised by the Centers for Disease Control and Prevention (CDC) (www.cdc.gov/growthcharts) [2]. Most of the data used to construct these charts comes from the National Health and Nutrition Examination Survey (NHANES), collected from 1971 to 1994, and includes all ethnic and racial groups, and both breastfed and formula-fed infants [3]. An innovation in the current growth charts is the inclusion of body mass index (BMI) values for age and gender for children aged 2–20 years. BMI provides an objective measure of weight in relationship to height to assess the degree of adiposity.

Interpretation of growth chart plots is an important function of primary care clinicians. Children require evaluation for underweight if their weight and/or height for-age falls below the 5th percentile. Crossing over 2 percentiles with weight loss or, when weight or linear growth plateaus on the growth chart requires further medical and nutritional evaluation. Remaining between the

5th and the 85th percentile (within ±2 percentile lines) represents a normal growth pattern. Children falling between the 85th percentile and the 95th percentile should be considered overweight [4]. Children falling above the 95th percentile are considered obese [4]. Growth charts for premature infants have been developed and should be used for very low birth weight infants (less than 1500 g), available on the CDC website [2].

Initially, during acute malnutrition the child's weight decreases or the rate of weight gain slows or plateaus. After 4 to 6 months the condition becomes chronic resulting in slowing of linear growth. Chronic malnutrition harms brain growth in children under three years old, which may result in abnormal head circumference growth.

Plotting a child's growth is a sensitive, noninvasive tool to identify relatively normal physiologic function [5]. The early detection of abnormal growth patterns in well child visits allows for effective preventive and therapeutic interventions. Therefore, it is critical to accurately measure and plot children's weight, height, and head circumference using current growth charts measurement of children and the plotting of their growth cannot be overstated [5]. Inaccurate measurements may result in growth failure not being identified, or a child with a normal growth pattern being referred for unnecessary evaluation. Gilluly, Johnson, and Rossiter have reported a study of 878 children measured in 55 pediatric and family primary care practices in seven US cities [5]. Baseline results indicated that only 30% of children were measured accurately. It is strongly recommended that a recumbent length-board be used to measure infants and young children from birth to 36 months. A stadiometer should be used to measure height in standing 2–18 year olds. BMI is not calculated until a standing height can be measured.

Energy and protein requirements

Energy requirements vary throughout childhood and correspond to the varied normal rate of weight gain seen from birth through adolescence. The energy and nutrient requirements of children are proportional to their resting energy expenditure plus the energy needs of activity and normal growth. The Food and Nutrition Board, Institute of Medicine, National Academy of Science Dietary Reference Intake (DRI) values for energy and protein are shown in Table 4.1 [6]. For more details on estimating individual energy requirements (EER) in children from birth to 18 years, see the National Academy of Science, National Academies Press website www.NAP.edu.

Calculation of calories and protein consumed by an individual child, best performed by a nutrition professional, can be of use when weight gain falls below or exceeds average rates for individual ages. An emphasis on calorie levels in guiding families toward good nutrition and adequate intake should be avoided. It is better to help families understand nutritional requirements for children of various ages and the importance of serving age-appropriate sizes and balanced diet based on the food guide pyramid. In addition to the assessment of a child's growth curve to determine that growth and weight gain

Table 4.1 Energy and protein requirements.

Age	Energy (kcal/day)		Protein (g/day)	
	Males	Females	Males	Females
0–6 months	570	520	9.1	9.1
7–12 months	743	676	11.0	11.0
1–2 years	1046	992	13	13
3–8 years	1742	1642	19	19
9–13 years	2279	2071	34	34
14–18 years	3152	2368	52	46

*RDA for protein uses ages 1–3 years (13 grams) and 4–8 years (19 grams).
Source: Adapted from [6].

are within normal ranges, Table 4.2 provides information on normal growth rates by age and gender for younger children.

Deviations in normal growth
Failure to thrive
Failure to thrive describes the child not gaining weight appropriately due to inadequate calorie intake, malabsorption and/or increased nutrient needs [8]. (see Table 4.3). Commonly used criteria include children whose (1) weight (or weight-for-height) is less than two standard deviations below the mean (5th percentile) for sex and age; and/or (2) weight curve has crossed more than two percentile lines (channels) on the National Center for Health Statistics/CDC growth charts after having achieved a previously stable pattern [1].

Evaluation of a child with growth failure should begin with a thorough history and physical exam, including a nutritional assessment. In the majority of cases sufficient information will be obtained to determine the etiology. Non-organic growth failure is the most common cause presenting in the U.S.; therefore simple, non-invasive screening for medical problems should be undertaken [9]. Many children with poor growth suffer from behavioral and developmental problems, as well as social and economic disadvantages. When

Table 4.2 Recommendations for weight and length gain in healthy children.

Age	Weight (g/day)	Length (cm/month)
<3 months	25–35	2.6–3.5
3–6 months	15–21	1.6–2.5
6–12 months	10–13	1.2–1.7
1–3 years	4–10	0.7–1.1
4–6 years	5–8	0.5–0.8
7–10 years	5–12	0.4–0.6

Source: Adapted from [7].

Table 4.3 Selective differential diagnosis of failure to thrive

---

Inadequate caloric intake
Incorrect preparation of formula (too diluted, too concentrated)
Unsuitable feeding habits (food fads, excessive juice)
Behavior problems affecting eating
Poverty and food shortages
Neglect
Disturbed parent-child relationship
Mechanical feeding difficulties (oromotor dysfunction, congenital anomalies, central nervous
    system damage, severe reflux)

Inadequate absorption
Celiac disease
Cystic fibrosis
Cow's milk protein allergy
Vitamin or mineral deficiencies (acrodermatitis enteropathica, scurvy)
Biliary atresia or liver disease
Necrotizing enterocolitis or short-gut syndrome

Increased metabolism
Hyperthyroidism
Chronic infection (human immunodeficiency virus or other immunodeficiency, malignancy,
    renal disease)
Hypoxemia (congenital heart defects, chronic lung disease)

Defective utilization
Genetic abnormalities (trisomies 21, 18, and 13)
Congenital infections
Metabolic disorders (storage diseases, amino acid disorders)

Source: [8].

further medical evaluation is warranted, laboratory assessment should include complete blood count, comprehensive metabolic panel, thyroid function tests and celiac panel. Other tests such as HIV, sweat testing, and inborn errors of metabolism should be performed as indicated by the history and physical findings.

Overweight and obesity
The epidemic of childhood overweight and obesity represents a dramatic setback in the progress toward assuring the future health of the US population. This epidemic is occuring nationwide, in young children as well as adolescents, across all socio-economic status (SES) and among all ethnic groups. Specific subgroups, particularly those of lower SES, African Americans, Hispanic and Native Americans, are disproportionately affected [4]. Over the past three decades, the rate of obesity has more than doubled for preschool children aged 2–5 years and adolescents aged 12–19 years, and more than tripled for children aged 6–11 years [4]. The medical complications associated with obesity in children include sleep apnea, hypertension, hyperlipidemia, insulin resistance, type 2 diabetes, orthopedic problems (such as slipped capital femoral epiphysis), pseudo tumor cerebri and psychosocial problems [10,11].

Etiology of obesity: genetics and environment

A strong genetic component has been found in studies comparing the BMI of children to that of their biologic and adoptive parents [12]. According to current estimates, a child with two obese biological parents has an 80% chance of becoming obese. The proportion drops to 40% of children with only one obese parent [10]. Acknowledging the strong genetic predisposition to obesity, environmental influences determine its expression.

Enviornmental and lifestyle changes correlate with the epidemic of childhood obesity over the last 30 years. These changes include both parents working outside the home, increased food marketing aimed at children, changes in the school environment (more high-fat foods and sugary beverages, as well as decreased physical activity) and more meals eaten outside the home, particularly fast food. Increased television viewing, as well as time devoted to sedentary activities, such as computer and video games, are also major contributing factors. Direct marketing to children through television commercials has influenced the foods they desire and eat, including fast food and sodas, often in "super-sized" portions.

Treatment of the overweight child

Comprehensive treatment programs that include behavior modification have been shown to be moderately effective in the treatment of childhood obesity. The best outcome of weight loss programs is achieved when the entire family works together to improve their diet and physical activity level. For overweight children, weight maintenance during continued linear growth in height is a reasonable approach in pre-pubertal children. Clearly, the most effective way to address the epidemic of obesity in children is through prevention.

Prevention issues

Preventing children from becoming overweight involves providing adequate calories to support growth and development, while ensuring enough physical activity to prevent inappropriate weight gain [4]. Health care providers should be able to identify those at risk for the development of obesity using growth charts and family history. At-risk groups include those who have one or both parents who are overweight or low socio-economic status, or are from certain ethnic groups. Mexican–Americans have the highest incidence of obesity followed by African–Americans. Maternal factors which increase a child's risk of obesity include formula-feeding instead of breastfeeding, excessive maternal weight gain during pregnancy (>15.9 kg), large-for-gestational-age infant and gestational diabetes [11]. It is extremely difficult to overfeed a breastfed child, making breastfeeding promotion an important part of obesity prevention.

Health care providers can identify high risk children by reviewing family history of overweight and obesity, assessing maternal weight gain during pregnancy, monitoring growth over time, including BMI, and tracking growth percentiles. The health care provider has a unique opportunity to guide families in their efforts to raise healthy, normal weight children. They can guide parents with knowledge and tools to provide nutritious foods at mealtimes while avoiding over-restriction. Children have the responsibility to decide which of these foods and quantities they will consume. Establishing this practice starting from infancy will support self-regulation, a key to life-long weight control.

Infant nutrition

Nutrition for the premature infant

Optimal nutrition is critical in the management of small, preterm infants [1]. Although no standard exists for the precise nutritional needs of infants born prematurely, current recommendations are developed to simulate the inutero growth rate. Breast milk or fortified breast milk is considered ideal for the preterm infant. Human milk fortifiers can be added to breast milk for the preterm infant to provide additional calories, protein, zinc, calcium phosphorous DHA and folic acid, and powdered formula can be used to fortify breast milk once the infant is discharged home. Breast milk provides many advantages to preterm infants in the form of growth factors, immunity to infection, support for the developing gastrointestinal tract, and enhanced calcium and phosphorus profiles. Infants who are formula-fed should receive specialized preterm formulas in the nursery and be discharged on preterm follow-up formulas to allow continued catch-up growth and improvement in bone mineral density during the first year of life [12]. It is suggested that these special formulas be used until 9–12 months corrected age (based on estimated date of confinement (EDC), not birth date).

Iron should be supplied to human milk-fed preterm babies at 1 month of age (2 mg/kg/day) until one year [1]. Formula-fed preterm infants may also benefit from an iron supplement (1 mg/kg/day) in addition to the iron present in preterm infant formulas, through the first year of life [1]. All infants who are breastfed should be supplemented with vitamin D (400 IU/kg/day) to support bone formation. Human milk powdered fortifiers and special formulas for preterm infants supply between 200–400 IU/day vitamin D. Babies who are breastfed alone require 200 IU/day of vitamin D [1,13]. Preterm infants are at high risk for rickets of prematurity due to inadequate calcium intake early in life thus, alkaline phosphatase, calcium and phosphorous levels should be monitored. When plotting the preterm infant on the NCHS growth chart after discharge from the hospital, correction for gestational age should be continued until age 2 years for linear growth and until age 3 years for weight and head circumference.

Nutrition for the term infant

Advocating breastfeeding

The World Health Organization (WHO) and American Academy of Pediatrics (AAP) strongly recommend exclusive breastfeeding for the first six months of life. Successful lactation depends on the knowledge and supportive attitude of clinicians in pediatric and obstetric services, hospital policies and practices conducive to the initiation and maintenance of breastfeeding. Many mothers will require support to successfully breastfeed their infants. Breast milk is the most complete form of nutrition for infants, with positive impacts on health, growth, development and immunity. Benefits include a reduction in the number of cases and severity of diarrhea, respiratory infections, and ear infections. Breastfeeding also has been shown to improve maternal health, promote faster maternal weight loss to pre-pregnancy weight, and decrease the risk of maternal breast cancer. *Healthy People 2010* (www.healthypeople.gov), target goals state that 75% of mothers should breastfeed their babies in the early postpartum period, 50% breastfeed their infants at 6 months of age and 25% breastfeed at one year [14]. Improvements have been made over time in reaching these goals. Results of the 2002 National Immunization Survey, which collected data on initiation and duration of breastfeeding, indicated that 71.4% of infants are breastfed at birth, 42.5% are exclusively breastfed at 3 months (51% receive some breastfeeding), 13% are exclusively breastfed at 6 months (35% receiving some breastfeeding), and 16.1% received some breast milk at 1 year [15].

What makes breastfeeding best for infants?

Human milk is unique in its components and dynamic nutrient composition. Composition changes throughout lactation and provides a higher protein more digestible mixture to preterm infants. Its whey : casein ratio of 70 : 30 makes it more digestible than the 18 : 82 content of cow's milk. Human milk contains the omega-3 fatty acids : arachidonic acid (ARA) and docosahexanoic acid (DHA) which may improve visual function and neurodevelopment in infants. Carbohydrates, in the form of lactose and oligosaccharides, are easily digested, supported by the presence of the digestive enzyme, lactase. Calcium and phosphorus, though in lower levels than cow's milk formulas, are more bioavailable in breast milk and support bone growth. Other micronutrients are adequate to meet the infant's nutritional needs until age 6 months when iron-fortified infant cereal should be introduced. Human milk contributes to the maturation of the gastrointestinal tract and provides a host of bioactive factors, including secretory IgA, lactoferrin, lysozyme, nucleotides, all supporting the immunity of the child [8]. Human milk protects against Crohn's disease, lymphoma and type 1 diabetes mellitus. Exclusive breast feeding in the first half-year of life may prevent the early development of allergic disease in early childhood [16].

How to know if an infant is eating enough?

The best way to be sure that babies are receiving adequate amounts of breast milk is to monitor their growth and development, so all infants should be seen regularly by their clinician. Milk production works on the principle of supply and demand. The more frequently an infant nurses, the more milk is produced. Frequent nursing in the first few days of life (every 1–3 hours), helps to stimulate initial milk production.

A baby who has at least six wet diapers a day and a minimum of three stools per day if they are breastfeeding, or two-to-three stools per day if they are drinking formula, and who is gaining weight appropriately (at least 7 ounces per week), is consuming enough milk. Although breastfed infants consume less milk than formula-fed infants over a 24-hour period and therefore have a lower energy intake, they are more energy efficient. By year three, breastfed infants have a lower percentage of body fat and are rarely overweight. The breastfed infant can control the flow of milk by alternating sucking and stopping, and this may help to explain why breastfed infants are less likely to overfeed than formula-fed infants. The breastfed infant adjusts feeding quantity according to its hunger and level of satiety, while bottle-fed infants are often fed until the bottle is empty. Mothers who breastfeed rely on the infant to self-regulate intake, an ability that helps a growing child eat enough, but not excessively, which may improve self-regulation of energy intake later in childhood. Breastfeeding also promotes good jaw and tooth development in the infant [17].

For these reasons, human milk is considered the best source of nutrition for infants. Even so, there are some cautions that should be stated regarding breastfeeding. Women who are infected with HIV should not breastfeed [1]. A second area of caution involves a breastfeeding mother who is a strict vegetarian/vegan. Several cases have been reported in the literature of infants with vitamin B_{12} deficiency who were breastfed by vitamin B_{12}-deficient mothers with a extended history of vegan diets [18,19]. Infants of vegan mothers should be monitored for signs of vitamin B_{12} deficiency including lethargy, failure to thrive, developmental delay, or macrocytic anemia.

Formula feeding

Full-term infants who do not receive human milk can be adequately nourished with iron-fortified infant formulas during the first year of life. These formulas, designed to mimic human milk, have been greatly improved over the last 70 years [1]. Standard cow's milk-based formulas are the feeding of choice when breastfeeding is not used. Modification of the casein : whey ratio to increase the whey content has improved protein digestibility. Lactose is the major carbohydrate in human milk and in standard cow's-milk-based infant formulas.

Only iron-fortified formulas should be offered to infants. Iron has a critical role in brain growth in infants. In the past, low iron formulas were recommended for infants with constipation. However, well-controlled studies have consistently failed to show any increase in the prevalence of fussiness, cramping, colic or constipation with the use of iron-fortified formulas [1]. In 1999 the AAP stated there was "no role for the use of low-iron formulas in infant feeding and recommends that all infant formulas be fortified with iron" [1]. Standard infant formulas contain a caloric density of 67–70 kcal/dL (20 kcal/oz). The usual intake of 150–200 mL/kg/day will provide 100–135 kcal/kg/day. The fat composition of formula has changed with the recent addition of ARA and

DHA. Whether addition of these fatty acids will have a long-term effect on growth, visual development, information processing skills, or IQ, is not known [20].

Infant formulas other than standard cow's-milk-based may be indicated for some infants. Soy protein formulas are lactose-free and constitute approximately 25% of all formulas sold. Soy protein based formulas are not recommended for preterm infants of less than 1800 g to avoid risk of osteopenia [1]. Phytates in soy protein bind calcium resulting in decreased bioavailability for bone mineralization. Soy formulas are successfully used by vegetarians and indicated in infants with cow's milk allergy. Soy formulas are also appropriate for the rare infant with lactase deficiency or galactosemia. Soy formulas may be used for secondary lactose deficiency following a prolonged gastroenteritis. Infants with these symptoms should be rechallenged with their regular formulas within a month.

Special formulas have been developed for babies with unique requirements. Protein hydrolysate formulas provide nutrition for infants who cannot digest or are intolerant of intact cow's milk protein. These are the preferred formulas for infants with cow's milk and soy protein intolerance and for those with gastrointestinal or hepatobiliary diseases such as biliary atresia or protracted diarrhea. These formulas may contain varying amounts of medium-chain triglycerides (MCTs) to facilitate fat absorption. Formulas containing free amino acids are also available for infants with extreme protein hypersensitivity who cannot tolerate hydrolyzed formulas. These formulas are very expensive and should be used only when needed.

Cow's milk of any kind, as well as goat's milk, evaporated milk or other milks should *not* be used during the first 12 months of life. The protein in cow's milk can cause chronic gastrointestinal blood loss and subsequent iron deficiency anemia. The higher the content of protein, sodium, potassium and chloride in cow's milk, provides an inappropriately high renal solute load. The level of essential fatty acids, vitamin E, and zinc in cow's milk are inadequate for infants. Skim milk should not be given to infants younger than 2 years due to its excessive protein and inadequate fat content.

The wide variety of formulas available, both standard and specialized, are reviewed in Table 4.4.

Complementary foods

Recommendations for the introduction of complementary (solid) foods have changed over the years. In the past, health care professionals recommended that children be introduced to solid foods as early as the first month of life. The consensus among pediatric clinicians today is to delay introducing solid foods until the child is 4–6 months of age. This recommendation is supported by both the AAP and the WHO. Both organizations support exclusive breast milk use for the first 6 months.

Introduction of solid foods earlier than 4–6 months may result in the development of food allergies. Furthermore, infants are not physiologically ready

Table 4.4 Indications and types of infant formulas.

Formula	Indications	Unique properties	Examples
Milk-based	Breast milk substitute for term infants	+/− Iron Ready to feed, powder, or liquid concentrate Variable whey : casein (20 kcal/oz) Contains DHA/ARA	Enfamil Lipil Similac Advance Enfamil Lactofree Similac Lactose-free Enfamil AR (pre-thickened) Good Start Supreme contains
Soy-based	Breast milk substitute for infants with lactose intolerance or milk protein allergy*	Lactose-free, may contain sucrose, or corn-free (20 kcal/oz) May contain fiber	Prosobee, Isomil Good Start Soy Essentials Isomil DF
Premature	Breast milk substitute for low birth weight, hospitalized preterm infants	Low lactose Whey : casein 60 : 40 High calcium and phosphorus (20 and 24 cal/oz) Contains DHA/ARA	Enfamil Premature Lipil Similac SpecialCare Advance Similac HMF Enfamil HMF
Human Milk Fortifiers	Fortification of breast milk for preterm infants	Increases calorie, protein, and vitamin/mineral content of breast milk	Similac HMF Enfamil HMF
Premature– transitional	Breast milk substitute for preterm infants >2.5 kg or discharge formula for preterm infants	22 kcal/oz ready to feed or powder Contains DHA/ARA	Enfacare Lipil Neosure Advance
Older Infant	Transition to whole milk	Varies	Good Start Essentials 2 Enfamil Next Step, & w/Soy
Hypoallergenic	Milk or soy protein allergy	Hydrolyzed protein Sucrose-free Lactose-free	Nutramigen
Predigested	Malabsorption Short bowel syndrome Allergy	Lactose-free Hydrolyzed protein or free amino acids	Alimentum, Pregestamil Neocate Elecare
Fat-modified	Defects in digestion, absorption, or transport of fat	Contains increased % of kcals as MCT	Portagen (no longer recommended for infants) Alimentum Pregestamil
Carbohydrate- modified	Simple sugar intolerance	Requires addition of complex carbohydrate to be complete	RCF 3232 A
Amino acid-modified	Inborn errors of metabolism	Low or devoid of specific amino acids that cannot be metabolized	Multiple products
Electrolyte and/or mineral modified	Renal disease requiring decreased electrolyte and mineral content	Decreased potassium content Decreased calcium and phosphorus content	Similac PM 60/40

*Children allergic to milk protein may also be allergic to soy protein.
Source: Sue Konek, MA, RD, CNSD, CNS, Department of Clinical Nutrition, Children's Hospital of Philadelphia. 2007. Used with permission.

to accept solid foods from a spoon until the protrusion reflex becomes extinguished at approximately 4 months. The development of head and neck control and coordination of oral musculature at 3–4 months will also prepare the infant for solids at 6 months.

A firm consensus on the progression of complementary foods does not exist. Review of practices in developed countries reveals a wide variety of recommendation for beginning foods. Guidelines on how to feed infants as they transition to solid food, are found in Table 4.5.

What are young children eating?
Knowledge of current intake patterns can assist in providing guidance to families on how to feed their toddlers to improve their nutritional intake. The 2002 Feeding Infants and Toddlers Study (FITS) surveyed 3022 US families with infants and toddlers age 4–24 months to see how nutrition in these children compared with current recommendations and the Dietary Reference Intakes (DRIs) [21–25]. This randomized survey was conducted through phone interviews using a 24-hour recall. Findings included solid foods started at the appropriate time and early introduction of whole cows milk (<6 months) was uncommon. By 24-months some infants drank little or no milk. It was suggested that this might set the stage for decreased milk consumption into childhood and adolescence. Toddlers as a group had energy intakes greater than that recommended by the DRIs. Of concern, 18–33% of infants and toddlers between ages 7–24 months did not consume any servings of vegetables and 25% did not consume fruits [22]. French fries emerged as a commonly eaten vegetable, even in children as young as 9 months. Also of concern was the finding that almost 50% of 7–8 month old infants were already consuming sweets, desserts, and sweetened beverages which increased through 24 months. After the first year of life, family eating patterns came into play [21]. For this reason, family-based approaches to food guidance are needed. The researchers of the FITS study recommended that parents be encouraged to offer a wide variety of vegetables and fruits on a daily basis. This recommendation should emphasize inclusion of dark green, leafy and deep yellow vegetables as well as colorful fruits. Sweets and desserts should be offered only occasionally, instead offering nutrient-dense food for dessert such as fruit, cheese, yogurt and cereals. Beverages should consist of water, limited amounts of 100% fruit juice, and low-fat milk for children over two years of age. The practice of offering toddlers several snacks daily was commonly observed. Because toddlers received about 25% of their calories from snacks, the importance of providing planned nutrient-rich foods at snack time becomes apparent. Five servings of fruit and vegetables daily as well as three servings of dairy foods remains a goal for toddlers [26].

Introducing new foods (see Table 4.5)
In order to detect a potential food allergy, new foods should be introduced to infants one at a time over a three-day period. Dietary recommendations for

Table 4.5 How to feed your infant during the first year of life.

Age in months	Breast milk or iron-fortified infant formula*	Cereals and breads	Fruits and fruit juices†	Vegetables	Protein foods	Dairy foods
0–4	5–10 feedings/day 17–24 floz/day (510–720 mL/day)	None	None	None	None	None
4–6 months	4–7 feedings/day 24–32 floz/day (720–960 mL/day)	Rice or barley infant cereals (iron fortified). Mix cereal with formula or breast milk until thin. Start with 1 tbsp at each feeding for a few days, and increase to 3–4 tbsp/day. Feed with small baby spoon (don't expect baby to eat much at first).	None	None	None	None
7–8	4–5 feedings/day 24–32 floz/day (720–960 mL/day)	Single grain infant cereals–rice, oatmeal, barley (iron fortified) in the morning 3–9 tbsp/day, mixed with breast milk or infant formula. Two feedings a day. Oven-dried toast or teething biscuits, crackers, or toast strips.	Strained or mashed fruits (fresh or cooked), mashed bananas, apple sauce. Infant 100% fruit juices (4 oz/day) <4 oz/day mixed with water and served in a cup.	Strained or mashed, well-cooked: dark yellow or orange (not corn), dark green vegetables. Start with mild vegetables such as green beans, peas, or squash 1/2–1 jar or 1/4–1/2 cup/day.	Smooth preparations of single meats: lamb, veal, chicken, may be started in small quantities (up to 2 tbsp/day).	Cottage cheese, yogurt

8–9	3–4 feedings/day 24–32 floz/day (720–960 mL/day)	Infant cereals or plain hot cereals mixed with breast milk or formula. Toast, bagels, crackers, teething biscuits. Small pieces of cooked noodles, potatoes.	Peeled soft fruit wedges: bananas, peaches, pears, oranges, apples (skin removed). 100% fruit juices including orange and tomato juices 4–6 oz/day (120–180 mL).	Cooked, mashed vegetables.	Well cooked, strained, ground or finely chopped chicken, fish, and lean meats: 2–3 tbsp/day (remove all bones, fat, skin). Cooked dried beans. Egg yolks only, no whites.	Cottage cheese, yogurt, bite-size cheese strips
10–12	3–4 feedings/day 24–32 floz/day (720–960 mL/day) by cup or bottle	Infant or cooked cereals mixed with breast milk or formula. Unsweetened cereals, white/ wheat breads. Mashed potatoes, rice, noodles, spaghetti.	All fresh fruits peeled and seeded or canned fruits packed in water. 100% fruit juices 4–6 oz/day (120–180 mL).	Cooked vegetable pieces. Some raw vegetables: tomatoes, cucumbers.	Small tender pieces of chicken, fish or lean meat. Cooked beans, Pasta.	Cottage cheese, yogurt, bite-size cheese strips

*These are general guidelines. Feeding schedules vary somewhat between children.
†There is no specific need for juice in an infant's diet.
Source: Lisa Hark, PhD, RD and Diane Barsky, MD, University of Pennsylvania School of Medicine. 2007. Used with permission.

children in families with a history of food allergies or asthma suggest avoidance of dairy products until one year of age; avoid eggs until age 2; and avoid peanuts, tree nuts and fish/shellfish until age 3. High risk children are those with parents or siblings with any allergies, including hay fever or pet allergies [10]. The Food Allergy and Anaphylaxis Network (www.foodallergy.org) [27] is an excellent resource for families with food allergies. (See chapter 14).

When preparing foods, it is important that salt and sugar not be added, to prevent infants from developing a preference for these tastes. Babies often prefer foods warmed to room temperature. If a microwave is used to warm foods, the food should be mixed well to avoid burning the infant's mouth. Table 4.6 outlines important feed tips for infants and young children.

Although there is no consensus on the exact order for the introduction of complementary foods, the following order is commonly used.

Cereals In the US, the most common initial solid food is iron-fortified rice cereal. It is recommended that this and other foods not be started before 4 months of age. Rice cereal, fortified with iron, is unlikely to cause allergies and is usually well tolerated. It is common practice to give one or two tablespoons of rice cereal, mixed with breast milk or infant formula, in the morning, as this is a well tolerated introduction to solids. There is no absolute in regard to the introduction of solid foods. Various cultures and ethnic groups vary in this practice. The cereal should be mixed to a consistency similar to that of apple sauce, with adjustments made for the child's preference. Cereal should always be fed from a small spoon. Eating is a new skill which may take the infant a few weeks to master. The practice of putting cereal in a bottle of formula should

Table 4.6 Tips on feeding your infant.

- Avoid laying your baby down with a bottle to prevent ear infections and tooth decay.
- Introduce only one new food every three days to detect sensitivities or allergies.
- Avoid overfeeding. Stop feeding when baby turns away from food or shows disinterest.
- Use a baby spoon to feed cereal and other foods. Do not put cereal in the bottle.
- Feed only breast milk for the first 6 months, formula until 4–6 months – no solid foods.
- Throw away unused formula from a bottle after each feeding.
- Use formula or breast milk, not cow's milk, until your baby's first birthday.
- Limit juice intake to less than 4–6 oz/day beginning after 6 months and dilute with water.
- Avoid offering sweet desserts, candy, soft drinks, fruit-flavored or sweetened drinks, or sugar coated cereal to infants and children.
- Avoid adding sugar or salt to baby's food. Check labels for added sugar and salt
- Feed baby food from a bowl, not from the jar.
- Avoid hard and round pieces of food that can cause choking (whole grapes, raw carrots, popcorn, hot dogs, peanuts)
- At 1 year of age, initiate whole cow's milk. Encourage milk in a cup rather than a bottle.
- Consider offering vegetables before fruit to avoid setting up a preference for sweets.
- Avoid adding honey to baby food, as it may contain bacteria, which can cause botulism in infants. Honey may be used after one year of age.

Source: Diane Barsky, MD and Lisa Hark, PhD, RD, University of Pennsylvania School of Medicine. 2007. Used with permission.

be discouraged. Studies show this does not help children to sleep through the night and may lead to over-feeding and possibly choking, especially when a larger hole is cut into the nipple. Oat or barley infant cereal may be tried after allowing four days to detect any allergy present. Wheat and mixed infant cereals should not be used in young infants, as wheat is a common allergen. These cereals can be added later in the first year.

Vegetables Cooked, strained vegetables without salt or spices, either homemade or purchased baby food, are appropriate to start at 6–8 months of age. There is no evidence to support introducing foods in a particular order [1]. Even so, some practitioners believe that vegetables should be introduced before fruits to prevent the infant from developing a preference for sweets. Salt and spices should be avoided in infant feeding, especially for families preparing homemade infant foods. Raw vegetables that are soft may be introduced at one year. Some hard vegetables, such as carrots, should be avoided until the eruption of top and bottom molars, to prevent a choking hazard.

Fruits Cooked, strained, and pureed fruits, purchased as baby food or homemade, (without sugar) may be started after rice cereal. Fresh, mashed bananas can also be introduced at this time. Peeled, soft fruits such as pears and peaches may be cut into small pieces and started at 8–10 months of age. As with vegetables, hard fruits such as apples should be delayed until the child can easily chew harder foods. Juices, such as apple, made from 100% fruit, may also be offered, but in small quantities – less than 4–6 ounces/day until one year as recommended by the AAP [1]. Excess juice consumption can lead to diarrhea due to high fructose and sorbitol content of fruit juices, as well as excessive weight gain.

Eggs Cooked egg yolks may be introduced to infants over the age of 6 months. Egg whites should be delayed until one year of age because of the potential risk of inducing egg allergy in younger infants. (Allergy to egg may delay or limit administration of vaccines that are produced in eggs.)

Meats Ground and finely chopped chicken, meats and fish, either homemade or purchased as baby food, are generally introduced after fruits and vegetables are well tolerated. Meat is a rich source of iron and zinc, nutrients that become limiting in human milk alone.

Starch/carbohydrate Children enjoy pasta, spaghetti and dry cereals, and these can be added to the diet later in the first year. These foods should not be used in place of more nutrient-rich foods, such as fruits and vegetables. Suggest whole wheat breads and pastas and whole grain pastas to help children learn to acquire a taste for these early on.

Fats Children under 2 years of age need a high-calorie diet to help ensure normal brain development and to support rapid growth. Fat in the diet allows

Table 4.7 Foods to avoid before age 3–4 to prevent choking.

- Carrots (unless cooked until very soft)
- Chewing gum
- Chunks of meat
- Hard candy
- Nuts
- Popcorn
- Raw apples or pears
- Seeds
- Whole grapes (may be cut into small pieces)
- Whole or large sections of hot dogs

Source: Diane Barsky, MD and Lisa Hark, PhD, RD, University of Pennsylvania School of Medicine. 2007. Used with permission.

young children to achieve their caloric goals. Essential fatty acids are especially important for normal brain development. Therefore, the AAP recommends that dietary fat should not be limited prior to age 2 [1]. After 2 years of age, lower fat dairy products (1% or 2% milk and low-fat yogurt and cheese) and limited consumption of high fat foods (such as fried foods, ice cream, and pizza) is one strategy to help prevent children from becoming overweight.

Special care to avoid choking During the first year of life and up to age 4, foods should be prepared to promote swallowing without the risk of aspiration. In addition, parents should not leave children alone when eating meals or snacks to guard against choking events (Table 4.7).

Detecting Food Allergies

Food allergies, actually, food hypersensitivity reactions, occur in 2–8% of children less than 3 years of age [1]. Approximately 2.5% of infants will experience allergic reactions to cow's milk in the first 3 years of life, 1.5% to egg and 0.6% to peanuts. Approximately 85% of these will later become tolerant to milk and eggs (within the first 5 years of life). Even peanut allergy may be "outgrown" by 20% of children. The following terms, suggested by the American Academy of Allergy and Immunology Committee on Adverse Reactions to Foods, are those which more clearly define food reactions:

- *Adverse reaction*: clinically abnormal response believed to be caused by an ingested food or food additive.
- *Food hypersensitivity (allergy)*: immunologic reaction resulting from the ingestion of a food or food additive.
- *Food anaphylaxis*: classic allergic hypersensitivity reaction to food or food additives involving IgE antibody and release of chemical mediators.
- *Food intolerance*: general term describing an abnormal physiologic response to an ingested food or food additive; can include idiosyncratic, metabolic, pharmacologic, or toxic response.

The gradual introduction of new foods (one new food every three days) starting after the age of six months, may reduce allergy risk and allow for the identification of foods which fit the definition of food hypersensitivity. Parents should be aware that swelling of the lips and face, a skin rash, vomiting or diarrhea are symptoms associated with food allergy. Once identified, strict avoidance of an offending food is the only way to prevent the allergic response. The challenge of treating food allergies occurs when children are allergic to many foods, sometimes requiring avoidance of whole groups of foods [28].

Eight foods account for 90% of all food allergies: peanuts, tree nuts (such as walnuts or almonds), eggs, milk, fish, shellfish, soy and wheat. Allergy to milk, wheat or eggs require careful avoidance of many foods, as these ingredients may be "hidden" in many foods. Soy protein is also widely used in prepared foods. Children who are allergic to the foods that make up critical groups, such as dairy, may benefit from consultation with a dietitian to identify inadequacies and help plan a diet that meets all of their nutrient requirements while avoiding the offending foods. (See chapter 14)

Iron deficiency anemia

The prevalence of iron deficiency in the US has decreased over the last 20 years due to increased iron supplementation of infant cereals and formulas and supplemental food programs for low-income families, such as the Women, Infants and Children (WIC) program. Even so, *Healthy People 2010* [14] reported that 9% of children aged 1–2 years, and 4% of children aged 3–4 years are iron deficient. Altered behavior and brain function, including learning difficulties, have been reported in iron-deficient infants and toddlers. Some studies have questioned whether iron supplementation before 6 months would benefit breastfed infants. Friel and colleagues found better visual acuity in breast-fed infants who were supplemented with iron [29]. Even small amounts of iron may be of benefit to the developing brain. Though practice change is not warranted in this regard at present, it is critical that iron-rich foods be among the earliest complementary foods. These iron-rich foods, including iron-fortified cereals, red meat, dark-green leafy vegetables and dried fruit such as raisin and prunes, should be used regularly through childhood. Raisins should be soaked in hot water, cooled and mashed for young children to reduce the risk of choking.

Toddler and preschool nutrition

After the rapid growth spurt of the first year of life, the decrease in food intake of two-year-olds associated with a slowed growth rate may be a concern to parents. Toddlers' intake will vary depending on growth spurts. In order to meet the nutritional needs of children between 2 and 5 years, small nutrient-rich meals and snacks are needed. It is recommended that a small snack be given between each meal and at bedtime. Parents need to know that a smaller appetite, varying from day to day, is the norm at this age.

Importance of role modeling

Parents must realize the important role they play in shaping the food habits of their children. The influence of family eating patterns is seen in children aged 2–4 years and may become more pronounced with increasing age [30]. Parental modeling does impact children's food choices. A study by Galloway *et al.* showed that mothers who consumed a variety of fruits and vegetables had daughters who also ate a variety of fruits and vegetables [31]. Parents and caregivers who eat a variety of healthy foods in normal amounts most often will have children who do the same.

Family meals

Eating together as a family is important for many reasons: children learn that mealtime is a structured setting where healthy foods are served, and family meals help children to develop both communication skills and healthy eating habits. Meals eaten together are the perfect opportunity for parents to serve as role models for good nutrition. Habits such as eating nutritionally balanced meals can be more easily established when parents and children do this together. Meals also offer an opportunity to relate as a family and talk about the day's events.

Teaching children about food

Teaching children about food, how it is prepared and how it helps their bodies grow, can increase a child's interest in eating a varied diet. Taking children to the grocery store, farmers markets or to a working farm will increase their knowledge and curiosity about food and how it nourishes their bodies. Encourage parents to shop for and prepare healthy foods with their children. Even young children can help prepare snacks and learn new skills by spreading cheese spread, peanut butter and fruit spread on crackers and toast. Allowing children to help make smoothies, mini whole wheat pizzas and fruit for dipping in yogurt helps children enjoy these foods even more (Table 4.8).

Arrival of the "picky eater!"

The "picky eater" typically presents when a child is between the ages of one and three years, and can last up to age five. Picky eating during childhood is very common and usually does not lead to nutritional problems. Studies show that most toddlers who skip meals will meet their nutritional needs over one weeks time. From a developmental standpoint, preschool years help children individualize through learning. Parents should be advised that repeated exposures to new foods (between 5–10 times) may be needed for their acceptance. Offering a new food once is not enough. Parents must trust that the child can self-regulate energy intake. Parents' responsibility is to determine what foods will be presented and when [8]. During the second year of life, the decrease in growth velocity may result in appetites that seems to wax and wane. Children who are allowed to "graze" or drink juice between meals may not be hungry at mealtime. Snacks should be planned, leaving a reasonable time period before

Table 4.8 Encouraging healthy eating habits in preschool children.

- Serve fruits and vegetables every day, at meals and snacks. Keep canned fruit such as pineapple, peaches and mandarin oranges in their own juice on hand for quick snacks.
- Provide milk (low-fat for children over 2 years) and water for meals or snacks. Limit juice to 4–6 oz/day.
- Do not be afraid to say no to junk food, chips, soda, candy or sweets.
- Serve small portions on small plates and small cups. Let the child regulate his or her own intake. Serving large portions and insisting on a "clean plate" can lead to overeating and the loss of self-regulation.
- Do not use dessert as a reward ("finish your vegetables or you won't have dessert") – dessert is part of the meal and should be no more desired than the meal itself. Serve healthy desserts when possible.
- When a child says they have finished, allow them to take their plate to the sink and return to the table while parents finish. Appropriate activities or books will allow the child to enjoy this time.
- Keep a cabinet full of healthy snacks for the child's choosing at snack time.
- Try to dine as a family whenever possible.
- Limit TV/computer time to less than two hours a day.
- Encourage your child to be physically active (children need at least one hour of activity/day).
- Offer family activities to promote exercise.

Source: Diane Barsky, MD, University of Pennsylvania School of Medicine and Sue Konek, MS, RD, CNSD, CPS, The Children's Hospital of Philadelphia. 2007. Used with permission.

meals. (2–3 hrs.) It is important that caregivers realize that children have small stomachs. Portion sizes should be small, served on small plates with small cups. Food jags, in which only a few foods will be eaten over several weeks or months, are common. These periods are often a sign of increasing independence. The less pressure that parents impose for children to eat specific foods, the greater the likelihood that this phase will pass. Tips for coping with a picky eater are suggested in Table 4.8. Children that demonstrate difficulty gaining weight or decline in percentiles on the growth chart are a concern and require further medical evaluation.

Sample menu: 1–2 years old

Breakfast: 2 mini whole grain waffles with low-sugar syrup, 4 oz of fruited yogurt and 4 oz of dilute orange juice (half juice, half water)
Snack: $^1/_2$ cup fruit salad and 4 oz of whole milk
Lunch: $^1/_2$–1 cup of macaroni and cheese with green beans, 4 oz milk and $^1/_2$ banana
Snack: 2 graham crackers and 4 oz dilute apple juice
Dinner: 2 oz white-meat chicken with $^1/_2$ cup cooked brown rice, $^1/_2$ cup soft broccoli florets, 2 slices of cucumber and 4 oz of whole milk

(Note: At 2 years, low-fat milk may be used instead of whole milk.)

Source: Deen D. and Hark L. *Nutrition for Life*. DK Publishing. New York, 2005 [17].

When to be concerned

Primary care clinicians should be concerned about the picky eater when the child is not gaining weight or growing appropriately, or when significant food refusal continues for more than a month. If the diet is markedly restrictive so that macro- and/or micro-nutrient intake is very low (calcium, protein, iron), consultation with a registered dietitian may be useful to guide families and determine the need for supplementation. Those children that demonstrate difficulty gaining weight or decline in percentiles on the growth chart require further medical evaluation.

Food rules: setting the stage for healthy eating

The following food rules will help in establishing healthy eating for children.

Beverages

The healthiest drinks for young children over the age of 3 are low-fat milk (1%), and water. Many parents allow children to drink large amounts of fruit juice, fruit-flavored drinks, sweetened beverages or soda. This practice contributes to excessive weight gain, poor dental health, and inadequate vitamin and mineral intake. The AAP recommends limiting juice to 4–6 oz/day for 1–5-year-olds. Fresh fruits should be recommended, as fruit has added nutrients and fiber. Only pasteurized juices should be offered to children. Primary care clinicians should discourage the use of sweetened beverages, soda, sports drinks, and any fruit drinks that are not 100% juice.

Age-appropriate portions

To help parents gauge the amount of food and beverages to offer children, sample age-specific meal plans are provided on p. 75, 77.

Toddlerhood to preschool – supporting healthy self-regulation

At this stage in their development, children become increasingly aware of the environment in which they eat and the social aspects of eating. Fostering independence while promoting healthy eating habits becomes vitally important. In these formative years, the division of responsibility for nutrition should be set.

• The parents and caregivers are responsible for providing a varied and healthy diet, in age-appropriate amounts. This should be done in a consistent and calm setting and with minimal distraction (no TV). Whenever possible, children should eat with family members.

• The child is responsible for deciding how much to eat at a given meal and to select which of the foods presented to eat. After an adequate amount of

time (15–20 minutes) they should be allowed to leave the table and have an opportunity to eat again at the next planned meal or snack.
• Dessert and other sweets, should not be used as a bribe to get children to eat their vegetables or finish everything on their plate.

Sample menu: 3–5 years old

Breakfast: 1/2 cup low-sugar whole grain cereal with low-fat milk and 1/2 sliced banana
Snack: Apple with a slice of low-fat cheese and 8 oz of water
Lunch: Turkey slices on whole wheat bread and a peach with 6–8 oz low-fat yogurt
Snack: 4 graham crackers, mandarin oranges in own juice, and 4 oz low-fat milk
Dinner: 3 meatballs in tomato sauce with string beans and tomatoes and 4 oz low-fat milk
Snack: 1/2 cup seedless grapes

Source: Deen D. and Hark L. *Nutrition for Life*. DK Publishing. New York, 2005 [17].

Nutrition for school-age children

School-age children require enough fuel to get them through the day, to support attentiveness and brain development.

Serving sizes for school-aged children

School-age children need to eat three meals and at least one snack each day. Breakfast is important to start every day while lunch is most often the meal consumed outside the home. Review menu choices with children to help them with their selection of healthy meals. Packing lunch can also help children to select healthy food. Snack time is the perfect opportunity to serve fruits and vegetables to help children to achieve the goal of five servings per day. Dinner is an opportunity to allow children to select from a variety of healthy choices.

The Food Guide Pyramid, (www.mypyramid.com) provides excellent guidance regarding portion sizes of all foods and a wealth of information on meal planning for people of all ages, based on age, sex and activity level [26].

The Food Guide Pyramid guidelines for children 6–12 are as follows:
• Grains: 5–6 oz/day – make half wholegrains
• Vegetables: 2–21/2 cups/day
• Fruits: 11/2–2 cups/day
• Dairy: 3 cups/day
• Meat and beans: 5–51/2 oz/day

Sample menu: 6 years old

Breakfast: 1 cup low sugar whole grain cereal with $\frac{1}{2}$ cup 1% milk, $\frac{1}{2}$ banana sliced onto cereal and 4 oz orange juice

Snack: $\frac{1}{2}$ whole wheat bagel with 1 teaspoon margarine (soft tub) and 4 oz apple juice

Lunch: 1 cup cheese ravioli with sauce, 1 slice whole wheat bread with margarine, 6 baby carrot sticks with low-fat ranch dressing, 4 oz fruit cocktail, canned in its own juice, and $\frac{1}{2}$ cup 1% milk

Snack: 4 graham cracker pieces and 1 cup 1% milk

Dinner: 1 baked chicken leg, 1 baked potato with margarine, $\frac{1}{2}$ cup steamed broccoli, 1 slice whole wheat bread, $\frac{1}{2}$ orange sliced in quarters, and 1 cup 1% milk

Source: Deen D. and Hark L. *Nutrition for Life*. DK Publishing. New York, 2005 [17].

Physical activity

The Centers for Disease Control and Prevention recommends at least 60 minutes of moderately intense physical activity most days of the week for all children and adolescents. The role of physical activity in balancing the energy equation cannot be overstated in order to prevent children from becoming overweight. As with food and eating, parents must set a positive example by leading an active lifestyle, and making physical activity part of the family's daily routine. Physical activity should be fun and can include team sports, individual sports, walking, running, skating, bicycling, swimming, jumping rope and playground activities. Activity should be age-appropriate and safety should be ensured with helmets, wrist pads and kneepads, as appropriate.

The AAP recommends restricting sedentary activity to 2 hours or less each day. Children under the age of 2 years should not watch televison. By limiting television time, children have been shown to engage in active play. Active play will help children lose weight, if this is a newly adopted practice.

Teen nutrition

Children aged 11–18 years have increased needs for nutrients as they progress through the second major growth period of life: puberty. During puberty energy needs increase to allow attainment of the individual's growth potential. Though boys and girls have different energy requirements, both need extra protein, calcium and iron.

The greater influence of peers with varied dietary patterns, the increased frequency of meals consumed away from home, and the adolescent need for control profoundly impacts the adolescent's food choices. Not surprisingly, teen boys are the highest consumers of junk food and sweetened beverages. It is therefore important that good nutritional habits be developed before adolescence.

Risk of calcium deficiency

Adolescents with a poor diet may be at increased risk for vitamin and mineral deficiencies, most notably riboflavin, calcium and iron. Bone mineral content peaks in adolescence and young adulthood, then declines with age. Maximizing peak bone mineral density early in life can help prevent osteoporosis with advancing age [10]. Many teenage girls are not meeting their calcium requirement during adolescence – 1300 mg per day. The inclusion of four servings of low-fat dairy foods each day in a teen's diet should be discussed with a parent and the patient themselves. (See Appendices G and H – Food Sources of Calcium.)

Risk of iron deficiency

The rapid growth rate during puberty increases iron requirements for males and females. Vigorous exercise, such as running and dancing, further increases requirements. Teenage girls require additional iron due to menarche, with those from ages 12–18 requiring 15 mg of iron daily. To achieve this intake, clinicians should encourage consumption of lean red meat, iron rich fruits such as dried fruits, vegetables such as fresh spinach salad, and iron-fortified breakfast cereal. Vitamin C enhances non-heme iron absorption when consumed together with iron-rich foods. (See Appendix L – Food Sources of Iron.)

Teens and exercise

The teen athlete will require increased calories and protein, dependent on the activity. With normal appetites, most adolescents will eat enough to meet their energy requirements. The most essential and often neglected nutrient requirement in an athlete's diet is water [1]. Hydration is especially important for those involved in endurance sports during hot weather. An athlete exercising in hot/humid weather may lose more than $1.0 \, L/m^2/h$ through sweating. Water with simple sugars (2.5–5%) or glucose polymers is sufficient to restore fluid losses from sweat [1]. Cold fluids have the advantage of helping to cool the body and may be more readily consumed. Recommended fluid intake during exercise is about 4–8 oz for every 15 minutes of physical activity. Small amounts of electrolytes, mostly sodium and chloride, may be lost in sweat during exercise. Most of these losses can be replaced in the diet. Sports drinks may be used, but salt tablets should be avoided as they can induce hypernatremia and increase the need for additional free water [1].

Weight loss in athletes

Female teens involved in gymnastics, ballet, cross-country running, diving and figure skating, and males involved in wrestling, may feel pressure to reduce weight. If appropriate, this can be accomplished, but gradual loss (no more than 2–3 pounds per week) should be a goal to achieve a healthy body weight-for-height. Further effort to reduce weight may result in loss of muscle tissue. Too much emphasis on weight loss and exercise can lead to an eating disorder.

Eating disorders: anorexia nervosa and bulimia

While overweight and obesity are a growing problem among children and adolescents, for some adolescent girls undernutrition is a serious concern. Studies suggest that about 20% of teenagers engage in abnormal eating behavior, while about 5% of high-school-aged girls have a diagnosed eating disorder.

Eating disorders primarily occur in adolescents and college-aged women. These disorders are more often found in industrialized cultures, and occur in all socio-economic levels and across all major ethnic groups. Dancers, long-distance runners, figure skaters, actors, models, wrestlers, gymnasts and jockeys are at higher risk for the development of eating disorders.

Teenagers with anorexia nervosa typically have an altered perception of their own body image that causes them to see themselves as overweight. This altered perception leads to severe restriction of calories and a drop in body weight to below-normal levels for age and height (less than 85% expected weight). (See Table 4.9)

A second type of eating disorder, bulimia nervosa, is characterized by frequent episodes of binge-eating followed by purging (self-induced vomiting or ingestion of laxatives or cathartics to induce diarrhea or vomiting). Adolescents with bulimia nervosa tend to be of normal or increased weight. Purging behavior may be associated with both anorexia nervosa and bulimia nervosa. (See Table 4.10)

Treatment recommendations for eating disorders

Treating eating disorders requires a team approach that combines medical management, psychological interventions, and nutritional counseling. Eating disorders are psychiatric conditions, but can lead to physical complications and

Table 4.9 Warning signs signaling anorexia nervosa.

- Refusal to maintain body weight at or above the lower limit of normal or failure to make expected weight gain during growth, which leads to a BMI <17.5.
- Intense fear of gaining weight or becoming fat, despite being thin.
- Disturbance in the way in which one's body weight or shape is experienced, undue influence of body shape and weight on self-evaluation, or denial of the seriousness of current low body weight.
- In females, absence of at least three consecutive menstrual cycles when otherwise expected to occur. This condition is referred to as amenorrhea.
- People who have anorexia are also classified as restrictive type or binge eating purging type (see below).

Restricting type During the episode of anorexia nervosa, the person *does not* regularly engage in binge eating or purging behavior (i.e. self-induced vomiting or the misuse of laxatives or diuretics)

Binge eating/purging type During the episode of anorexia nervosa, the person regularly engages in binge eating or purging behavior (i.e. self-induced vomiting or the misuse of laxatives or diuretics)

Source: [32].

Table 4.10 Warning signs signaling bulimia nervosa.

- Recurrent binge eating at least twice a week for a minimum of 3 months.
- Binge eating refers to eating in a discrete period of time (e.g. within any 2-hour period an amount of food that is definitely larger than most people would eat during a similar period of time in similar circumstances; and, having a sense of lack of control over eating during the episode, such as a feeling that you cannot stop eating or control what or how much you are eating).
- May compensate for overeating by self-inducing vomiting; misusing laxatives, diuretics, or other medications; fasting or exercising excessively.
- Excessive preoccupation with body weight or shape.
- The disturbance does not occur exclusively during episodes of anorexia nervosa.

Source: [32].

even death. Patients identified early can improve when managed appropriately by an experienced care team. More severe cases with medical and nutritional issues require the involvement of a multidisciplinary specialty team working through the outpatient, inpatient or day program settings.

Assessment and treatment by a psychologist or psychiatrist familiar with eating disorders is crucial in establishing a diagnosis, evaluating the risk of suicide, and assessing the severity of the psychological symptoms as well as other related conditions such as depression, anxiety, substance abuse, or personality disorders. To improve, a teenager with an eating disorder needs to recognize the problem, improve his/her perceived body image and set and achieve nutritional and weight goals. To complete the treatment team, a dietitian experienced with eating disorders should provide guidance for nutritional rehabilitation and education and a physician must monitor the patient for medical complications.

Vegetarianism

Many adolescents choose to adopt a vegetarian dietary pattern. The decision to become a vegetarian may be influenced by health-related or philosophical reasons. Vegetarianism is the accepted dietary practice of many cultures in the world and can be healthful when appropriately planned to be nutritionally adequate. A vegetarian diet is defined as one that does not include meat, fish or fowl and for some, may exclude dairy foods. Nutrients that may become deficient include: protein, iron, zinc, calcium, vitamin D, riboflavin, vitamin B_{12}, vitamin A, omega-3 fatty acids, and iodine. There are two distinct patterns of vegetarianism: lacto–ovo vegetarians, and vegans.

Lacto–ovo vegetarians

Lacto–ovo vegetarians eat vegetable products, dairy foods, and eggs. A diet including dairy and eggs allows the inclusion of most nutrients.

Vegans

Vegetarians who are vegans omit all animal products from the diet. Removing dairy and eggs from the diet decreases the availability of many important

Table 4.11 Meeting nutrient needs in vegan diets.

Protein Legumes, whole grains, soy products, nuts and seeds, fruits, and all vegetables.
Iron Iron-fortified breakfast cereals, iron-fortified grain products, dried beans, and peas. (Eat with food high in vitamin C to increase absorption.) Iron supplement.
Zinc Yeast-fermented whole grain breads and zinc-fortified cereals.
Calcium Calcium-fortified soy products, calcium-fortified cereals and orange juice, dark leafy green vegetables (chard, broccoli, kale and mustard greens), nuts, calcium-set tofu, and calcium supplements.
Vitamin D Cod liver oil and menhaden oil if these are acceptable and vitamin/mineral supplements containing vitamin D. Soy products that are supplemented with vitamin D.
Riboflavin B-vitamin fortified grain products and cereals.
Vitamin B$_{12}$ Supplement for vegans.
Vitamin A Supplementation or inclusion in the diet of Beta-carotene in the form of yellow vegetables.
Omega-3 fatty acids Available in flax and other seeds, as well as walnuts and soybeans.
Iodine Iodine-fortified salts, sea salts.

Source: Diane Barsky, MD, University of Pennsylvania School of Medicine and Sue Konek, MA, RD, CNSD, CPS, Children's Hospital of Philadelphia. 2007. Used with permission.

nutrients, most notably vitamin B$_{12}$. These diets require the inclusion of a wide variety of vegetables, fruits, grains and oils. It may be necessary to include grain products that are fortified, especially with iron, on a regular basis. Supplementation with B$_{12}$, is recommended for all vegans. Vitamin B$_{12}$ supplements come in the form of sublingual daily pills, monthly injections or nasal spray. Soy milk, fortified with vitamin B$_{12}$, could also be recommended on a daily basis. Achieving adequate calcium intake is also a challenge for many vegans. Calcium needs can be met with the inclusion of fortified soy products (fortified soy milk/tofu) as well as calcium-fortified juices. Calcium supplements can augment daily intake to meet nutritional requirements. A varied diet is the key to adequate nutrition for all vegetarians with examples listed in Table 4.11.

Do children need vitamin and mineral supplements?

If children eat a varied diet, they should not require supplements. A very picky eater may benefit from a daily multi-vitamin/mineral supplement. At certain times during childhood a few vitamins and minerals may be insufficient including calcium, vitamin D, vitamin K, fluoride and iron.

• *Calcium:* Children who consume the recommended amounts of dairy foods for their age (milk, yogurt, cheese) will receive adequate calcium. Those who do not consume 3 servings of dairy foods everyday may require a calcium supplement. Calcium needs are particularly high for adolescents who increase height by 20% and gain 50% of adult skeletal mass during this period. (See Appendices G and H).

• *Vitamin D:* The AAP recommends that all babies, including those who are exclusively breastfed, receive vitamin D within the first two months of life.

Infant formulas provide adequate vitamin D. Breastfed infants should receive 200 IU/daily in a supplement. Vitamin D intake through the use of fortified dairy products should continue through childhood, and especially adolescence, to support development of a healthy skeletal structure. (See Appendix B)

• *Vitamin K:* Newborn babies are given vitamin K, in injection form, soon after birth for prophylaxis against hemorrhagic disease of the newborn, now called vitamin K deficiency bleeding (VKDB) (See Appendix D).

• *Fluoride:* A supplement of fluoride is recommended for infants 6 months or older who are breastfed or living in an area without fluoridated water. Infants 7–12 months require 0.5 mg/day, 1–2 years: 0.7 mg/d, 3–8 years: 1 mg/d. Primary care clinicians should determine fluoride levels in their communities to guide adequate dosing of fluoride for children.

Conclusion

Primary care clinicians have the unique opportunity to support and guide families in the health and normal growth of their children. These practitioners are among the first to note deviations from normal growth patterns and can provide early intervention to allow correction to the norm. Referral to specialists, when indicated including RDs, will provide families the support they require to achieve normal growth and development of their children.

References

1 Kleinman RE (Ed). *Pediatric Nutrition Handbook*, fifth edition. American Academy of Pediatrics, Committee on Nutrition; AAP, Illinois 2004.

2 Centers for Disease Control and Prevention. National Center for Health Statistics 2000 CDC Growth charts: United States. www.cdc.gov/growth charts.

3 Centers for Disease Control and Prevention. National Center for Health Statistics. National Health and Nutrition Examination Survey (NHANES). www.cdc.gov/nchs/nhanes.htm.

4 Koplan JP, Liverman CT, Kraak VI (Eds). *Preventing Childhood Obesity: Health in the Balance*. Institute of Medicine. The National Academies Press: Washington DC. 2005.

5 Gilluly K, Johnson L, Rossiter K. Effect of educational preparation on the accuracy of linear growth measurement in pediatric primary care practices: results of a multicenter nursing study. *J Pediatr Nurs* 2005;20(2):64–74.

6 Institute of Medicine Food and Nutrition Board, Institute of Medicine. Dietary Reference Intakes for energy and protien. National Academy of Science. National Academies Press, Washington, DC 2000.

7 Fomon SJ, Haschke F *et al.* Body composition of reference children from birth to age 10 years. *Am J Clin Nutr* 1982;35:1169.

8 Krugman DS, Dubowitz H. Failure to Thrive. *Am Fam Physician* 2003; 68:879–886.

9 Markowitz R and Duggan C. Failure to thrive: malnutrition in the pediatric outpatient setting, in Walker, Watkins, Duggan: *Nutrition in Pediatric*, 3rd Ed., 2003, BC Decker Inc, Hamilton, London.

10 Tershakovec AM, Van Horn L. Infants, Children and Adolescents In: *Medical Nutrition and Disease: A Case-Based Approach*. Third edition. Hark L, Morrison G (Eds). Blackwell Publishing: Boston. 2003.

11 Owen CG, Martin RM, Whincup pH, Smith GD, Cook DG. Effect of infant feeding on the risk of obesity across the life course: a quantitative review of published evidence. *Pediatrics* 2005;115:1367–77.

12 Carver JD, Wu P, Hall RT, Ziegler EE, Sosa R, *et al.* Growth of preterm infants fed nutrient enriched or term formula after hospital discharge. *Pediatrics* 2001:683–689.

13 Gartner LM, Greer FR. Section on Breastfeeding and Committee on Nutrition. American Academy of Pediatrics. Prevention of rickets and vitamin D deficiency: new guidelines for vitamin D intake. *Pediatrics* 2003;111(4 Pt 1):908–10.

14 *Healthy People 2010:* Department of Health and Human Services www.healthypeople.gov.

15 Li R, Darling N, Maurice E, Barker L, Grummer-Strawn LM. Breastfeeding rates in the United States by characteristics of the child, mother or family: the 2002 national immunization survey. *Pediatrics* 2005;115:e31–e37.

16 Kull I, Wickman M, Lilja G, Nordvall SL, Pershagen G. Breast feeding and allergic diseases in infants – a prospective birth cohort study. *Arch Dis Child* 2002;87:478–81.

17 Hark L. and Deen, D *Nutrition for Life*. DK Publishing: New York. 2005.

18 Roschitz B, Plecko B, Huemer M, Biebl A, Foerster H, Sperl W. Nutritional infantile vitamin B_{12} deficiency: pathobiochemical considerations in seven patients. *Arc Dis Child* 2005;90:F281–FF282.

19 Zschocke J, Schindler S, Hoffman GF, Albani M. Nature and nurture in vitamin B_{12}. *Arch Dis Child* 2002;87:75–6.

20 Thorpe M. Infant formula supplemented with DHA: Are there benefits? (Editorial.) *J Am Diet Assoc* 2003;103:551–2.

21 Dwyer JT, Suitor CW, Hendricks K. FITS: New Insights and Lessons Learned. *J Am Diet Assoc* 2004:104:(1 Suppl 1):S5–S7.

22 Fox MK, Pac S, Devaney B, Jankowski L. Feeding infants and toddlers study: What foods are infants and toddlers eating? *J Am Diet Assoc* 2004;104(1 Suppl 1):S22–S30.

23 Briefel RR, Reidy K, Karwe V, Jankowski L, Hendricks K. Toddlers' transition to table foods: impact on nutrient intakes and food patterns. *J Am Diet Assoc* 2004;104:S38–S44.

24 Skinner JD, Ziegler P, Pac S, Devaney B. Meal and snack patterns of infants and toddlers. *J Am Diet Assoc* 2004;104:S65–S70.

25 Devaney B, Ziegler P, Pac S, Karwe V, Barr SI. Nutrient intakes of infants and toddlers. *J Am Diet Assoc* 2004;104:S14–S21.

26 United States Department of Agriculture. *2005 Food Guide Pyramid.* www.mypyramid .gov

27 The Food Allergy and Anaphylaxis Network. www.foodallergy.org.

28 Khakoo GA, Lack G. Introduction of solids to the infant diet. (Commentary.) *Arch Dis Child* 2004;89:295.

29 Friel JK, Aziz K, Andrews WL, Harding SV, Courage ML, Adams RJ. A double-masked, randomized control trial of iron supplementation in early infancy in healthy term breast-fed infants. *J Pediatr* 2003;243:554–6.

30 Berkowitz, RI, Stallings VA, Maislin G, Stunkard AJ. Growth of children at high risk of obesity during the first 6 y of life: implications for prevention. *Am J Clin Nutr* 2005;81:140–6.

31 Galloway AT, Fiorito L, Lee Y, Birch LL. Parental pressure, dietary patterns and weight status among girls who are "picky eaters". *J Am Diet Assoc* 2005;105:541–8.

32 American Psychiatric Association. *Diagnostic and Statistical Manual of Mental Disorders,* Fourth Edition Text Revision. American Psychiatric Association, Washington, DC, 2000. Lipman TH, Hench KD, Benyi T, Delaune J, Gilluly K, Johnson L, *et al.* Arch Dis Child 2004;89, 342–343.

CHAPTER 5

Feeding the mother-to-be

**James M Nicholson, Catherine Sullivan and
Morghan B Holt**

Introduction

While adequate nutrition is important throughout the life span, it is especially crucial for pregnant and lactating females, whose nutrient and energy demands are substantially increased by the nutritional requirements of developing fetuses. It is important for pregnant and lactating women and their health care providers to be aware of the changes in nutritional requirements throughout pregnancy, during the post-partum period and during lactation. Understanding the changing nutritional demands of pregnancy and lactation will allow health care providers to make informed recommendations regarding diet alterations and supplementation for their pregnant and lactating patients. If the increased dietary demands during pregnancy and lactation are not adequately met, both the mother and her baby risk developing nutritional deficiencies. Recent research demonstrates maternal nutrition affects not only the health and development of the newborn but also the subsequent health of the child as it grows, even into adulthood [1,2]. Adult risks for chronic diseases are increasingly being linked to fetal nutritional environment [3]. It is important for health care providers to recognize risk factors for deficiencies or excesses during pregnancy and lactation, understand the implications of these for both the mother and her fetus, and know how to safely and effectively prevent and treat deficiencies or excesses throughout pregnancy and lactation. Avoiding nutritional deficiencies during pregnancy promotes optimal outcomes for both mother and baby; avoiding nutritional deficiencies during lactation promotes prolonged breastfeeding, maternal health and satisfaction, and optimal infant development.

Physiological and biochemical impact of pregnancy

The physiological and biochemical changes which occur during pregnancy are primarily designed to accommodate and promote the growth and development of the fetus. Physiological changes during pregnancy include the development and growth of the feto–placental unit, increased maternal blood volume, increased maternal adipose tissue, decreased gastrointestinal (GI) motility and breast enlargement to prepare for lactation. Throughout pregnancy, hormonal alterations create maternal insulin resistance and increase the uptake of fatty acids in extrauterine tissues, both of which promote transportation of glucose to the developing fetus. In order to support the additional energy requirements of their developing fetuses, women must adjust their daily caloric intake throughout pregnancy; the amount of adjustment will depend upon pre-conception body mass index (BMI), maternal developmental stage (adolescence versus adulthood), and the developmental stage of pregnancy. Additionally, as fetuses depend on maternal dietary consumption to support their nutritional, as well as metabolic, needs, it is crucial that pregnant women increase their intake of various nutrients to ensure that their own resources are not depleted and that fetal daily requirements are adequately met.

Current nutritional recommendations during pregnancy

Energy and protein

The Dietary Reference Intakes (DRI) provides daily recommendations for calories and protein for pregnant and lactating women. Basal requirements should be determined based on maternal age, stature, activity level, pre-conception weight, BMI and gestational weight gain goals [2, 4–6]. During the first trimester, total energy expenditure does not change greatly and weight gain is minimal, therefore, additional energy intake is recommended only in the second and third trimesters. An additional 340 kcal/day is recommended during the second trimester and 452 kcal/day is recommended during the third trimester [6]. Lactating women should consume an additional 500 kcal/day for the first 6 months and an additional 400 kcal/day for 7 to 9 months. Additional protein is needed during pregnancy for fetal, placental and maternal tissues to develop during the second and third trimesters. Protein recommendations are therefore increased from 46 g/day for an adult, non-pregnant woman to 71 g/day for a pregnant woman. Protein requirements for lactating women are also recommended at 71 g/day [6].

Vitamins and minerals

Maternal blood volume begins to increase at about 16 weeks age of gestation (AOG) preceeding increased maternal erythropoesis, which begins about about 28 weeks AOG. This results in dilutional anemia, characterized by decreased values for hemoglobin and hematocrit. The decrease begins at 16–24 weeks AOG and continues until 24–36 weeks AOG. The levels begin to rise around term (approximately 38 weeks AOG), and should be normal by 6 weeks postpartum.

Iron

In many pregnant women, nutritional anemia accompanies the normal dilutional anemia. Nutritional anemia is usually the result of inadequate iron intake. The hemoglobin levels of approximately 40% of women who do not receive iron supplements drop below 11 g/dL. In the presence of iron supplementation, hemoglobin levels this low are rare. Nutritional megaloblastic anemia secondary due to folate deficiency also occurs during pregnancy, but it is less common and can also be treated effectively with folate or vit B_{12} supplementation.

Iron requirements increased during pregnancy, and maintaining adequate iron stores is important, as iron-deficiency anemia increases the risk of maternal and infant death, preterm delivery, and low neonatal birth weight. Patients should be screened for anemia prior to pregnancy (if possible) and during each trimester for high risk individuals. Hemoglobin levels less than 11 g/dL or hematocrit levels below 33% in the first or third trimester indicate anemia. Hemoglobin levels less than 10.4 g/dL or hematocrit levels below 32% in the second trimester indicate anemia [7]. As the significant increase in maternal blood volume during pregnancy typically reduces hemoglobin levels, ferritin levels and mean corpuscular volume, should also be used as a diagnostic criteria as these measures are not affected by the increased blood volume. Serum ferritin is also useful in assessing the post gastric bypass pregnant patient. A serum ferritin level of <15 ng/mL warrants aggressive treatment and may require intramuscular injection rather than oral supplementation.

Throughout pregnancy, maternal blood volume increases 20–30%, and erythropoeisis under such conditions requires that an additional 450 mg of iron be delivered to the maternal marrow. The fetus and the placenta require 350 mg of iron, and approximately 250 mg of iron is lost in blood at delivery. A total iron increase of approximately 1000 mg is required during pregnancy [8]. It is difficult for many women to meet the iron requirements of pregnancy by altering their diets. Prenatal care providers generally recommend iron supplementation in the form of a daily supplement of 30 mg of elemental iron in the form of simple salts, beginning around the twelfth week of pregnancy for women who have normal pre-conception hemoglobin measurements [2]. The RDA for iron is 27 g/day in pregnancy and 9 g/day lactation. For women who are pregnant with multiple fetuses or have low pre-conception hemoglobin measurements, a supplement of between 60–100 mg/day of elemental iron is recommended until hemoglobin concentrations are normal. Once previously-anemic women's hemoglobin concentrations become normal, they may decrease their supplemental iron intake to 27 mg/day. Iron supplementation can have gastrointestinal side effects specific to pregnancy which should be taken into account when prescribing the course of treatment. During the first trimester, nausea is a common problem and can be exacerbated by oral iron supplements; physicians may elect to defer supplementation until the second trimester, when iron requirements increase and nausea has waned. Nausea resulting from iron supplements can be minimized by taking the supplement following a meal; however, iron absorption may be inhibited if the supplement is ingested immediately following a meal. Oral iron supplements can also cause constipation, which can be effectively treated with bulk laxatives. Antacids impair iron absorption and should not be taken concurrently; this is of particular importance during the third trimester, when gastroesophogeal reflux is common. Iron is better absorbed if the maternal diet contains adequate amounts of vitamin C. Occasionally, pregnant women develop pica, craving for non-food substances such as clay, dirt or ice. Iron-deficiency has been postulated to cause pica but there are also cultural beliefs that lead to these practices. Pregnant women with iron deficiency should be asked about pica, and women experiencing pica should be tested for iron deficiency. Pica is mostly of concern if it prevents the mother from consuming nutrient-rich foods.

Folate

Folic acid deficiency is the most common vitamin deficiency during pregnancy, with well know associations to birth defects (see chapter 11). Severe folate deficiency commonly manifests as megaloblastic anemia. The increased demand for folic acid during pregnancy is the result of increased maternal erythropoesis. Maternal erythropoesis increases most significantly during the second and third trimesters, but adequate maternal folic acid intake is crucial throughout pregnancy and even prior to conception. Folic acid supplementation of 0.4 mg/day before and during the first four weeks of pregnancy has been repeatedly associated with a drastically reduced incidence of neural tube defects. As embryonic neural tube closure is complete by 18–26 days after conception, it is especially crucial that pregnant women consume adequate levels of folic acid before and during the first four weeks of pregnancy.

In 1992, the Centers for Disease Control and Prevention issued the recommendation that all women of childbearing age take 0.4 mg/day of supplemental folic acid, in order to ensure that pregnancy, whether intended or not, occurs at a time during which adequate levels of folate are present. Folic acid antagonists, such as phenobarbitoal, phenytoin, primidone, carbamazepine, trimethoprim and triamterene, taken during the second or third month following the last menstrual period doubles the relative risk for fetal cardiovascular and urinary tract defects and oral clefts. Folic acid antagonists taken before or after this time period seem to have no adverse effects, which illustrates the particular importance of adequate folate levels during early pregnancy. The RDA for folate in women of childbearing age is currently 0.4 mg/day, and the RDA for folate in pregnant women is 0.6 mg/day [2]. A healthy diet should contain approximately 0.7 mg/day of folate, of which about half is bioavailable. Women with a history of neural tube defects may be advised to consume higher doses. Typically the diet in the U.S. is lacking folate-rich food sources and a patient might be deficient in folate.

In 1997, the US began the folic acid fortification program. Grains, such as cereals, pastas, rice and breads are now fortified with folic acid. Good dietary sources of natural folate include dark green leafy vegetables, green beans and lima beans, orange juice, fortified cereals, yeast, mushrooms, pork, liver and kidneys. Dietary folate is dramatically influenced by food storage and preparation; for instance, it is destroyed by boiling and canning. Folate stores are likely to be easily depleted among women who have folate-deficient diets, are alcoholic, or are of lower socio-economic status. Additionally, evidence exists to suggest that the long-term use of oral contraceptives inhibits folate absorption and enhances folate degradation in the liver. Therefore, folate stores may be more rapidly depleted in women who have used oral contraceptives, which may lead to a higher incidence of folate deficiency in such women if they become pregnant; providers should be sure to inquire about pre-conception contraceptive usage to inform supplementation decisions.

Calcium

In contrast to maternal iron and folate stores, which are relatively small and, therefore, easily depleted, maternal calcium stores are large and are mostly stored skeletally, allowing for easy mobilization as needed. Over the course of pregnancy, a single fetus requires between 25–30 g of calcium, which represents a mere 2.5% of total maternal stores. In the first half of pregnancy, the requirement is only an additional 50 mg/day. Most of the additional calcium requirement of pregnancy occurs during the final trimester, during which the fetus absorbs an average of 300 mg/day. Evidence has shown that calcium supplementation reduces the risk of developing hypertension during pregnancy, but only in women who did not have adequate calcium intakes prior to supplementation [9,10]. The recommended adequate intake (AI) for women 19–50 years old is 1000 mg/day; the AI for the adolescent female population age 9–19 is 1300 mg/day. The amount of additional calcium required during pregnancy remains debatable. Some professionals argue that non-adolescent pregnant women should increase their daily intake to 1200 mg/day, while others argue that the amount of calcium required by the fetus is negligible and easily satisfied if pregnant women consume the amount of calcium recommended for their non-pregnant counterparts. Others suggest that adolescents should increase their calcium intake during pregnancy, particularly since their own bones still require calcium deposition to ensure adequate bone density in adults.

Consuming an adequate intake of dietary calcium presents no problem for women who consume at least 3 servings of dairy foods every day. Even in women who limit their intake of dairy foods because of lactose intolerance, seem to be able to tolerate yogurt and cheese on a daily basis. Low fat varieties should be encouraged at least 3 servings/day. Additionally, many vegetables, also contain calcium and soy milk, orange juice, cereal and bread products fortified with calcium should also be suggested (See Appendices G and H).

In the US, calcium intake varies by race and geographical region. In the event that women consume inadequate dietary calcium during pregnancy, they should be encouraged first to increase their intake of calcium from various food sources as described above. If increased intake is not possible or effective, supplementation may be needed. Calcium carbonate, gluconate, lactate or citrate may provide 500–600 mg/day of calcium to account for the difference between the amount of calcium required and that consumed. Supplements must be carefully implemented, because the tolerable upper intake for calcium during pregnancy is 2500 mg/day. The standard prenatal vitamin contains 450 mg per serving. Multivitamins marketed to the non-pregnant population generally have less than 200 mg per serving. Calcium is generally thought to be absorbed in doses of 500 mg at one time making it unlikely that pregnant women would reach the upper tolerable limit.

The data concerning the role of calcium in controlling pregnancy-induced-hypertension or pre-eclampsia has been mixed. While calcium supplementation has been shown to decrease blood pressure and pre-ecalmpsia in smaller studies, larger trials have failed to show an effect [2,9]. It is prudent to make sure women are meeting the AI for their age.

Vitamins A and D

In order to ensure proper absorption of calcium, adequate vitamin D intake is essential. Vitamin D increases gastrointestinal calcium absorption and initiates parathyroid hormone activity. Vitamin D supplementation during pregnancy is not generally required. The AI for vitamin D during pregnancy is 5 μg/day, which is the same for non-pregnant and lactating women. Vitamin D deficiency can result from a very low dietary intake of vitamin in conjunction with limited exposure to ultraviolet light. In pregnancy, maternal vitamin D deficiency can result in fetal deficiency, which manifests as neonatal hypocalcemia. Supplementation of 5 μg/day can be considered for strict vegetarians or women who avoid sunlight or fortified milk. The needs of the breastfeeding infant will be discussed in the section on lactation. While the research is conflicting, some evidence indicates that excessive vitamin D intake resulting from large doses of supplements may cause fetal hypercalcemia. Higher doses of vitamin D have been used in breastfeeding mothers without evidence of toxicity to mother or baby [11]. The established tolerable upper intake for vitamin D is 50 μg/day.

As with calcium and vitamin D, severe vitamin A deficiency is rare in the United States, and an adequate intake of vitamin A is readily available in a healthy diet. Women with lower socio-economic status, however, may consume diets with inadequate amounts of vitamin A. Increasing dietary intake of vitamin A is quite simple, and should be encouraged before supplementation to avoid excessive intake, which has been reported to be teratogenic. Many commercially available vitamin supplements contain excessive doses of vitamin A and thus should not be used in pregnancy. Additionally, topical creams which contain retinol derivatives commonly used to treat acne should not be used in pregnancy. The tolerable upper intake for vitamin A is 3 mg/day (10,000 IU).

Magnesium and Vitamin C

Recommendations for magnesium intake increase by 40 mg/day during pregnancy (from 310–320 mg/day in non-pregnant adult women to 350–360 mg/day for pregnancy, and 400 mg/day in pregnant women younger than 18), although no experimental data directly support this recommendation. Similarly, no experimental data has been shown to support the need for increased vitamin C intake. Still, current recommendations indicate that pregnant women should consume 85 mg/day, rather than the 75 mg/day recommended for non-pregnant adult women, ostensibly to protect against depleted plasma vitamin C levels and to ensure that adequate vitamin C is transported to the developing fetus. Adequate vitamin C is also needed for iron uptake. However, because vitamin C is actively transported from the maternal to the fetal circulation, and no human studies have examined the effects of large doses of vitamin C on fetal growth and development, a tolerable upper intake has been set at 1800–2000 mg/day. Women who smoke have an increased need for vitamin C. Although only limited data exist to support the need for increased intake, the DRI's for riboflavin, niacin, vitamin B_{12}, zinc, copper, iodine and molybdenum are modestly increased during pregnancy.

Blood pressure

Circulating blood volume and tissue fluid increase substantially during pregnancy. Blood pressure, however, decreases during the second trimester and generally returns to preconception levels near term (38–41 weeks gestation). Pregnant women require substantial fluid intake to maintain blood pressure and flow to vital organs. Inadequate fluid intake could inhibit the necessary increase in circulating blood volume, which has been associated with preterm delivery, intrauterine growth retardation (IUGR) and hypertension. The AI for water in pregnancy is 3 L per day [6]. If the public water supply contains lead, pregnant women should drink bottled water, as excessive lead intakes can have deleterious neurological consequences for the developing fetus.

Contaminants and food borne illness

Food thought to be contaminated by heavy metals can have neurotoxic effects for the fetus. Most heavy metals are known teratogens. Specifically, methyl mercury, lead, cadmium, nickel and selenium are known to have dire consequences for developing fetuses. Mercury can be removed from vegetables by peeling or washing well with soap and water. Consumption of raw fish products and highly carnivorous fish (including tuna, shark, tilefish, swordfish and mackerel) should be limited or avoided during pregnancy [12]. All foods should be handled in a sanitary and appropriate manner to prevent bacterial contamination. All dairy foods and juices consumed during pregnancy should be pasteurized. *Listeria monocytogenes* contamination results in food poisoning during and outside of pregnancy. In pregnancy, however, it can develop into a blood borne, transplacental infection that can cause choriamniontis, premature labor, spontaneous abortion, or fetal demise. To avoid listeriosis, pregnant women should wash vegetables and fruits, cook meats, avoid processed, precooked meats (cold cuts) and soft cheeses (brie, blue cheese, camabert, Mexican caso-blanco).

Substance abuse

Nicotine consumption during pregnancy has been consistently associated with low neonatal weight. If women who smoke become pregnant, they should discontinue cigarette use for the sake of their fetuses. Heavy alcohol consumption during pregnancy is also associated with low neonatal weight, as well as deficiencies in B vitamins, folate and protein. Maternal alcoholism contributes to fetal nutritional deficiencies because it inhibits maternal absorption of nutrients, and it poses a toxic threat to the developing fetus. Fetal alcohol syndrome (FAS) has been identified as resulting from heavy maternal drinking throughout pregnancy and manifests in such deformities as microcephaly, cleft palate and micrognathia. While it is certain that heavy maternal drinking is harmful to developing fetuses, the issue of whether more modest amounts of alcohol consumption are acceptable during pregnancy remains controversial. Currently, no defined intake level which can be consumed without increased risk exists for alcohol. The National Institute of Alcohol Abuse and Alcoholism advises non pregnant women against drinking more than 1 oz of alcohol (i.e., 24 oz of beer, 10 oz of wine or 2 oz of liquor) each day. Alcohol should be avoided entirely throughout the first trimester. Although the debate remains as to whether mild to moderate drinking affects fetal development in the latter trimesters of pregnancy, the Council on Scientific Affairs of the American Medical Association recommends abstinence from alcohol throughout pregnancy [2]. The CDC recommends that clinicians identify women at risk in the preconception period and provide education and support for cessation [13].

The effect of caffeine consumption on fetal development is unclear. Recent studies have found an association between the caffeine level present in two cups of coffee consumed each day and spontaneous abortion during the first trimester. The current recommendation advises pregnant women to reduce their caffeine intake from all sources, including tea, cocoa and soda. Total intake should be minimized to 150–300 mg/day [2].

Assessing nutritional status during pregnancy

Assessing nutritional status during pregnancy is useful in identifying women with nutritional risk factors that could adversely affect their health or the health of their fetuses. Maternal nutritional status at conception influences how nutrients are partitioned between the mother and the fetus. In severe deficiencies, maternal nutrition is preferred; in the absence deficiencies or in modest deficiencies, fetal nutrition is favored. It is important to identify deficiencies and risk factors of nutritional depletion in the early stages of pregnancy in order to implement timely treatment and prevent potential maternal and fetal complications. Very recent data suggest that the impact of maternal nutritional status during pregnancy may not be immediately observed; maternal nutrition during pregnancy may impact the developing fetus covertly and manifest as disease states or risks for disease states into adulthood [2]. Growing evidence suggests that maternal nutritional status during pregnancy may alter the epigenetic state of the fetal genome, causing fetal programming for adult disease risk [3]. Both undernutrition and overnutrition have been shown to have undesirable effects. Maintaining proper nutrition throughout pregnancy is therefore of increasing importance. Evaluation of nutritional status during pregnancy includes clinical, dietary and laboratory measures. The first of these measures is a thorough review of patient medical history.

Obstetric history

For each pregnant patient, a detailed obstetric history should be recorded and reviewed, as the events during and outcomes of previous pregnancies have implications for the current pregnancy. Many of the items included in the obstetric history will provide insight into the current nutritional status and needs of the patient. The obstetric history should include the total number and dates of prior pregnancies and describe maternal and fetal outcomes and complications. In evaluating the nutritional requirements during pregnancy it is important to assess nutritionally significant outcomes (e.g., severe anemia) of previous pregnancies. The obstetric history should also include information about previous deliveries of low birth-weight (<2500g) or high birth-weight (>400 g), or small-for-gestational-age infants (<10th or >90th percentile for gestational age), stillbirths (≥20 weeks), spontaneous abortions (<20 weeks) and neonatal deaths, as well as previous weight-gain patterns during pregnancy, prior history of nausea, vomiting or hyperemesis during pregnancy, gestational diabetes, eclampsia, anemia, PICA, weight status (BMI) and patterns of contraception use. Previous breastfeeding experience should be assessed as well as the intention to feed in this pregnancy.

The medical history should also identify maternal risk factors for nutritional deficiencies and chronic diseases with nutritional implications (e.g., absorption disorders, eating disorders, metabolic disorders, infections, diabetes mellitus, PKU (phenylketonuria), sickle cell trait, or renal disease). Closely spaced pregnancies (i.e., less than a year between pregnancies) are at increased risk of having depleted nutrient reserves. Maternal nutrient depletion may be associated with the increased incidence of preterm birth, IUGR and maternal mortality/morbidity among women with closely spaced pregnancies. Caffeine, tobacco, alcohol and recreational drug consumption should also be quantified in the medical history, as should any vitamin or herbal supplementation or alternative pharmacological therapies. A history of medication use should also be obtained to evaluate the extent to which past or present medications may affect nutrient absorption.

In addition to the medical history, specific questions regarding professional, social, economic and emotional stresses and religious practices (including dietary restrictions and fasting) should be included in the assessment to account for any impact they may have on the patient's nutritional status. Some work environments adversely impact dietary intake, as they may provide inadequate time during the day to eat proper meals or permit direct access to only nutritionally marginal food; for this reason, pregnant patients should be asked about the conditions of their employment, and identified limitations and potential solutions should be reviewed with the patient. For women who have identified themselves as of lower socioeconomic status, it is important to inquire about access to nutritious food and the ability to store and prepare food; referral to food assistance programs (e.g., Women, Infants and Children) may be appropriate.

In specifically evaluating dietary practices, patient interviews and written questionnaires are effective and appropriate. The evaluation should address issues of both current and past appetite, meal patterns, dieting regimens, cultural dietary practices, vegetarianism, food allergies, and cravings/aversions. Current dietary practices can be evaluated using the 24-hour recall, usual intake or food frequency questionnaire.

If a patient has identified nutritional risk factors, she may benefit from referral to a registered dietitian for nutrition education. During and just before pregnancy, nutritional issues have increased explicit significance for the expecting or hopeful mother. Therefore, preconception (in planned pregnancies) and the early stages following conception are ideal times to encourage development of good dietary practices in order to prevent future medical problems (e.g., obesity, diabetes, hypertension, osteoporosis) [3].

Appropriate weight gain during pregnancy

A crucial element of the clinical nutritional evaluation is the determination of the preconception BMI, which can be calculated using the patient's preconception weight and height, or can be derived from a published BMI table. A patient's BMI is an important tool in evaluating preconception weight status, and it should be shared with and explained to the patient when discussing weight-gain goals. Preconception weight should be determined from clinical records obtained immediately before reported pregnancy whenever available. At each prenatal visit, the patient's weight should be measured, and her rate of weight gain should be determined. Research studies are beginning to document adverse neo-natal outcomes based on materal weight gain. It is thought that both excessive and insufficient weight gain may have detrimental outcomes [14].

The Institute of Medicine issued recommendations in 1990 that stated that women with low pre-pregnancy body mass indices (BMI <19.8) should increase their caloric intake substantially to attain a weight gain between 28 and 40 pounds during the course of pregnancy [4,5,13,16], women with normal pre-pregnancy BMI (19.8–26.0) should increase their caloric intake moderately to gain between 25 and 35 pounds during the course of pregnancy, and women with high BMI (>26.0–29.0) should increase their caloric intake in a limited fashion, to gain between 15 and 25 pounds during the course of pregnancy [4,13,16]. An area of controversy is the weight gain needs of the obese woman. Women with a BMI greater than 29 are considered obese and should gain 15 pounds during the pregnancy [4]. Women who are short (<62 inches) should strive for weight gain patterns similar to those recommended for women with high pre-pregnancy BMI to avoid excess fetal weight gain leading to the potential for cephalo–pelvic disproportion, one of the most prevalent indications for cesarean section delivery. Pregnant adolescents should strive for weight gain patterns similar to those recommended for women with low pre-pregnancy BMI, as adolescents need to fulfill the energy requirements of their developing fetuses as well as the nutritional requirements of their own continued growth and development [17].

Low preconception BMI (underweight)

Women with low preconception BMI (<19.8) are at risk for delivering low birth weight infants and/or developing toxemia. If a woman who was underweight before conception does not gain adequate weight during her pregnancy, these risks are further increased. As with general nutritional assessment and treatment, the optimal time for evaluating and treating underweight women is prior to conception. However, the March of Dimes has determined that approximately half of all pregnancies are unplanned, making this an unrealistic option in many cases. A woman with a BMI of less than 19.8 who is considering pregnancy should be encouraged to gain weight before conceiving. If an underweight woman has conceived without gaining adequate weight, she should be encouraged to gain between 28 and 40 pounds over the course of her pregnancy. Protein–calorie supplementation may assist in correcting preconception nutritional deficits and provide adequate nutrients for fetal development.

Inadequate weight gain (<2 lb/month during the second and third trimesters) is associated with low birth weight, IUGR and fetal complications. Inhibited fetal growth usually correlates with inadequate weight gain. Discrepancy in gestational age versus uterine size or biparietal diameter of the fetal head as measured by sonography are signs of IUGR. Women with inadequate weight gain or weight loss should have repeated and thorough nutritional evaluations. Careful diet histories should be taken to determine the adequacy of dietary intake, and supplementation should be provided as necessary.

Overweight and obesity

Women with high preconception BMIs (>26) are at risk for developing diabetes, hypertension and thromboembolic events, and for delivering macrosomic infants. Although there is considerable controversy regarding the management of pregnancy in obese women, the current guidelines calls limited maternal weight gain of up to 15 pounds [4,5,16]. Despite preconception obesity, severe caloric restriction during pregnancy should not be considered, as caloric restriction is linked to inadequate intake of important micro- and macronutrients [15]. Even in severe obesity carbohydrate recommendations are 175 g/day. Adequate consumption of calcium, iron, folate, B vitamins and protein is particularly crucial during pregnancy, regardless of maternal weight. If caloric intake is inadequate, ingested proteins are catabolized for energy needs and are therefore unavailable for maternal/fetal protein synthesis. An estimated 32 kcal/kg/d is necessary for optimal use of ingested protein. Severe restriction of caloric intake paired with severe restriction of carbohydrate intake can result in ketosis, which in studies of diabetic women have shown to be detrimental for developing fetuses. Studies have also suggested an association between ketosis and reduced uterine blood flow. Ketone bodies are concentrated in amniotic fluid and absorbed by the developing fetus. The mental development of children whose mothers have had ketonuria during pregnancy has been shown to be stunted, although the direct causal link between fetal ketosis and inhibited mental development has yet to be definitively established. To avoid inadequate intake of crucial nutritional components, which can adversely impact both mother and fetus, pregnant women with high preconception BMIs should limit their weight gain during the course of their pregnancies, but they should not severely restrict their caloric intake such that the nutrients required to sustain a healthy pregnancy are insufficient.

Rapid, excessive weight accumulation is usually the result of fluid retention, which is associated with, but does not cause, toxemia. Fluid retention in the absence of hypertension or proteinuria is not an indication for salt restriction or diuretic therapy, but women who retain fluid should be monitored for other signs of toxemia. Edema in the lower extremities is cause by the accumulation of interstitial fluid secondary to obstruction of the pelvic veins and commonly occurs during the later stages of pregnancy. Edema can be treated by elevating the legs and wearing support hose.

Excessive weight gain during pregnancy may also be caused by fat deposition. As excessive weight gain is associated with both maternal and fetal morbidities, weight gain that exceeds the recommendations corresponding to preconception BMI should be monitored. A careful dietary history should be taken to determine the source of excess fat deposition, and recommendations for dietary changes should be offered accordingly.

The adolescent patient

Nutritional assessment of pregnant adolescents is particularly important, as their own growth and development may increase the demand for caloric and nutrient intake. Younger adolescents may need to gain additional weight (above the amount recommended for their preconception BMIs) in order to support their own normal growth during the course of their pregnancies. Both the pattern of weight gain and the total weight gain are especially significant among pregnant adolescents. Inadequate weight gain before 24 weeks-AOG, regardless of total pregnancy weight gain, has been associated with low birth weight among infants born to adolescent mothers. Recent research on adolescent pregnancy has demonstrated that dietary intake also directly impacts neonatal birth weight. Pregnant adolescents who consume diets which consist of large amounts of carbohydrates and limited amounts of protein and fat seem to have reduced risk of delivering low-birth-weight infants or preterm infants as compared to pregnant adolescents who consume diets lower in carbohydrates. The nutritional assessment of pregnant adolescents should involve thorough evaluation of their dietary habits and direct recommendations for any nutritional changes necessary for optimal pregnancy outcomes.

Pregnancy-related caloric demands are negligible during most of the first trimester, but increase dramatically at the end of the first trimester, and remain consistently amplified until after delivery. Weight gain patterns during pregnancy should reflect the increased energy requirements for each phase of pregnancy. That is, women should gain most of their weight during the latter half of pregnancy. Adequate weight gain during the second trimester is of particular importance, as it seems to have a protective effect on fetal and neonatal weight even if weight gain during the first or third trimesters is inadequate. Appropriate weight gain over the course of pregnancy is also important, as low maternal weight gain is a risk factor for low birth weight, IUGR and preterm birth; while excessive maternal weight gain is a risk factor for hypertension, preeclampsia, gestational diabetes, prolonged labor, macrosomia, cephalo–pelvic disproportion, cesarean section delivery, and, paradoxically, IUGR.

Recent evaluations of national birth data suggest that fetal birth weight and maternal weight gain are lower for African–American women than for Caucasian women, and that the incidence of low birth weight is higher in African–American infants than in infants of other racial and ethnic groups. In an attempt to alter this trend, the Institute of Medicine recommends that African–American women gain toward the higher end of the weight-gain range recommended for their preconception BMI. It is important to remember, however, that African–American women are more likely to retain more weight gain post partum over their Caucasian counterparts. This should be monitored closely to reduce the risk of obesity [8]. No adjustments to the weight gain recommendations have been made for pregnant women from other ethnic minorities.

Illnesses with nutritional significance during pregnanacy

Gestational diabetes

Women with type 1 diabetes mellitus (DM) must be diligent to avoid both hypoglycemia and hyperglycemia with ketosis during pregnancy. Additionally, women with pre-diabetes or type 2 diabetes who become pregnant may develop a resistance to insulin and may require increased insulin to manage their diabetes. Fetal glucose utilization may also cause maternal fasting hypoglycemia. Therefore, it is especially important that women who enter pregnancy with type 1 DM be aware of the critical significance of frequent blood glucose monitoring.

When maternal insulin secretion cannot accommodate normal pregnancy-induced glucose intolerance, the result is gestational diabetes mellitus (GDM). GDM occurs in approximately 7% of all pregnancies (200,000 cases annually) [18]. GDM is usually diagnosed during the second or third trimester of pregnancy, at which time insulin-antagonist hormone levels increase, usually resulting in insulin resistance. After delivery, approximately 90% of all women with GDM become normoglycemic, but they remain at increased risk of developing type-2 diabetes.

GDM has been associated with increased fetal morbidity. Therefore, clinicians believe all pregnant patients should be screened for GDM at 24–28 weeks

Time	mg/dL	mmol/L
Fasting	95	5.3
1-h	180	10.0
2-h	155	8.6
3-h	140	7.8

Table 5.1 Normal ranges of serum glucose values in pregnancy.

Source: American Diabetes Association [4].

AOG; risk factors alone may fail to identify up to 50% of patients with GDM. According to the American Diabetes Association women with low-risk status do not require glucose testing. This category is highly limited to women under the age of 25, normal pregravid weight, low-risk ethnicity, no known diabetes in a first degree relative, no history of abnormal glucose tolerance and no history of poor obstetric outcome [18]. High-risk patients, for example those who have a personal history of abnormal glucose tolerance, who are from ethnic groups with high prevalence of GDM (African–American, Native American, Southeast Asian, Pacific Islander, Hispanic), who are obese, who have first-degree relatives with Type-2 diabetes, who have a history of glucosuria, or who have obstetric histories consistent with diabetes (past macrosomia, fetal anomalies or neonatal hypoglycemia) should be screened by 16 weeks AOG. Screening for GDM is a two-step approach. The first measure is performed one hour after a 50 g oral glucose load. A threshold level greater than or equal to 130 mg/dL for the one-hour screen should be used. Roughly 20% of patients will test positive, and these patients will require a second screening during a three-hour, 100 g, glucose load. The diagnosis of GDM is appropriate when two or more serum glucose values are outside of the normal range proposed by the American Diabetes Association (see Table 5.1).

Medical nutritional therapy for GDM aims to provide energy levels for appropriate gestational weight gain, achievement and maintenance of normoglycemia and absence of ketone bodies. Individualized meal plans are recommended, as both the ideal percentage and the ideal type of carbohydrate are controversial. Monitoring blood glucose, urine or blood ketones, appetite and weight gain is crucial in individualizing and adjusting meal plans. Generally, 40–45% of total energy intake should be from carbohydrates, distributed throughout the day in three small or moderately sized meals and two to four snacks [18,19]. An evening snack prevents accelerated ketosis overnight. Carbohydrates are not well-tolerated at breakfast, possibly as a result of increased levels of cortisol and growth hormones. The initial meal plan should therefore limit carbohydrate intake at breakfast to 30 g, and adjustments made according to blood glucose monitoring results. To satisfy appetite and meet fetal needs, high-protein foods, which do not impact blood glucose, should be added to the main meals.

Patients with serum glucose levels consistently above recommendations require insulin therapy to achieve normoglycemia. These recommendations include initiating insulin therapy in patients that fail to maintain a fasting plasma glucose ≤105 mg/dL, or 1-hour postprandial plasma glucose ≤155 mg/dL, or 2-hour postprandial plasma glucose ≤130 mg/dL [18]. Recent data evaluating the use of second-generation sufonylureas (e.g., glyburide) are encouraging but the use of these agents is not FDA approved for the treatment of gestational diabetes [18].

The US Preventive Services Task Force found fair to good evidence that screening, combined with diet and insulin therapy can reduce the rate of fetal macrosomia in women with gestational diabetes [20].

Whether or not insulin therapy is implemented, the goal of therapy should be to prevent the maternal and fetal complications that have been associated with GDM. All women with GDM should receive medical nutrition therapy counseling as standard of care [4]. Maternal complications include fetal macrosomia and resultant delivery complications (e.g., increased risk of cesarean section, operative vaginal delivery, shoulder dystocia). Fetal complications include possible increased incidence of fetal demise and ketonemia, which has been associated with lower average IQ scores at 2–5 years of age. The data remain inconclusive as to whether the complications are entirely preventable using the currently accepted therapies.

Following delivery, patients who developed GDM should be re-screened for type 2 diabetes, as the risk of development is increased by 50% over the 15–20 years following a pregnancy complicated by GDM. Promotion of breast-feeding to diabetic mothers is especially important as recent research shows that there may be a protective effect in preventing diabetes in both mothers and babies [21–23].

Common side effects

Nausea and vomiting are associated with increased levels of the pregnancy hormone human chorionic gonadotropin (hCG). hCG doubles every 48 hours in early pregnancy, peaking at about 12 weeks of gestation. Nausea affects about 60% of pregnant women. Of those women who experience nausea during early pregnancy, a small number require hospitalization for severe hyperemesis gravidarum. There are many strategies for alleviating nausea and vomiting in pregnancy; the success of any specific strategy varies between individuals. Eating foods high in carbohydrates (e.g., crackers, bread or dry cereal) immediately upon waking and before rising in the morning may help. Eating small, low-fat meals and snacks (e.g., fruits, pretzels, crackers, low-fat yogurt) slowly and frequently, avoiding strong food odors, drinking fluids between meals, and avoiding foods that cause stomach irritation (e.g., caffeine, fatty foods, spicy foods, tomato-based foods) may also assist in alleviating nausea and vomiting. Some clinicians recommend using ginger, sea-bands and vitamin B$_6$ as adjunctive therapy. In severe cases of hyperemesis gravidarum, total parental nutrition must be considered.

Reflux esophagitis is common in pregnancy as a result of increased abdominal pressure caused by the enlarging uterus. Hormonal changes may relax the cardiac sphincter, permitting chyme to be redirected into the esophagus.

Managing reflux esophagitis in pregnant patients is similar to management in nonpregnant patients. Recommendations for alleviating the symptoms of heartburn in pregnancy include: elevating the head of the bed four inches; avoiding meals or snacks two to three hours before reclining; avoiding alcohol entirely; avoid acidic fruits, caffeine, carbonation and peppermint, eating small, frequent meals; and taking antacids as needed. Antacids do inhibit iron absorption, however, and should be used sparingly and only when all other management strategies have proven ineffective. The amount of calcium from antacids should be taken into consideration when assessing total calcium intake.

Constipation is common during pregnancy as a result of abdominal pressure from the enlarging uterus, hormonal changes and iron supplementation. Smooth muscle relaxation and increased water reabsorption in the large intestine during pregnancy result in decreased gastrointestinal motility, compounding the problem of constipation. Constipation during pregnancy can cause marked discomfort, including bloating, and aggravation of hemorrhoids. Strategies for managing constipation include increased fluid intake (to two or three quarts daily), increased low-impact physical activity (e.g., walking or swimming), increased dietary fiber intake to the AI of 14 g/1000 calories/day through food (e.g., in the form of high-fiber cereals, whole grains, legumes, fruits or vegetables), or the use of a supplemental psyllium or polycarbophil preparation.

Women with a history of previous gastric bypass should be monitored closely for nutrient malabsorption and malnutrition [21]. There is one case report in the literature of maternal and fetal death post gastric bypass due to a intestinal infarction [22]. Most clinician's recommend that women of child bearing age be committed to avoid pregnancy for at least one year after gastric bypass. Adjustable Gastric Banding (AGB) for women planning conception is often the recommended procedure because of the importance of vitamin and mineral nurture during pregnancy [4,23]. For patients who have had a Roux-en-Y procedure, laboratory values such as vitamin B_{12}, CBC and comprehensive metabolic panels should be checked monthly. To reduce the risk of dumping syndrome, screening for gestational diabetes is done using 2-hour post prandial blood glucose measures rather than a one hour glucola or 3 hour oral glucose tolerance tests. Many patients require folate in doses up to 2 g/day. In the normal adult a vitamin B_{12} less than 200 pg/mL is of concern. The normal range for vitamin B_{12} during pregnancy is 80–120 pg/mL. If B_{12} and iron levels consistently drop below normal levels (serum ferritin <15 µg/L) and are not improved with oral supplements, intramuscular injections are used. More research is needed to develop guidelines.

Breastfeeding goals and recommendations

Human breast milk is the optimal food for human infants and has been shown to decrease the risk of postneonatal death in the US [18]. It has been recommended as the "gold standard" for infant feeding by all professional medical groups. In 2005 the American Dietetic Association, American Academy of Pediatrics and the International Lactation Consultants Association all published revised detailed position statements on breastfeeding [27,29,30]. Currently these associations recommend that babies be exclusively breastfed until 6 months of age. Starting at 6 months solid foods may be incorporated into the infants' diet but mothers are encouraged to continue to breastfeed until 12 months of age or as long as mutually desirable for mom and baby [27–33]. The World Health Organization recommends breastfeeding until 24–30 months of age or as long as mutually desirable. The current *Healthy People 2010* goal is to have 75% of mothers initiate breastfeeding at hospital discharge. Duration goals set by *Healthy People 2010* are to have 50% exclusively breastfeeding until 6 months and 25% at one year [31]. During the *Mid-Course Review for Healthy People 2010* [32] additional breastfeeding objectives have been added. Exclusive breastfeeding is now listed as a separate goal for *Healthy People 2010*. The goals are to have 60% of women exclusively breastfeeding until 3 months of age and 25% exclusively breastfeeding until at least 6 months of age [32].

Breast milk contains an overwhelming numbers of unique dietary components and host resistance factors that cannot be replicated in conventional commercial infant formulas. Most women in the US are fully capable of breastfeeding their infants adequately. Although some problems (e.g., difficulty latching on, mastitis) may be encountered during the course of lactation, most informed nurses and physicians can readily manage and provide support to overcome these obstacles. Referral to an International Board Certified Lactation Consultant (IBCLC)/Registered Lactation Consultant (RLC) can ensure continued lactation when problems are more complex.

Benefits of breastfeeding

Breast milk contains leukocytes (specifically, macrophages), immunoglobins (secretory IgA, IgG, IgM and antiviral antibodies), bifidus factor (to support *Lactobacillus bifidus*), lysozymes (to promote bacterial lysis), interferon, lactoferrin (to bind whey protein and inhibit *E. coli* colonization), lactadherin (to protect against symptomatic rotavirus infections), growth factors and cytokines (bFGF, EGF, NGF, TGF, G-CSF, interleukins, TNF-alpha and others), prostaglandins, hormones (pituitary, hypothalamic and steroid), gastrointestinal peptides (VIP, gastrin, GIP) and other unique components (e.g., complement factors, glutamine, oligosaccharides, nucleotides, long-chain polyunsaturated fatty acids). Many of these components work alone or in combination to minimize risk of infection in the nursing infant [34].

Breastfed infants are hospitalized less frequently during the first six months of life. Significant health care cost savings from the decreased incidence of lower respiratory infections, otitis media and gasteroenteritis are associated with breastfeeding [29,30,33]. Strong evidence suggests that human milk also decreases the incidence and severity of diarrhea, bacteremia, bacterial meningitis, urinary tract infections and necrotizing enterocolitis. Many studies have demonstrated the protective effect of breast milk against immune- or autoimmune-related diseases (e.g, chronic and inflammatory bowel diseases, type-I diabetes mellitus, allergic diseases). Breast milk may also prevent against sudden infant death syndrome (SIDS) and cancers such as leukemia and lymphoma. Breastfeeding promotes jaw and tooth development in the infant, and the act of breastfeeding enhances maternal fetal bonding [28,29,30,33].

Breastfeeding mothers experience earlier return to pregravid weight, decreased accumulation of adipose tissue, delayed return of ovulation with increased pregnancy spacing, improved bone remineralization upon resumption of menses, and reduced risk of ovarian and premenopausal breast cancer. Breast milk also offers the added benefit of convenience; it is at the proper temperature, and requires neither preparation nor storage.

Composition of breast milk

Breast milk comes in three forms: colostrum, transitional and mature. Colostrum is produced during the later stages of pregnancy and is present in highest concentration during the first few days of lactation. It is high in protein, immunoglobins, beta-carotene, sodium, potassium, chloride, fat-soluble vitamins, minerals and unique hormones. Colostrum promotes growth of bifidus flora, maturation of the gastrointestinal tract and meconium passage. Transitional milk is produced 7–10 days post partum to 2 weeks post partum. It is higher in fat and lactose and lower in protein and minerals than colostrum. Mature milk is usually produced by the fifteenth day of lactation through the termination of lactation. It is composed of emulsified fat and lactose, and it provides 20–22 calories/ounce and is nutritionally optimal.

Breast milk is rich in nutrients and other substances essential to growth and development during the first six months of life. When breastfeeding, women should encourage their infants to suckle at each breast for as long as the infant shows signs of hunger usually this is 10–15 minutes per breast [28,33,29]. It is important to teach nursing mothers signs of hunger. Crying is a very late sign. If a child makes sucking movements, brings their hands to their mouth, makes sucking movements, displays rapid eye movements, makes soft cooing or sighing sounds or is restless they are showing sings of hunger [29]. Mothers should be encouraged to feed at least 8 times each 24 hours as breast milk is easily digested and clears the gut faster than formulas.

The total amount of fat in breast milk is constant, but its specific composition varies. Initially, breast milk has relatively low fat content. Following the first let-down reflex, breast milk becomes higher in fat and calories. The fat content of breast milk provides 50% of the infant's total energy requirements in readily absorbable form.

Breast milk contains whey and casein proteins. Whey protein accounts for roughly 70% of the total protein in breast milk, mainly in the form of alpha-lactalbumin, lactoferrin and secretory IgA. Casein protein accounts for the remaining 30% of breast milk's total protein composition and forms micelles that enhance absorption of calcium, phosphorous, iron, zinc and copper [36].

The total protein concentration is relatively low, but it is the optimal concentration for infant nutrition.

The primary carbohydrate source in breast milk is disaccharide lactose. Small amounts of glucose and immunologically active oligosaccharides and glycoproteins are also present.

Some breastfed infants are at risk for vitamin D deficiency because breast milk contains only small quantities of this nutrient. The risk is enhanced for dark-skinned infants of mothers with decreased vitamin D levels resulting from dietary deficiencies and/or minimal sun exposure. Currently, the Academy of Pediatrics recommends that all exclusively breastfed infants receive 200 IU of vitamin D daily by two months of age regardless of skin color [33,35]. However, vitamin D supplementation remains an area of controversy. Breast milk contains only small traces of vitamin K. However, supplementation is generally unnecessary, as most infants receive vitamin K injections immediately following delivery to prevent hemorrhagic disease of the newborn. All breastfed infants should receive 1.0 mg of Vitamin K oxide intramuscularly after the first feeding is completed. This should be within the first 6 hours of life [33].

Physiological and biochemical impact of breastfeeding

During early pregnancy, breasts enlarge in response to hormones generated by the pituitary gland and the corpus luteum. By 16 weeks' gestation the branching stage has produced epithelial strips that will become the secretory alveoli [36]. The lacteal cells differentiate in preparation for milk production. Stage 1 lactogenesis starts about 12 weeks before delivery. As the breast undergoes these preparatory changes, the areola darkens and expands, and the skin over the nipple increases in elasticity and erectness to facilitate suckling. The abrupt decrease in progesterone and estrogen levels following birth is believed to initiate lactogenesis by increasing prolactin synthesis. As the infant suckles, receptors in the nipple and areola are stimulated, sending nerve impulses to the hypothalamus. The hypothalamus responds by stimulating the synthesis and release of prolactin and oxytocin from the anterior and posterior pituitary glands, respectively. Prolactin stimulates milk production, and oxytocin stimulates myoepithilial cells around the milk ducts to contract and eject milk from the alveolus. The initial influx of oxytocin commonly occurs three to five days postpartum and the sensation is referred to as "let down." Milk accumulates in the milk ducts beneath the areola and is released when the areola is compressed between the suckling infant's tongue and palate. Many factors may influence milk production. They include, but are not limited to, the timing of initial nursing (optimal timing is within the first hour postpartum), the schedule of nursing (feeding on demand 8–12 feeds per 24 hours), the infant's weight and maturity, the presence of illnesses which impede suckling in the infant, maternal age and parity, maternal stress, maternal fluid intake (3.8 L/day), and maternal use of cigarettes, alcohol and oral contraceptives (all of which impair milk production).

Nutritional recommendations during breastfeeding

Maternal nutritional status is not related to milk volume in developed countries. Average milk volumes (750–800 mL/day) are comparable regardless of maternal weight. Exercise does not appear to affect milk volume. The nutritional quality of human milk is not usually impacted by modest deficiencies in maternal nutrition. The mother often loses a small amount of weight gradually during lactation. Even milk from malnourished women generally provides nursing infants with adequate amounts of calories, proteins, vitamins and minerals. Most nutrient levels in human milk are maintained at the expense of maternal stores. Maternal dietary intake does not affect the general macronutrient content of milk, but the types of fatty acids available in the milk are influenced by maternal intake. The calcium, phosphorous, sodium, potassium and magnesium levels of milk are not altered by the maternal diet, but the iodine and selenium levels of breast milk reflect maternal intake. The concentrations of vitamins in breast milk depend on maternal stores and dietary intake. However, within usual dietary intake levels, the differences observed are not practically significant. The levels of pyridoxine and vitamins A, D and B_{12} in breast milk are the most likely to be adversely impacted by long-term maternal malnutrition.

The Dietary Reference Intake (DRI) for most nutrients, except vitamin D, magnesium and iron, are somewhat greater for lactating women than for non-lactating women. An additional caloric intake of 500 calories each day is usually recommended to sustain lactation. The Institute of Medicine recommends an additional 330 calories in the first six months of lactation and 400 calories for the second six months of lactation [6]. Protein needs are the same as pregnancy with an additional 25 g/day above the non-pregnant recommendation for adults of 46 g/day. An additional 530 µg/day of vitamin A, 4 mg/day of vitamin E, 35 mg/day of vitamin C, 0.2 mg/day of riboflavin, 0.1 mg/day of vitamin B_6, 0.2 mg/day of vitamin B_{12} and 1 mg/day of zinc is recommended to maintain optimal micronutrient content of breast milk above that in pregnancy. Folate needs drop to 500 µg and niacin drops to 17 mg/day from pregnancy. Increasing maternal nutrient intake beyond the RDA level usually does not result in correspondingly high nutrient levels in breast milk, except for the levels of iodine, selenium, vitamin D and pyroxidine.

The iron requirements of the lactating woman are decreased to 9 mg per day because the amount of iron secreted in breast milk is less than that normally lost during menstruation. However, it is common obstetric practice to prescribe an iron supplement during the course of lactation.

Nutritional assessment during breastfeeding

Lactating women should be educated to obtain adequate nutrition from a healthful diet rather than through the use of nutritional supplements. Women with specialized dietary practices (e.g., vegans) should receive nutritional advice from trained professionals to ensure optimal nutritional health for their infants. No data exist that discourage women with specialized dietary practices from breastfeeding their infants. Appropriate dietary advice should be supplied and, if necessary, supplementation should be offered to provide those nutrients which are consumed in limited quantities. Women who have had gastric bypass or breast surgery are able to lactate but will likely need professional help in achieving and maintaining adequate milk supply for optimal infant growth. Mothers of multiples are able to provide enough nutrition for their growing infants. Referral to a registered dietitian and/or a lactation consultant is appropriate if there are any signs of malnutrition in mother or baby.

Women who are HIV-positive should not breastfeed their infants. The main route of transmission of HIV from mother to child is breastfeeding; transmission of the virus can be prevented by encouraging use of commercial formulas and discouraging breastfeeding for infants of HIV-positive mothers. In some developing countries, the mortality risks of not breastfeeding outweigh the morbidity and mortality risks associated with possible transmission of maternal infections. Other contraindications for breastfeeding in the United States are infants with classic galactosemia, mothers with active, untreated tuberculosis, or who are positive for human T-cell lymphotropic virus type I or II, mothers receiving exposure to radioactive isotopes (review timing of exposure), mothers on specific antimetabolite or chemotherapeutic agents, and mothers using drugs of abuse. Mothers with herpes simplex lesions that are on the breast should not feed on the affected breast. They may however feed off an unaffected breast. It is important to note that there are many conditions for which mothers have been told to avoid breastfeeding that are indeed compatible with breastfeeding. Cytomegalovirus (CMV) is not a contraindication for breastfeeding in the term baby. The clinician must weigh the risk benefit of breastfeeding in the premature infant born to a mother with CMV. Neither Hepatitis B or C is a contraindication to breastfeeding [27–31,33].

Substance abuse and the use of recreational drugs should be actively discouraged during lactation. Addicted women should be encouraged to enter appropriate treatment programs and should be drug free before lactation is initiated. Lactating women should not smoke but this is not a contraindication to breastfeeding. In addition to the long-term health risks, smoking decreases milk volume. Smoking is associated with shortened exclusive and total breastfeeding duration [29]. Modest consumption of coffee and alcohol (i.e., less than one to two cups/drinks daily) is not known to affect lactation or infant health adversely. Alcohol does pass readily into breast milk so caution should be used.

Medications can pass through human milk to the infant. It is best to evaluate each medication individually before making a decision about use. Considerations are molecular weight of the drug, peak concentration, protein binding, half life, relative infant dose (RID), infant age, dose, risk/benefit to mother and baby and alternative medication options. Drugs pass into human milk if they are highly lipid soluble, have a low molecular weight (<500), low protein binding, are in high concentration in maternal plasma and pass into the brain easily [37]. There are several resources available to help you make decisions about medication use. The Academy of Pediatrics has a position statement entitled The Transfer of Drugs and Other Chemicals Into Human Milk which is included in *Breastfeeding Handbook for Physicians* (2005) [28]. Discussion about contraception should include the risk of milk supply depletion with all hormone related forms of birth control. The lactational amennorhea method (LAM) is the ideal form of contraception if all of the following criteria are met: no menstrual bleeding, exclusive breastfeeding and infant age under 6 months [38].

Promotion and support of breastfeeding

As healthcare professionals it is our ethical and professional responsibility to promote, protect and support breastfeeding. Women should be informed of not only the benefits of breastfeeding but the inherent risks of not breastfeeding. Position papers published in 2005 by the Academy of Pediatrics, American Dietetic Association and the International Lactation Consultants Association [27,29,33] provide guidance for clinicians in supporting breastfeeding efforts. The Academy of Family Physicians also has clear guidelines on the clinical management of breastfeeding [30] but also on medical and residency education. Breastfeeding infants should be monitored closely for their growth and observation of the mother infant dyad should be a routine part of post partum care. Breast milk is the optimal food source for infants.

References

1 Barker DJ. The developmental origins of adult disease. *Eur. J Epid* 2003;18(8):733–6.
2 Kirkham C, Harris S, Grzybowski S. Evidence-Based Prenatal Care: Part I. General Prenatal Care and Counseling Skills. *Amer Fam Phys.* 2005;71(7): 1307–1316.
3 Godfrey KM and Barker PJD. Fetal nutrition and adult diseases. *AM J Clin Nutr.* 2000; 71:13445–13525.
4 American College of Obstetricians and Gynecologists Committee Opinion Number 315. Obesity in Pregnancy. *American College of Obstetricians and Gynecologist* 2005;106:671–5.
5 Institute of Medicine. *Nutrition During Pregnancy: Weight Gain, Nutrient Supplements.* National Academy Press, Washington, DC, 1990.
6 Food and Nutrition Board Institute of Medicine. Dietary *Reference Intakes for Energy, Carbohydrate, Fiber, Fat, Fatty Acids, Cholesterol, Protein, and Amino Acids.* National Academies Press, Washington, DC, 2002.
7 Mahomed K. Iron supplementation in pregnancy. *Cochrane Database of Systematic Reviews.* 2005;1.
8 Gillen-Goldstein J, Edmund FF, Roqué. Nutrition in Pregnancy. UptoDate 2006.
9 Solomon CG, Seely EW. Hypertension in Pregnancy. *Endocrinology and Metabolism Clin North Ameri.* 2006;35:157–71.
10 Atallah AN, Hofmeyr GJ, Duley L. Calcium supplementation during pregnancy for preventing hypertensive disorders and related problems. Cochrane Database of Systemic Reviews 1, 2006.

11 Basile L, Taylor S *et al*. The Effect of High-Dose Vitamin D Supplementation on Serum Vitamin D Levels and Milk Calcium Concentration in Lactating Women and Their Infants *Breastfeeding Medicine* 2006;1:27–35.

12 Environmental Protection Agency. Mercury Fish Advisories. www.epa.gov/mercury/advisories.htm (Accessed April 14, 2006).

13 CDCMMWR. Recommendations to Improve Preconception Health & Health Care – United States. 2006;55(RR06); 1–2.

14 Stotland NE, Chang YW, Hopkins LM, Caughey AB. Gestational weight gain and adverse Neonatal outcomes among term infants. *Obstet Gyncol* 2006; 108(3):635–43.

15 Kramer MS. Energy/protein restriction for high weight-for-height or weight gain during pregnancy. Cochrane Database of Systemic Reviews. 1, 2006.

16 Institute of Medicine. *Nutrition During Pregnancy and Lactation*. National Academies Press, Washington, DC, 1992.

17 Story M, Stang J. Nutrition and the Pregnant Adolescent: A Practical Reference Guide, Maternal and Child Health Bureau, Rockville, MD, 2000.

18 American Diabetes Association. Position Statement: Gestational Diabetes Mellitus. *Diabetes* Care 2004; 27(Suppl. 1):S88–S90.

19 Thomas AM, Gutierrez YM. *American Dietetic Association Guide to Gestational Diabetes Mellitus*. American Dietetic Association, 2005.

20 US Preventive Services Task Force. *The Guide to Clinical Preventive Services 2005*. Department of Health and Human Services. Washington, D.C.

21 Chen A. Rogan WJ. Breastfeeding and the risk of postneonatal death in the United States. *Pediatrics*. 113(5):e435–9, 2004 May.

22 Taylor JS. Kacmar JE. Nothnagle M. Lawrence RA. A systematic review of the literature associating breastfeeding with type 2 diabetes and gestational diabetes. *J Am Coll Nut*. 24(5):320–6.

23 Stuebe AM. Rich-Edwards JW. Willett WC. Manson JE. Michels KB. Duration of lactation and incidence of type 2 diabetes. *JAMA* 2005;294(20):2601–10.

24 Woodard, CB. Pregnancy Following Bariatric Surgery. *The Journal of Perinatal and Neonatal Nursing* 2004;18(4):329–40.

25 Moore K, Ouyang D, Whang, E. Maternal and Fetal Deaths after Gastric Bypass Surgery for Morbid Obesity. *The New England Journal of Medicine* 2004;351(7):721–2.

26 Skull AJ *et al*. Laparoscopic Adjustable Banding in Pregnancy: Safety, Patient Tolerance and Effect on Obesity-Related Pregnancy Outcomes. *Obesity Surgery* 2004;14:230–5.

27 American Dietetic Association, Position of the American Dietetic Association: Promoting and Supporting Breastfeeding. *Journal of the American Dietetic Association*. 2005;105(5):810–18.

28 American Academy of Pediatrics, American College of Obstetricians and Gyncecologists. *Breastfeeding Handbook for Physicians*. 2005.

29 International Lactation Consultant Association. Clinical Guidelines for the Establishment of Exclusive Breastfeeding, 2005.

30 American Academy of Family Physicians. Breastfeeding (Position Paper). http://aafp.org/policy/x1641.xml.

31 Department of Health and Human Services. *HHS Blueprint for Action on Breastfeeding*. Washington, D.C., 2000.

32 *Healthy People 2010*. Department of Health and Human Services. Washington, D.C. www.healthypeople.gov.

33 American Academy of Pediatrics. Breastfeeding and the Use of Human Milk. *Pediatrics* 2005;115(2);496–506.

34 Hanson, LA. *Immunology of Human Milk: How Breastfeeding Protects Babies.* Pharmasoft Publishing, Amarillo Texas, 2005.
35 Gartner LM, Greer FR. Clinical Report: Prevention of Rickets and Vitamin D Deficiency: New Guidelines for Vitamin D Intake. *Pediatrics* 2004;111(4):908–10.
36 Lawrence, Ruth and Robert. *Breastfeeding: A Guide for the Medical Profession.* Elsevier Mosby, 2005.
37 Hale, Thomas. *Medications and Mother's Milk.* Pharmasoft Publishing, 2006.
38 Academy of Breastfeeding Medicine Protocol Committee. ABM Clinical Protocal #13: Contraception During Breastfeeding. Breastfeeding Medicine 2006 1(1):43–51.

Further reading

Godfrey, KM, Barker DJ. Fetal nutrition and adult disease. *American Journal of Clinical Nutrition* 2000;71:1344S.

Guise *et al.* The Effectiveness of Primary Care-Based Interventions to Promote Breastfeeding: Systematic Evidence Review and Meta-Analysis for the US Preventive Services Task Force. Annals of Family Medicine 2003:1(2):70–8.

Institute of Medicine. *Nutrition Services in Perinatal Care.* National Academy Press, Washington, DC, 1992.

Kramer MS, Kakuma R. Optimal duration of exclusive breastfeeding. *Cochrane Database of Systemic Reviews.* 1, 2004.

Langer O, Conway DL, Berkus MD, Xenakis EM, Gonzales O. A Comparison of glyburide and insulin in women with gestational diabetes mellitus. *NEJM* 2000;343(16).

Li R, Jewell S, Gremmer-Strawn L. Maternal Obesity and Breast-Feeding Practices. *Am J Clin Nutr.* 2003;77(4):931–6.

Mason G, Ronolt S. 2006. Promoting Protecting and Supporting Breastfeeding & North Carolina. Blueprint for Action. North Carolina Division of Public Health, Raleigh, NC.

US Preventive Task Force. Behavioral Interventions to Promote Breastfeeding: Recommendations and Rationale. *Annals of Family Medicine* 2003;1(2):79–89.

World Health Organization. WHO Expert Consultation on the Optimal Duration of Exclusive Breastfeeding: Conclusions and Recommendations. Vol. 20 01: WHO 2001.

CHAPTER 6

Staying healthy in later life

Connie Watkins Bales and Heidi K White

The inevitable result of "successful aging" and declining birth rates is the dramatic increase in the elderly population, currently at an all time high in the US of 13% of the population. This trend is predicted to continue throughout the developing world for several decades and the future focus of primary care practice will be on a predominately elderly patient population. Prevention of the development and progression of chronic diseases will be a major challenge for the primary care practitioner. This chapter reviews the impact of aging on nutritional needs and details appropriate interventions for many of the most important nutrition-related geriatric concerns, including depression, cachexia, dementia, dysphagia, and nutritional frailty.

Alterations in nutrient requirements and nutritional status

A variety of social, economic, and psychological factors affect dietary intakes and thus influence nutritional status. Alterations in nutritional needs of older adults occur due to the physiologic and metabolic changes associated with normal aging. In addition, physiologic requirements for certain nutrients are altered with aging [1]. The Dietary Reference Intakes (DRIs) for known essential nutrients for individuals age 51–70 years and greater than 71 years are shown in Tables 6.1 and 6.2 [2].

Fluids and hydration

Dehydration is a common presenting problem in the elderly, particularly for those with impaired cognition. Poor thirst responses and limited access to fluids contribute to dehydration. The potential negative effects of excessive water consumption, leading to dilutional hyponatremia (water intoxication) and increased nocturia have also been identified as concerns in older adults. Six to eight glasses of fluid per day will provide sufficient hydration for healthy elderly people except during situations likely to greatly increase fluid loss [3]. Recommending additional drinks, such as tea, juices and even sports drinks may be helpful to older adults who need to take in more fluids.

Table 6.1 Dietary reference intakes for adults aged ≥51 years: Macronutrients and minerals.

Gender Age (y)	Protein[1] (g)	Carbohydrate (g)	Fiber (total)[2] (g)	Calcium[2] (mg)	Magnesium (mg)	Iron (mg)	Zinc (mg)	Copper (μg)	Chromium[2] (μg)	Selenium (μg)
Men										
51–70 y	56	130	30	1,200	420	8	11	900	30	55
>70 y	56	130	30	1,200	420	8	11	900	30	55
Women										
51–70 y	46	130	21	1,200	320	8	8	900	20	55
>70 y	46	130	21	1,200	320	8	8	900	20	55

All values represent the RDA unless otherwise noted.

[1] 0.80 g/kg/day for the reference body weight.

[2] Adequate Intakes (AIs) represent the recommended average daily intake level based on observed or experimentally determined approximations. AIs are used when there is insufficient information to determine an DRI.

Source: [2, 10]

Table 6.2 Dietary reference intakes for adults aged ≥51 years: Vitamins.

Gender Age (y)	Vitamin A (µg RAE)[1]	Vitamin D[2] (µg)/(IU)	Vitamin E (mg)/(IU)	Vitamin K[2] (µg)	Vitamin C (mg)	Thiamin (mg)	Riboflavin (mg)	Niacin (mg)	Folacin (µg)	Vitamin B$_6$ (mg)	Vitamin B$_{12}$ (µg)
Men											
51–70 y	900	10/400	15/22	120	90	1.2	1.3	16	400	1.7	2.4
>70 y	900	15/600	15/22	120	90	1.2	1.3	16	400	1.7	2.4
Women											
51–70 y	700	10/400	15/22	90	75	1.1	1.1	14	400	1.5	2.4
>70 y	700	15/600	15/22	90	75	1.1	1.1	14	400	1.5	2.4

All values represent the RDA unless otherwise noted.

[1] RAEs – retinol activity equivalents.

[2] Adequate Intakes (AIs) represent the recommended average daily intake level based on observed or experimentally determined approximations. AIs are used when there is insufficient information to determine an DRI.

Source: [2,10]

Vitamins

Vitamin A

No evidence exists that the requirement for vitamin A increases with age. Body retention of this vitamin is likely enhanced with aging, especially in older individuals who consume large amounts from supplements and fortified foods [4]. Excessive accumulation of vitamin A is of particular concern in the elderly since recent studies have linked high levels of this vitamin with increased risk of osteoporotic fractures of the hip [5].

Vitamin D

There is clearly an increased need for vitamin D in older adults due to a number of age-related changes. These include decline in skin photosynthesis, impaired renal conversion of 25-hydroxyvitamin D to the active form, and reduced gut responsiveness to $1,25(OH)_2D$. Vitamin D deficiency results not only in impaired bone metabolism, but also muscle weakness predominantly of the proximal muscle groups. Recent studies have investigated whether vitamin D supplementation in the elderly would preserve and possibly improve muscle strength and subsequent functional ability. From experimental studies it was found that vitamin D metabolites directly influence muscle cell maturation and functioning through a vitamin D receptor. Vitamin D supplementation in vitamin D-deficient, older adults improved muscle strength, walking distance, and functional ability and resulted in a reduction in falls and non-vertebral fractures [6]. Recent studies have also found a protective relationship between sufficient vitamin D status and lower risk of colon cancer [7,8]. The evidence suggests that efforts to improve vitamin D status, for example by vitamin D supplementation, could reduce cancer incidence and mortality at low cost, with few or no adverse effects [9].

When these roles are added to the well-known role of the vitamin in bone health via the regulation of calcium and phosphorus metabolism, it exemplifies the critical importance of vitamin D for the health and function of older persons. Since only a few common foods (e.g., oily fish, fortified dairy products) contain substantial amounts of vitamin D, it may be difficult for older adults to fully meet their vitamin D requirements from dietary sources (see Appendix B).

Skin synthesis is not a dependable source of vitamin D in the elderly due to reduced sun exposure and decreased skin synthesis rates of vitamin D. Moreover, the current Adequate Intake level (10 μg/day or 400 IU/day for 51–70 years and 15 μg/day or 600 IU/day for ≥71 years) may not be sufficient for all individuals. Thus, supplements of 10–20 μg/day (400 to 800 IU) have been recommended for individuals at risk of deficiency [10].

Vitamin E

While absorption and utilization of vitamin E do not change with age, dietary intake of vitamin E has been shown to be below recommended levels in studies of older adults [1,10]. Possible explanations include avoidance of high-fat food sources containing vitamin E (e.g., vegetable oils, nuts, peanut butter) or under-reporting of such foods (see Appendix C). While high intakes of vitamin E have been associated with the prevention of chronic diseases in some studies, especially heart disease, a recent meta-analysis indicates that high doses of supplemental vitamin E (>150 IU/day) are actually linked with increased all-cause mortality and thus, supplementation exceeding this amount should be avoided [11].

Vitamin C

Intake of vitamin C is highly variable among older adults. While most consume generous amounts of vitamin C and achieve nutritional adequacy, some groups have been identified as having increased risk of deficiency, including those with dental problems, dementia, and those in hospitals and nursing homes [12]. Aging does not alter the absorption or metabolism of vitamin C, so low status is generally attributed to poor intake or increased requirements (see Appendix E).

Thiamin, riboflavin and niacin

Thiamin, riboflavin and niacin function as coenzymes in energy metabolism; thus it might be expected that requirements for these vitamins would diminish in parallel with declining energy expenditures in older adults. But available evidence indicates that the requirements of these nutrients are unchanged by age. The intakes and status of these B vitamins are variable. Mean intakes of all three vitamins were reported to be adequate in elderly subjects participating in NHANES III; however, low blood levels of thiamin and riboflavin have been reported in some sub-groups. Potential causes of low blood levels include chronic alcohol use (thiamin) and low consumption of dairy products (riboflavin). Niacin status is likely to be adequate, although elderly subjects with food insecurity have reported low intakes [13].

Folate

Requirements for folate do not change with age; however, inadequate folate status contributes to hyperhomocysteinemia which may increase the risk of coronary disease, as well as other chronic diseases common in older adults. Starting in the late 1990s, to reduce the risk of neural tube birth defects associated with folate deficiency, the Food and Drug Administration mandated folate fortification of all grain products. Thus folate intake for all adults has actually increased to the point of raising concerns about excessive intake in the elderly who consume a large amount of fortified foods such as breakfast cereals, breads and products made from enriched flours, as this may mask a vitamin B_{12} deficiency (see Appendix F).

Vitamin B_{12}

Requirements for vitamin B_{12} are not increased with age but low stomach acid secretion due to atrophic gastritis could seriously impair the absorption of vitamin B_{12} in older adults over age 50 [14]. To assure nutritional adequacy, adults over age 50 are advised to take supplements containing vitamin B_{12} or eat food products fortified with vitamin B_{12}, such as soy milk and cereals [14]. The masking of a vitamin B_{12} deficiency by high folate consumption is a serious concern [15] and thus, it is recommended that when supplementing folate, vitamin B_{12}, supplements are prescribed as well, especially in elderly patients.

Minerals

Calcuim

The essential role of calcium in bone health is well recognized; in addition, the mineral may also have beneficial effects in the prevention of colon cancer and hypertension. Calcium intake has been shown to be inadequate for much of the adult population and decreases progressively with age [16]. According to the NHANES III, more than 70% of men and 87% of women had low calcium intakes. The disparity between the dietary requirement for calcium and the amount that is actually being consumed by the adult population is probably the most dramatic of any known essential nutrient. There is an urgent need to address this inadequacy in all older adults, and especially in older women (see Appendices G, H).

Magnesium

Working in conjunction with vitamin D and calcium, magnesium is an essential nutrient for bone health, as well as for other critical roles such as nerve and muscle function. Magnesium status has been linked to bone mineral density in both men and women [17]. With age, magnesium absorption decreases, urinary losses increase, and low magnesium intake is often observed [2,17] (see Appendix K).

Zinc

While inadequate dietary intake of zinc is commonly reported, the lack of a good zinc status indicator for the mineral has limited our understanding of the exact role of zinc in human health [2,16]. Its potential impact on immune function and wound healing underscore the need for further study of this essential trace mineral. Aging effects on zinc requirements are not well understood but it is likely that zinc needs are increased with age. Reduced zinc status in older subjects has been linked with decreased immunity and poor response to vaccinations. Zinc supplementation reduces susceptibility to infections and in older adults, has been shown to enhance wound healing [18]. Supplemental doses of zinc should not exceed 40 mg/day unless patients are under regular medical supervision, as high doses can induce copper deficiency and/or immune suppression.

Macronutrients

Energy

It is well established that food and calorie (energy) intakes decrease with age in response to reductions in metabolic rate, loss of lean body mass, and lower energy expenditure from physical activity [16]. In middle age, the decrease in calorie intake is generally offset by the aforementioned decrements in energy requirements. However, in late life, negative energy balance (calorie malnutrition) is a concern for a substantial subset of the elderly population.

Protein

The current RDA for protein (0.8 g/kg/day) is the same for adults of all ages, although there is evidence that a higher protein intake could help counteract sarcopenia (loss of muscle mass) by enhancing hypertrophic response to strength conditioning in the elderly [19]. The oldest age groups are most at risk for protein deficiency, especially when health problems or other stresses are manifested and when institutionalization (hospital or long-term care) occurs.

Lipids, carbohydrates and fiber

With age, there is a decrease in the intake of fat and cholesterol, as well as a reduction in the percentage of calories coming from fat. While absolute intakes of carbohydrate typically decrease with age, carbohydrate as a percent of calories increases slightly due to the reduction of calories coming from fats. Most adults, including the elderly, consume less fiber than the recommendation of 21–30 g/day. Increasing dietary fiber to the recommended levels could help prevent constipation as well as age-related chronic diseases such as coronary heart disease (see Appendix O).

Identifying individuals at risk for malnutrition

Most older adults living independently in the community exhibit adequate nutrition; however, the prevalence of malnutrition does increase over the age of 70 years [20]. In a group of older (>65 years) veterans seen in an outpatient clinic, the incidence of involuntary weight loss greater than 4% of body weight was more than 10% per year [21]. Malnutrition is a known risk for older adults who are hospitalized for serious illnesses and for the homebound elderly. Overweight and obesity can also have pronounced detrimental effects on the health and quality of life of the elderly [22]. Achieving the optimal balance of energy and nutrient needs presents a considerable challenge to the physician providing primary care to elderly patients.

Health professionals may feel unprepared to diagnose and treat malnutrition in older adults, as well as feel unsure of the potential benefits of doing so. Thus malnutrition often goes unrecognized and untreated, yet it can have a profound effect on overall health status [23,24]. Evidence is growing that nutritional interventions can improve overall function and quality of life in a cost-effective manner for older adults [25].

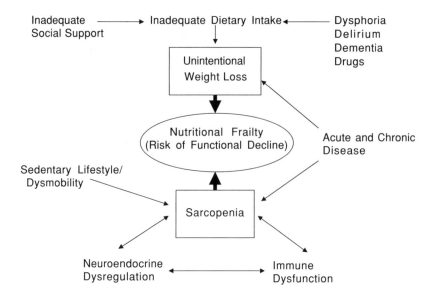

Figure 6.1 Dimensions of nutritional frailty.
Source: Adapted from [27]. Connie Bales, PhD, RD and Heidi White, MD, Duke University Medical Center. 2007. Used with permission.

Nutritional frailty

Defined as a disability that occurs among older adults due to loss of lean body mass (sarcopenia) and rapid, unintentional loss of body weight, nutritional frailty is a relatively new conceptualization of malnutrition that brings together the pathophysiology and resultant impairments seen among older adults. Sarcopenia is the loss of muscle mass and strength that occurs with aging and results in functional limitations [19,26]. Disease processes, drugs and deconditioning can play a role in the development of nutritional frailty. The interplay of factors that contribute to nutritional frailty is illustrated in Figure 6.1.

Nutrition assessment in older adults

Purpose

The purpose of the brief nutrition assessment is to identify patients at risk for poor or excessive nutritional intake resulting in malnutrition, overweight, obesity and/or chronic diseases (chapter 2). The elements of the nutrition assessment include past medical history, family history, social history, diet and exercise history, vital signs, review of systems, physical exam, and biochemical data. The following section focuses on the specific issues relevant to elderly patients.

Screening tool for older adults

Recognizing individuals who are at risk for malnutrition may be a greater challenge than it is to diagnose the condition once it has occurred. For this reason, various screening tools have been developed to help clinicians identify individuals at risk for malnutrition. In addition to these measurements, the Nutrition Screening Initiative (NSI) has developed a brief screening tool that can be filled out by the patient and used not only to identify those at risk, but also potential contributing factors for malnutrition (Fig. 6.2). NSI is a broad, multidisciplinary effort of the American Academy of Family Physicians, The American Dietetic Association, and a coalition of more than 25 national health, aging, and medical organizations with the goal of promoting the integration of nutrition screening and intervention into health care for older adults.

Another well-known and commonly utilized screening measure for older adults is the Mini Nutritional Assessment (Fig. 6.3). This is completed by health care professionals while interviewing patients or family members and making some brief measurements. If the screening portion indicates possible malnutrition, the assessment portion can be used to identify potential causes and provide a score that can be followed to monitor subsequent changes in nutritional status.

Physical examination

The first and most important way that primary care practitioners can screen their patients is to systematically measure weight at each office visit. For older adults this may require having a scale that they can easily mount or even a scale that will allow weight measurement in a chair. Height should also be measured so that body mass index (BMI) can be calculated.

Percent weight change

Weight loss is very common in hospitalized and nursing home patients. Weight loss is also frequently seen in older adults with significant appetite changes due to chronic illnesses, such as cancer, gastrointestinal problems, or secondary to surgery, chemotherapy or radiation therapy. If weight loss is identified in the medical history or review of systems, it is essential to take a diet history and determine the percent weight change over that period of time using the patient's current body weight and usual weight. Malnutrition is generally defined by clinically significant unintentional weight loss or the status of being underweight. A 5% involuntary weight loss in a 6–12 month period is generally considered a clinically significant loss that should prompt further evaluation.

$$\text{Percent weight change} = \frac{\text{Usual weight} - \text{Current weight}}{\text{Usual weight}} \times 100$$

BMI

BMI (weight (kg) / height (m)^2) is a measure of weight in relationship to height that identifies individuals who are underweight or overweight. The association

The Warning Signs of poor nutritional health are often overlooked. Use this Checklist to find out if you or someone you know is at nutritional risk.

DETERMINE YOUR NUTRITIONAL HEALTH

Read the statements below. Circle the number in the "yes" column for those that apply to you or someone you know. For each "yes" answer, score the number in the box. Total your nutritional score.

	YES
I have an illness or condition that made me change the kind and/or amount of food I eat.	2
I eat fewer than 2 meals per day.	3
I eat few fruits or vegetables or milk products.	2
I have 3 or more drinks of beer, liquor or wine almost every day.	2
I have tooth or mouth problems that make it hard for me to eat.	2
I don't always have enough money to buy the food I need.	4
I eat alone most of the time.	1
I take 3 or more different prescribed or over-the-counter drugs a day.	1
Without wanting to, I have lost or gained 10 pounds in the last 6 months.	2
I am not always physically able to shop, cook and/or feed myself.	2
TOTAL	

Total Your Nutritional Score. If it's –

0-2   **Good!** Recheck your nutritional score in 6 months.

3-5   You are at moderate nutritional risk. See what can be done to improve your eating habits and lifestyle. Your office on aging, senior nutrition program, senior citizens center or health department can help. Recheck your nutritional score in 3 months.

6 or more   You are at high nutritional risk. Bring this Checklist the next time you see your doctor, dietitian or other qualified health or social service professional. Talk with them about any problems you may have. Ask for help to improve your nutritional health.

Remember that Warning Signs suggest risk, but do not represent a diagnosis of any condition. Turn the page to learn more about the Warnings Signs of poor nutritional health.

These materials are developed and distributed by the Nutrition Screening Initiative, a project of:

AMERICAN ACADEMY OF FAMILY PHYSICIANS
THE AMERICAN DIETETIC ASSOCIATION
THE NATIONAL COUNCIL ON THE AGING, INC.

 The Nutrition Screening Initiative • 1010 Wisconsin Avenue, NW • Suite 800 • Washington, DC 20007
The Nutrition Screening Initiative is funded in part by a grant from Ross Products Division of Abbott Laboratories, Inc.

Figure 6.2 DETERMINE Checklist from the Nutrition Screening Initiative.
Source: Nutrition Screening Initiative: [28].

between BMI and mortality follows a U-shaped curve, with increased mortality being associated with BMIs both above and below the ideal range. The nadir of the U-shaped curve increases with age, thus the best weight for older adults is higher than the best weight for younger adults [30]. Taking this into account, a BMI of less than 22 indicates that an elderly patient is underweight and further

NESTLÉ NUTRITION SERVICES

Nestlé

Mini Nutritional Assessment
MNA®

Last name:		First name:	Sex:	Date:
Age:	Weight, kg:	Height, cm:	I.D.Number:	

Complete the screen by filling in the boxes with the appropriate numbers.
Add the numbers for the screen. If score is 11 or less, continue with the assessment to gain a Malnutrition Indicator Score.

Screening

A Has food intake declined over the past 3 months
due to loss of appetite, digestive problems,
chewing or swallowing difficulties?
0 = severe loss of appetite
1 = moderate loss of appetite
2 = no loss of appetite ☐

B Weight loss during last months
0 = weight loss greater than 3 kg (6.6 lbs)
1 = does not know
2 = weight loss between 1 and 3 kg (2.2 and 6.6 lbs)
3 = no weight loss ☐

C Mobility
0 = bed or chair bound
1 = able to get out of bed/chair but does not go out
2 = goes out ☐

D Has suffered psychological stress or acute
disease in the past 3 months
0 = yes   2 = no ☐

E Neuropsychological problems
0 = severe dementia or depression
1 = mild dementia
2 = no psychological problems ☐

F Body Mass Index (BMI)(weight in kg)/ (height in m)^2
0 = BMI less than 19
1 = BMI 19 to less than 21
2 = BMI 21 to less than 23
3 = BMI 23 or greater ☐

Screening score (subtotal max. 14 points) ☐ ☐

12 points or greater   Normal – not at risk –
no need to complete assessment

11 points or below   Possible malnutrition – continue assessment

Assessment

G Lives independently (not in a nursing home or hospital)
0 = no   1 = yes ☐

H Takes more than 3 prescription drugs per day
0 = yes   1 = no ☐

I Pressure sores or skin ulcers
0 = yes   1 = no ☐

J How many full meals does the patient eat daily?
0 = 1 meal
1 = 2 meals
2 = 3 meals ☐

K Selected consumption markers for protein intake
• Atleast one serving of dairy products
(milk, cheese, yogurt) per day?   yes ☐   no ☐
• Two or more serving of legumes
or eggs per week?   yes ☐   no ☐
• Meat, fish or poultry every day   yes ☐   no ☐
0.0 = if 0 or 1 yes
0.5 = if 2 yes
1.0 = if 3 yes   ☐ ☐

L Consumes two or more servings
of fruits or vegetables per day?
0 = no   1 = yes ☐

M How much fluid (water, juice, coffee, tea, milk…)
is consumed per day?
0.0 = less than 3 cups
0.5 = 3 to 5 cups
1.0 = more than 5 cups   ☐ ☐

N Mode of feeding
0 = unable to eat without assistance
1 = self-fed with some difficulty
2 = self-fed without any problem ☐

O Self view of nutritional status
0 = view self as being malnourished
1 = is uncertain of nutritional state
2 = views self as having no nutritional problem ☐

P In comparison with other people of the same age,
how do they consider their health status?
0.0 = not as good
0.5 = does not know
1.0 = as good
2.0 = better   ☐ ☐

Q Mid-arm circumference (MAC) in cm
0.0 = MAC less than 21
0.5 = MAC 21 to 22
1.0 = MAC 22 or greater   ☐ ☐

R Calf circumference (CC) in cm
0 = CC less than 31   1 = CC 31 or greater ☐

Assessment (max. 16 points) ☐ ☐ ☐

Screening score ☐ ☐

Total Assessment (max. 30 points) ☐ ☐ ☐

Ref.:   Guigoz Y, Vellas B and Garry PJ. 1994. Mini Nutritional Assessment: A practical assessment tool for
grading the nutritional state of elderly patients. Facts and Research in Gerontology. Supplement
#2:15-59.
Rubenstein LZ, Harker J, Guigoz Y and Vellas B. Comprehensive Geriatric Assessment (CGA) and
the MNA: An Overview of CGA, Nutritional Assessment, and Development of a Shortened Version
of the MNA. In: "Mini Nutritional Assessment (MNA):Research and Practice in the Elderly". Vellas
B, Garry PJ and Guigoz Y , editors. Nestlé Nutrition Workshop Series. Clinical & Performance Pro-
gramme, vol. 1. Karger, Bâle, in press.

® Société des Produits Nestlé S.A., Vevey, Switzerland, Trademark Owners

Malnutrition Indicator Score

17to 23.5 points   at risk of malnutrition ☐

Less than 17 points   malnourished ☐

Figure 6.3 Mini Nutritional Assessment tool for screening and assessment.
Source: Mini Nutrition Assessment [29].

assessment may be warranted. BMI can be difficult to accurately measure and interpret in frail older adults because of alterations in height due to conditions such as osteoporotic kyphosis or the inability to stand for measurement. This underscores the importance of systematic monitoring of body weight.

Other signs and symptoms

In addition to measuring height and weight, the physical exam may reveal many conditions that contribute to malnutrition, as well as signs of frank malnutrition. Muscle wasting and, in particular, temporal muscle wasting (sunken temples) are signs of cachexia. Broken, missing or loose teeth, ill-fitting dentures, mouth sores or abscesses may limit oral intake. Physical examination is of particular importance in patients with cognitive impairment who may not be able to verbally report conditions such as constipation, urinary retention, or abdominal discomfort. A brief cognitive screening test, such as the mini-mental status examination, will help to uncover cognitive deficits that may be contributing to malnutrition. Figure 6.4 provides an algorithm to aid the primary care provider to identify, assess and treat weight loss and nutritional frailty in older adults living in the community.

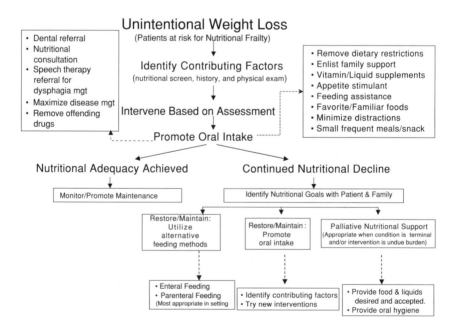

Figure 6.4 Algorithm to guide primary care providers as they identify, assess, and treat weight loss and nutritional frailty in older adults living in the community.
Source: Connie Bales, PhD, RD and Heidi White, MD, Duke University Medical Center. 2007. Used with permission.

Laboratory data

Protein–energy malnutrition in the elderly is typically the result of metabolic responses that increase requirements for energy and protein. It is generally diagnosed by a serum albumin level less than 3.0 g/dL and often occurs in the setting of acute illness, however albumin is also influenced by other factors.

Etiology/causes of malnutrition

Decreased oral intake

Poverty, poor dentition, gastrointestinal obstruction, abdominal pain, anorexia, dysphagia, depression, social isolation, and pain from eating are some of the many possible causes of decreased oral intake.

Increased nutrient loss

Glycosuria, bleeding in the digestive tract, diarrhea, malabsorption, nephrosis, a draining fistula, and protein-losing enteropathy can all result in nutrient losses.

Increased nutrient requirements

Any hypermetabolic state or excessive catabolic process can result in increased nutrient requirements. Common examples of situations that can dramatically affect nutrient requirements include surgery, trauma, fever, wound healing, burns, severe infection, malabsorption syndromes, and critical illness.

Chronic diseases

Chronic medical illness is an important risk factor for malnutrition. It is important to recognize and address malnutrition as a separate treatable condition from the chronic illness.

Cancer cachexia has been largely related to the effects of pro-inflammatory cytokines on metabolic processes, causing excessive muscle turnover and wasting [31]. Reversal of these processes is often difficult even with adequate nutritional support. Tumor burden, including location and size, can cause symptoms such as dysphagia, early satiety, abdominal pain, and intestinal obstruction that negatively impact nutritional status as well. Cardiac cachexia is marked by the loss of lean body mass and metabolic disturbances that may result from altered cytokine levels [32]. Reduction in BMI may be modest, in part due to extracellular fluid accumulation, but also due to a shift in body composition to a higher proportion of fat, compared to lean, mass. As recently outlined by Gray-Donald and Saudny-Unterberger, weight loss is a common clinical feature of chronic obstructive pulmonary disease (COPD) [33]. This is likely related to increased resting energy expenditure from the increased work of breathing and total daily energy expenditure, despite the apparent inactivity associated with the disease process. Similarly to cancer and cardiac cachexia, patients with COPD can have elevated cytokine levels and catabolic processes that lead to muscle wasting. Specific symptoms, such as dyspnea and fatigue, may also interfere with caloric intake. Corticosteroids used in the treatment of COPD contribute to reduced muscle mass, reduced bone density, and negative nitrogen balance.

Those suffering with chronic illness may also be experiencing depression. Rates of major depression are particularly high among hospitalized patients with acute illness or those living in nursing homes. This condition often goes unrecognized and untreated and can affect nutritional status by either increasing or decreasing appetite.

Cognitive dysfunction may be another important cause of unintentional weight loss and malnutrition among older adults. Numerous studies have confirmed the tendency for patients with Alzheimer's disease to lose weight even early in the disease process [34]. Weight loss and subsequent malnutrition in Alzheimer's disease can lead to serious consequences, including increased mortality [35]. Early in the disease process, inadequate access to food and the inability to prepare food may contribute to weight loss. Furthermore, anorexia or alterations in appetite perception contribute to early weight loss in Alzheimer's disease.

There are two primary physiologic mechanisms that might explain anorexia and therefore decreased caloric intake in Alzheimer's disease: taste and smell dysfunction, and the effect of inflammatory mediators (e.g. cytokines) on appetite [36]. Taste and smell alterations has been well established in early Alzheimer's disease. Alterations in cytokine levels have not been studied in detail but may contribute to anorexia. Other types of cognitive dysfunction such as delirium may also contribute to weight loss and malnutrition in older adults.

Medications

Medication use can have a profound impact on nutritional status. Many older adults living in the community use multiple prescription and non-prescription medications. For example, in one study of women over the age of 65, 23% were using five or more prescription medicines [34]. The extent of multi-drug regimens is even higher among nursing home residents. Medications may affect nutritional status in a variety of ways, including alteration or loss of taste and smell, nausea, anorexia, dry mouth, diarrhea, reduced feeding ability, or increased appetite. Non-prescription and recreational drugs should not be overlooked. Even relatively small quantities of nicotine can suppress appetite.

Social, economic and functional considerations

Social and environmental factors strongly influence diet quality and nutritional adequacy [38]. Economic hardship may limit financial resources for adequate nutrition. Reduced social contact and eating meals alone impacts dietary intake (protein, calories, fiber and calcium), as will inadequate assistance with shopping and preparing food. Many older adults who eat alone make poor decisions and eat the same foods day after day. The old adage about little old ladies subsisting on tea and toast is frequently the reality. These risk factors may go unrecognized by health care providers, family, and friends.

Dysphagia

Dysphagia should not be overlooked as a factor contributing to weight loss among frail older adults. Oropharyngeal dysphagia is often due to cricopharyngeal incoordination, which can be the result of numerous neurological conditions. Esophageal dysphagia is more often due to mechanical abnormalities such as stricture, webs, carcinoma, or extrinsic compression. Esophageal dysmotility can result from numerous conditions including diabetes, scleroderma, dermatomyositis, and myasthenia gravis. Symptoms of dysphagia usually include coughing, watery nose and eyes with eating (coryza), and aspiration pneumonia. It is important for a clinician not only to ask about difficulty swallowing but also coughing or watering eyes with meals and intolerance of solids or liquids.

Interventions for malnutrition and nutritional frailty

Primary care practitioners caring for elderly patients in the community need to be knowledgeable about the potential benefits, risks, and costs of specific interventions for nutritional frailty. Much of the research and guideline development for assessing and managing nutritional frailty in older adults to date has been done in the context of nursing homes. In the nursing home environment we have the ability to closely monitor nutritional status and the resources to intervene, including the availability of dietitians. However, as discussed in the following sections, much of what has been learned in the nursing home can be applied in the outpatient primary care setting.

Dietary modifications

When calorie and protein intake are inadequate, it is appropriate to remove traditional dietary restrictions related to disease processes, a position strongly supported by the American Dietetic Association [39]. Low sodium and low cholesterol diets have a profoundly negative impact on the taste and smell of food, thus limiting overall caloric intake. Similarly, adding flavor enhancement has been shown to increase food intake and maintain weight in nursing home residents [40]. Furthermore, having someone else to eat with has been shown to significantly increase food consumption among homebound older adults [38].

In older adults with dysphagia, altering food and liquid consistency can minimize the risk of aspiration and help limit weight loss. When crycopharyngeal dysfunction is the issue, semi-solid consistencies are generally tolerated better than liquids. Potentially helpful techniques to minimize the risk of aspiration include positioning the patient upright during meals and for 30 minutes after meals, tucking the chin during swallowing, swallowing multiple times with each bolus, and keeping the bolus to less than 1 teaspoon. A speech pathologist can be helpful, not only in diagnosing dysphagia and other eating problems, but also in developing the treatment plan and providing education for patients or caregivers.

Nutritional supplements

When adequate nutrient intake cannot be achieved from ad libitum meals, commercially prepared (usually liquid) nutritional supplements are often prescribed, with the goal of increasing total nutrient and calorie intake. These products provide a good source of shelf-stable nutrients in appropriate amounts. However, some products may be low in protein and/or fiber content and they may be misused as meal replacements rather than taken in addition to a meal. Timing of liquid nutrition supplements can be a major determinant of their effectiveness. When given too close to meals, they may simply result in lower food intakes at mealtime and thus no net gain in daily calorie consumption. Elderly patients with urinary incontinence may refuse these products in an effort to limit fluid intake. The chance of electrolyte and carbohydrate overload in chronic renal insufficiency and diabetes, respectively, should also be considered [41]. A recent meta-analysis of 55 supplementation trials showed that hospitalized subjects (>65 years) and/or malnourished, benefited the most (fewer complications and decreased mortality) from supplement use [42]. Protein/calorie supplements have also been linked to better outcomes for elderly patients recovering from hip fracture [43].

In the community setting, liquid protein/calorie supplements have the most to offer for patients with limitations in their oral food intake, such as food intolerances, inability, or unwillingness to eat. Additionally, these supplements are beneficial in situations where having the patient do their own food preparation is prohibited or unsafe [41]. They have the most benefit in the case of acute catabolic events or severe malnutrition.

Whenever dietary deficiencies are a concern, micronutrient (multivitamin and mineral) supplements that provide approximately 100% of the DRI should be considered. While these supplements will not directly benefit protein and weight status, indirect benefits could be substantial since correcting micronutrient deficiencies could lead to better food intake by enhancing appetite, immune response, and cognition.

Appetite stimulants and antidepressants

In an effort to enhance food intake, orexigenic agents are often considered in the treatment of weight loss and malnutrition in older adults with anorexia. Megestrol acetate has been studied in undernourished older adults as a means to improve oral nutrition. In a group of nursing home patients with anorexia and cachexia who had lost 5% of their weight over the previous 3 months or had a body weight 20% lower than their ideal body weight, it provided an improved sense of well-being and appetite [44]. At the end of 3 months of treatment there was no significant change in weight compared to the placebo group. However, 3 months after treatment was discontinued there was a significant weight gain in the treatment group compared to the placebo group. A reduction in cytokine levels was also noted in the treatment group [45]. The effects of megestrol may be related to changes that take several months to have an effect on appetite and weight status. Careful studies of megestrol acetate in other patient populations, such as those with cancer and AIDS, have found an increase only in fat mass but no significant increase in lean body mass. No survival advantage has been demonstrated. Side effects include adrenal suppression, fluid retention, deep vein thrombosis, confusion, and impotence. Other agents that have been used to stimulate appetite, but for which there are little data regarding their use, include cyproheptadine, dronabinol, testosterone, growth hormone, oxandrolone, and steroids.

When considering the use of an orexigenic agent, the etiology of the weight loss and the goals of care need to be carefully defined. If dysphagia is the primary issue hindering caloric intake, then appetite stimulation may only serve to make the patient's condition more uncomfortable. The disease process is also important to consider when making this decision since benefits may be less in certain conditions such as advanced dementia than in other disease processes where an improved sense of well being has been a meaningful and measurable outcome with orexigenic agents. Patients with advanced dementia are not likely to experience an improved sense of well-being, since they cannot appreciate the importance of their nutritional health.

Although alcohol is touted as an appetite stimulant and potential benefit to cardiovascular health, it should rarely be recommended to frail older adults. Reasons for this include the potential for abuse and other deleterious effects such as cognitive dysfunction, vitamin deficiencies, falls, insomnia, osteoporosis, and drug interactions.

In the situation of otherwise unexplained weight loss, the diagnosis of depression must be considered; even when the diagnosis is uncertain, a trial of an antidepressant medication may be reasonable. Although tricyclic antidepressants frequently result in weight gain for younger patients who consider this an unpleasant side effect, they may not produce weight gain in frail older adults [46]. Side effects that include constipation, dry mouth, orthostatic hypotension, and urinary retention make tricyclic antidepressants less desirable with the advent of selective serotonin reuptake inhibitors (SSRIs, e.g., sertraline, citalopram). Initial concern that SSRIs may produce weight loss in older adults has not been substantiated [46]. Mirtazapine, a multireceptor agonist, has been associated with increased appetite and weight gain in younger patients in comparison to SSRIs. However, effectiveness of this agent in producing significant weight gain in frail older adults is unknown. In many instances weight gain may represent improvement in depression.

Feeding tubes

Enteral feeding tubes and peripheral/central parenteral nutrition were developed for and have been primarily used in the treatment of acute reversible illness; specifically, this applies to limited periods of time when oral intake is not possible or not adequate. Even so, in the situation of dysphagia post-acute stroke, the largest randomized controlled study to date found no benefit of enteral feeding with regard to mortality or functional status [47]. However, the availability of these feeding mechanisms has led to more widespread consideration of use in the setting of nutritionally deficient patients with chronic illness despite a lack of evidence to support this clinical practice.

Placement

Unless a patient has a feeding tube placed surgically during another abdominal procedure, most feeding tubes are percutaneous endoscopically-placed gastrostomy (PEG) tubes. These tubes are generally placed by gastroenterologists or radiologists and do not require general anesthesia. Jejunostomy tubes are placed past the Ligament of Treitz for the theoretical purpose of further minimizing tracheal aspiration. Such tubes are rarely appropriate for long-term use due to difficulty maintaining these small caliber tubes and the absolute necessity of administering the feeding in small increments with a pump. Gastrostomy tubes are more durable and more easily replaced when they become dysfunctional. They provide more flexibility and options for administration.

Formulas

Standard formulas provides 1.0–1.2 kcal/mL and calorie dense formulas provide 1.5–2.0 kcal/mL. The osmolality of standard formulas is well tolerated and previous practices of diluting tube feeding have been abandoned. Most standard formulas are lactose and gluten free. Specialized products to meet the needs of patients with particular diseases such as Crohn's disease, diabetes, renal disease, lung disease, and hepatic encephalopathy are available but are expensive and should not be used unless the patient has not tolerated more conventional formulations. Whenever possible, a registered dietitian should be involved in the prescription and administration of enteral feedings. Their involvement has been associated with better outcomes in the sub-acute setting [48].

Administration

The initial feeding rate or bolus size is increased gradually to a set goal by the second or third day of use. The patient's torso should be elevated 30–45° during and for at least 30 minutes after feeding. Mild bloating and loose bowel movements are common initial adverse effects that generally resolve with time. Feeding should be discontinued and evaluation pursued if more serious problems such as nausea, vomiting, diarrhea, or high gastric residual feedings should occur. Feeding administration should meet not only the nutritional but also the social and physical needs of the patient. In a home situation, the capabilities of the caregiver should also be considered. Feedings can be administered as boluses by intermittent gravity feeding at meal times or continuously at night time using a pump.

Since meals are a significant part of typical social interaction, it can be extremely difficult for cognitively intact individuals to completely give up oral intake. If not eating is having a detrimental effect on quality of life, the clinician should discuss the risks and benefits of "pleasure eating" with the patient and family. Patients and their families should be instructed in the safest consistencies and the signs of overt (e.g. cough, gag) or silent aspiration (runny nose, course breath sounds) that should signal them to abort the meal.

Monitoring

Feeding prescriptions should be based on calculated caloric and protein goals. In the outpatient setting, most patients can be monitored infrequently except when they become ill. Electrolytes, blood urea nitrogen (BUN), creatinine, glucose, albumin may be monitored every 1–3 months in stable patients. Weight is an important guide for feeding adjustment. When patients become ill, special attention to fluid status is needed to provide adequate hydration in the face of emesis, diarrhea, fever, or drains.

Avoiding a clogged tube can be very important in long-term use. Tubes should be flushed with water whenever feeding is stopped or medication is administered. Even unused feeding tubes that are left in place should be flushed daily. Medications are a particular risk for clogging. Even liquid medications that are syrup consistency can clog tubes as residue accumulates. Solid medication must be crushed into very fine powder and suspended in liquid for administration. Enteric coated, sustained release or extended release preparations cannot be altered and should not be administered through a feeding tube. Alternative routes of administration such as rectal absorption (e.g. suppositories) or sublingual absorption may be necessary.

Percutaneous gastrostomy and jejunostomy tubes can become dislodged. Patients who are cognitively impaired may unintentionally pull the tube out. Mechanisms for retaining the tube, such as stitches to the skin or an inflated bulb in the stomach, can break. Any percutaneous tube that becomes dislodged must be replaced immediately or the tract may close.

When a patient is transitioning back to an oral diet, careful monitoring is needed. Tube feeding will need to be gradually decreased and administered in a way that does not interfere with appetite for meals, such as night-time continuous feeding.

Use in patients with dementia

Both physicians and patients' surrogate decision makers tend to have high expectations for feeding tube placement to improve nutrition, functional status, and quality of life [49]. In the case of advanced dementia, these high expectations for improved nutritional and health status are not supported by current research. There have been no randomized clinical trials comparing tube feeding with oral feeding in patients with severe dementia. A review of existing literature by Finucane and colleagues [50] found no evidence to support that tube feeding (gastrostomy or jejunostomy) prevents aspiration pneumonia. In fact, tube feeding does nothing to prevent the aspiration of oral secretions, nor can it prevent aspiration from regurgitated gastric contents. Additionally, these researchers did not find evidence to support prevention of other infections, the consequences of malnutrition, or pressure ulcers, nor any evidence to support a survival benefit, improved functional status, or greater patient comfort [50]. In general, adverse events associated with feeding tubes include aspiration pneumonia, tube occlusion, leakage, and local infection. The mortality during percutaneous endoscopic gastrostomy (PEG) tube placement is low (0–2%), but perioperative mortality ranges from 6–24%.

Palliative nutritional care

In circumstances where careful hand feeding has not provided adequate nutrition and has resulted in pneumonia or other complications of malnutrition, consideration should be given to palliative nutritional care. With this type of care, food and liquid are provided as tolerated, allowing a natural death to occur without enteral or parenteral feeding. It is important for health care providers to initiate conversations early with patients and their families regarding care at the end of life in any chronic or terminal disease process, when cognitive abilities will still allow a meaningful discussion. Many states allow individuals to specify in advance directives their desire to forgo alternative feeding mechanisms such as feeding tubes. In the nursing home setting, federal regulations should not be seen as a barrier to forgoing alternative feeding mechanisms as long as the eating problems are identified and properly assessed, and reasonable efforts to hand feed are being made [51]. Careful documentation by physicians and other healthcare providers should indicate that nutritional decline is not preventable because of the patient's advanced dementia, terminal disease, or advanced chronic disease process.

Conclusions

Primary care providers are in a unique position to influence the health and well-being of their older adult patients by recognizing threats to nutritional adequacy and intervene to maximize nutritional health. Primary care providers should be aware of alterations in nutrient requirements for older adults and often need to discuss these requirements with patients and family members to optimize nutrient intake and avoid excessive consumption of calories. Even the status of hydration, protein, carbohydrates, lipids and fiber needs cannot be assumed or ignored, especially in frail older adults with multiple chronic illnesses. Assessing nutritional status can be incorporated into routine office practice. The primary care provider should partner with other professionals to optimize nutritional health by involving dietitians, speech pathologists, dentists, and other healthcare providers. Most of all, primary care providers can assist their patients in setting realistic goals for their nutritional health and support them in achieving these goals.

References

1 Bales CW, Ritchie CS. Nutritional Needs and Assessment During the Life Cycle: The Elderly. In Shils ME *et al.*(eds). *Modern Nutrition in Health and Disease* 10th edition. Baltimore MD: Lippincott Williams and Wilkins, 2006:843–58.

2 Food and Nutrition Board, Institute of Medicine. Dietary Reference Intakes (DRI) for Energy, CHO, Fiber, Fat, Protein. National Academies Press. Washington, DC. 2002.

3 Lindeman RD, Romero LJ, Liang HC, Baumgartner RN, Koehler KM, Garry PJ. Do elderly persons need to be encouraged to drink more fluids? *J Geriatr* 2000;55A:M361–M365.

4 Russell RM. The aging process as a modifier of metabolism. *Am J Clin Nutr* 2000;72(Suppl):529S–32S.

5 Penniston KL, Tanumihardjo SA. Vitamin A in dietary supplements and fortified foods: Too much of a good thing? *J Am Diet Assoc* 2003;103:1185–7.

6 Janssen HCJP, Samson MM, Verhaar HJJ. Vitamin D deficiency, muscle function, and falls in elderly people. *Am J Clin Nutr* 2002;75:611–5.

7 Garland CF, Garland FC, Gorham ED *et al.* The role of vitamin D in cancer prevention. *Am J Public Health* 2006;96:2:252–61.

8 Garland CF, Garland FC. Do sunlight and vitamin D reduce the likelihood of colon cancer? *Int J Epidemiol* 2006 April;35(2):217–20. Epub 2005 Nov 22.

9 Giovannucci E. The epidemiology of vitamin D and colorectal cancer: recent findings. *Curr Opin Gastroenterol* 2006;22:24–9.

10 Food and Nutrition Board, Institute of Medicine. Dietary Reference Intakes (DRIs) for Vitamins, Minerals and Trace elements. National Academies Press. Washington, DC. 1997–2004.

11 Miller ER, Pastor-Barriuso R, Dalal D, Riemersma RA, Appel LJ, Guallar E. Meta-analysis: high-dosage vitamin E supplementation may increase all-cause mortality. *Ann Intern Med* 2005;142:1:37–46.

12 Sheiham A, Steele JG, Marcenes W *et al.* The relationship among dental status, nutrient intake, and nutritional status in older people. *J Dent Res* 2001;80:408–13.

13 Lee JS and Frongillo EA Jr. Nutritional and health consequences are associated with food insecurity among U.S. elderly persons. *J Nutr* 2001;131:1503–9.

14 Ho C, Kauwell GP, Bailey LB. Practitioners' guide to meeting the vitamin B$_{12}$ recommended dietary allowance for people aged 51 years and older. *J Am Diet Assoc* 1999;99:725–7.

15 Weir DG, Scott JM. Brain function in the elderly: role of vitamin B$_{12}$ and folate. *Br Med Bull* 1999;55:669–82.

16 Wakimoto P, Block G. Dietary intake, dietary patterns, and changes with age: an epidemiological perspective. *J Gerontol A Biol Sci Med Sci* 2001;56:65–80.

17 Tucker KL, Hannan MT, Chen H, Cupples LA, Wilson PW, Kiel DP. Potassium, magnesium, and fruit and vegetable intakes are associated with greater bone mineral density in elderly men and women. *Am J Clin Nutr* 1999;69:727–36.

18 Zorilla P, Salido JA, Lopez-Alonso A, Silva A. Serum zinc as a prognostic tool for wound healing in hip hemiarthroplasty. *Clin Orthop Relat Res* 2004;420:304–8.

19 Evans WJ. Protein nutrition, exercise and aging. *J Am Coll Nutr* 2004;23:6:601S–609S.

20 Cornoni-Huntley JC, Harris TB, Everett DF *et al.* An overview of body weight of older persons, including the impact on mortality. *J Clin Epidemiol* 1991;44:8:743–53.

21 Wallace JI, Schwartz, RS, LaCroix AZ, Uhlmann RF, Pearlman RA. Involuntary weight loss in older outpatients: Incidence and clinical significance. *J Am Geriatr Soc* 1995;43:329–37.

22 Villareal DT, Apovian CM, Kushner RF, Klein S. Obesity in older adults: technical review and position statement of the American Society for Nutrition and NAASO, The Obesity Society. *Am J Clin Nutr* 2005;82:923–34.

23 Mowé M, Böhmer T. The prevalence of undiagnosed protein-calorie undernutrition in a population of hospitalized elderly patients. *J Am Geriatr Soc* 1991;39:1089–92.

24 Payette H, Coulombe C, Boutier V, Gray-Donald K. Weight loss and mortality among free-living frail elders: a prospective study. *J Gerontology MS* 1999;54A:M440–M445.

25 Kant AK, Schatzkin A, Graubard BI, Schairer C. A prospective study of diet quality and mortality in women. *JAMA* 2000;283:2109–15.

26 Sowers MR, Crutchfield M, Richards K *et al.* Sarcopenia is related to physical functioning and leg strength in middle-aged women. *J Gerontology MS* 2005;60A 4:486–90.

27 Ritchie CS, Bales CW. Sarcopenia and Nutritional Frailty: Diagnosis and Intervention. In Bales CW and Ritchie CS (eds): *Handbook of Clinical Nutrition and Aging*. Humana Press Inc., Totowa, NJ: 2004:309–33.

28 Nutrition Screening Initiative: www.aafp.org/x16081.xml.

29 Mini Nutrition Assessment (MNA). www.mna-elderly.com/index.htm.

30 Andres R, Elahi D, Tobin J *et al.* Impact of age on weight goals. *Annal Intern Med* 1985;103(6):1030–3.

31 Vickers SM, Nagi PA. Nutritional Requirements Following Cancer: Treatment/Surgery. In Bales CW and Ritchie CS (eds): *Handbook of Clinical Nutrition and Aging*. Humana Press Inc., Totowa, NJ: 2004:477–486.

32 Anker SD, Chua TP, Ponikowski P *et al.* Hormonal changes and catabolic/anabolic imbalance in chronic heart failure and their importance for cardiac cachexia. *Circulation* 1997;96:2:526–34.

33 Gray-Donald K, Saudny-Unterberger, H. Nutrition and Chronic Obstructive Pulmonary Disease. In Bales CW and Ritchie CS (eds): *Handbook of Clinical Nutrition and Aging*. Humana Press Inc., Totowa, NJ: 2004:457–473.

34 White H, Pieper C, Schmader K, Fillenbaum G. Weight change in Alzheimer's disease. *J Am Geriatr Soc* 1996;44:265–72.

35 White H, Pieper C, Schmader K. The association of weight change in Alzheimer's disease with severity of disease and mortality: A longitudinal analysis. *J Am Geriatr Soc* 1998;46:1223–7.

36 White H. Geriatric Syndromes: Nutritional Consequences and Potential Opportunities: Dementia In Bales CW and Ritchie CS (eds): *Handbook of Clinical Nutrition and Aging*. Humana Press Inc., Totowa, NJ: 2004:349–365.

37 Kaufman DW, Kelly JP, Rosenberg L, Anderson TE, Mitchell AA. Recent patterns of medication use in the ambulatory adult population of the United States: The Sloan survey. *JAMA* 2002:287–337.

38 Locher JL, Robinson CO, Roth DL, Ritchie CS, Burgio KL. The effect of the presence of others on caloric intake of homebound older adults. *J Gerontology MS* 2005;60A:1475–8.

39 American Dietetic Association. Position of the American Dietetic Association: Liberalization of the diet prescription improves quality of life for older adults in long-term care. *JADA* 2005;105:1955–65.

40 Mathey MF, Sieblink E, de Graaf C, Van Staveren WA. Flavor enhancement of food improves dietary intake and nutritional status of elderly nursing home residents. *J Gerontol A Biol Sci Med Sci* 2001;56A:4:M200–M205.

41 Johnson C, East JM, Glassman P. Management of malnutrition in the elderly and the appropriate use of commercially manufactured oral nutritional supplements. *J Nutr Health Aging* 2000;4:42–6.

42 Milne AC, Avenell A, Potter J. Meta-Analysis: Protein and energy supplementation in older people. *Ann Intern Med* 2006;144:37–48.

43 Schurch MA, Rizzoli R, Slosman D, Vadas L, Vergnaud P, Bonjour J-P. Protein supplements increase serum insulin-like growth factor-1 levels and attenuate proximal femur bone loss in patients with recent hip fracture: a randomized, double-blind, placebo-controlled trial. *Ann Intern Med* 1998;128:801–9.

44 Yeh SS, Wu SY, Lee TP *et al.* Improvement in quality-of-life measures and stimulation of weight gain after treatment with megestrol acetate oral suspension in geriatric cachexia: results of a double-blind, placebo-controlled study. *J Amer Geriatr Soc* 2000;48:5:485–92.

45 Yeh SS, Wu SY, Levine DM *et al.* The correlation of cytokine levels with body weight after megestrol acetate treatment in geriatric patients. *J Gerontol A Biol Sci Med Sci* 2001;56:1:M48–54.

46 Rigler SK, Webb MJ, Redford L, Brown EF, Zhou J, Wallace D. Weight outcomes among antidepressant users in nursing facilities. *J Am Geriatr Soc* 2001;49:49–55.

47 Dennis MS, Lewis SC, Warlow C. Effect of timing and method of enteral tube feeding for dysphagic stroke patients in hospital (FOOD): a multicentre randomised controlled trial. *Lancet* 2005;365:764–73.

48 Braga JM, Hunt A, Pope J *et al.* Implementation of dietician recommendations for enteral nutrition results in improved outcomes. *J Am Diet Assoc* 2006;106:281–4.

49 Cox CE, Lewis CL, Carey TS *et al.* Expectations and outcomes of feeding tube placement from the perspective of patients' surrogates and physicians. *J Gen Intern Med* 2002;17(S1):187. (Tracking ID#50915).

50 Finucane TE, Christmas C, Travis K. Tube feeding in patients with advanced dementia: a review of the evidence. *JAMA* 1999;282:14:1365–70.

51 Gillick, MR. Rethinking the role of tube feeding in patients with advanced dementia. *N Engl J Med* 2000;342:3:206–10.

Improving health by changing diet and lifestyle behaviors

CHAPTER 7

Dyslipidemia, hypertension and metabolic syndrome

Frances Burke and Philippe Szapary

Cardiovascular disease (CVD) is the number-one cause of morbidity and mortality in the US. Much of this burden of disease is linked to poor lifestyle habits, leading to overweight and obesity, and the aging of the population [1]. The National Cholesterol Education Program (NCEP) Adult Treatment Panel III (ATP III) emphasizes the importance of lifestyle modification to improve cardiovascular risk [2,3]. The US Preventive Services Task Force found that dietary counseling by a team that includes primary care clinicians and registered dietitians can improve the diet and health outcomes of patients with hyperlipidemia and other risk factors for CVD [4]. Primary care clinicians are well placed to screen for cardiovascular risk factors and to initiate treatment for lipid abnormalities.

Therapeutic lifestyle changes for CVD risk reduction

Low density lipoprotein (LDL) cholesterol has been identified by ATP III as the most atherogenic lipoprotein, making it the primary target for cholesterol lowering therapy. LDL goals have been established for diet and drug treatment of hyperlipidemia based on cardiovascular risk factors and the Framingham Risk scoring system (Table 7.1) [2].

Diet and physical activity are considered to be the cornerstones of effective treatment for dyslipidemia. ATP III has designated the term therapeutic lifestyle changes (TLC) to emphasize and reinforce a multifaceted approach to achieve LDL goals and cardiovascular risk reduction. This dietary approach includes restricting dietary fats that are more atherogenic and allowing moderate intake in those dietary fats that are less atherogenic (see Figure 7.1).

Medical Nutrition Therapy for dyslipidemia consists of the TLC diet (See Appendix Q). The following components of the TLC diet have been outlined in ATP III for achievement of LDL goals.
- Minimize LDL-raising nutrients:
  - reduce dietary intake of saturated fat and trans fat;
  - keep dietary cholesterol intake less than 200 mg/day;
  - substitute monounsaturated fat (MUFA) and polyunsaturated fat (PUFA) for saturated and trans fats.

Table 7.1 ATP III LDL-C goals and cut-points for therapeutic lifestyle changes (TLC) and drug therapy in different risk categories.

Risk category	LDL-C goal	Initiate TLC	Consider drug therapy[†]
High risk: CHD or CHD risk equivalents (10-year risk >20%)	<100 mg/dL (optional goal: <70 mg/dL)	≥100 mg/dL	≥100 mg/dL (<100 mg/dL: consider drug options)
Moderately high risk: 2 + risk factors (10-year risk 10–20%)	<130 mg/dL	≥130 mg/dL	≥130 mg/dL (100–129 mg/dL; consider drug options)
Moderate risk: 2 + risk factors (10-year risk <10%)	<130 mg/dL	≥130 mg/dL	≥160 mg/dL
Lower risk: 0–1 risk factor	<160 mg/dL	≥160 mg/dL	≥190 mg/dL (160–189 mg/dL: LDL-lowering drug optional)

Source: [2]

- Addition of dietary factors to enhance LDL lowering:
  - increase viscous fiber intake to 10–25 g/day;
  - include 2 g of plant stanol/sterol esters per day.
- Adjust total calories to maintain desirable body weight and prevent weight gain.
- Increase regular physical activity.

Macronutrient Content of the Therapeutic Lifestyle Change diet

The TLC diet is approximately 25–35% of energy from total fat, <7% saturated fat, up to 20% from monounsaturated fat, 10% from polyunsaturated fat, 15% of energy from protein and 50–60% of energy from carbohydrate. The 2001 ATP III report recommends ranges in total fat intake because it was recognized that some patients, such as those with metabolic syndrome, would benefit from diets higher in unsaturated fat and lower in carbohydrate [2]. For the patient with dyslipidemia, key questions relating to fat intake will help the clinician focus on the nutritional recommendations to reduce CHD risk. The effects of different fatty acids and other dietary components are discussed below.

Saturated fat

The effect of saturated fat on increasing both total and LDL cholesterol has been well documented. Compared to unsaturated fat, saturated fat decreases the synthesis and activity of LDL receptors. As LDL levels rise they become susceptible to oxidation and lead to the formation of foam cells which contribute to the growth of artherosclerotic lesions [5]. Several large-scale clinical

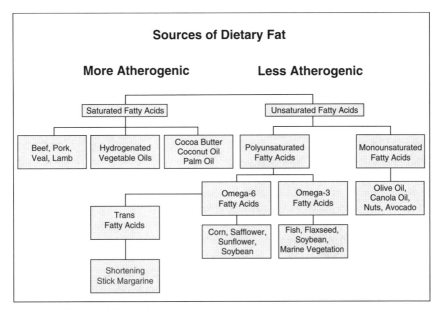

Figure 7.1 Sources of dietary fat.
Source: Linda Van Horn, PhD, RD, Northwestern University Feinberg School of Medicine. 2007.
Used with permission.

trials have conclusively demonstrated that reducing LDL reduces the number of acute cardiac events and deaths from coronary heart disease (CHD) both in patients with existing disease and those at risk due to elevated lipid levels [2]. An increase of 1% in LDL increases CHD risk by 1% [2].

According to the NHANES III data (1988 to 1994) approximately 11% of the calories in the American diet come from saturated fat. This amount has declined over the last several decades from 18–20% of total calories contributing to a decline in CHD rates [6]. Saturated fat is solid at room temperature and is found in animal products as well as palm and coconut oil. The major sources of saturated fat in the diet are red meat, butter, and whole milk (Table 7.2).

Table 7.2 Dietary CAGE questions for assessment of intakes of saturated fat and cholesterol.

C	Cheese (and other sources of dairy fats-whole milk, 2% milk, ice cream, cream, whole milk yogurt)
A	Animal fats (hamburger, ground meat, frankfurters, bologna, salami, sausage, fried foods, fatty cuts of meat)
G	Got it away from home (high-fat meals either purchased and brought home or eaten in restaurants)
E	Eat (extra) high-fat commercial products: candy, pastries, pies, doughnuts, cookies

Source: [2]

The decline in whole milk consumption is thought to account for most of the reduction in saturated fat [7]. Although there is some evidence that specific saturated fatty acids do not increase LDL levels (e.g. stearic acid found in chocolate) patients need to be reminded that eating too much of these foods can contribute to weight gain which raises cardiovascular disease (CVD) risk [5]. On average, adherence to a low saturated fat diet can be expected to reduce LDL cholesterol levels by 8–10% [2,6].

Trans fats

Trans fats are polyunsaturated fats whose double bond is in the trans configuration. Randomized clinical trials have shown that trans fatty acids raise LDL cholesterol and lower high density lipoprotein (HDL) levels when compared with naturally occurring cis-unsaturated fatty acids [2,8]. A high intake of trans fats has also been shown to increase plasma levels of lipoprotein a (Lpa) and triglycerides and may decrease endothelial function. Trans fatty acids have also been found to interfere with essential fatty acid metabolism by inhibiting the enzyme delta-6 desaturase [7]. The current US Department of Agriculture Dietary Guidelines advise eating as little trans fat as possible. The major source of trans fats are partially hydrogenated vegetable oils which are added to foods to prolong their shelf-life. Foods containing trans fats include stick margarine, French fries, cookies, crackers, and baked desserts. It is recommended that individuals use soft tub margarines that are trans fat free, canola oil, or olive oil. The Food and Drug Administration had mandated that information regarding trans fatty acids be listed on all food labels beginning January 2006 [9].

Cholesterol

Of the total body cholesterol pool, approximately 25% is dietary; the remainder is derived from hepatic synthesis [10]. Typically, foods high in saturated fat are also sources of dietary cholesterol, so reducing these foods provides the additional benefit of limiting cholesterol intake. Sources of cholesterol in the diet include egg yolks, shellfish and organ meats, however, these foods are relatively low in saturated fat. Several observational studies suggest that egg consumption is not associated with higher cholesterol levels and does not increase risk of CHD among healthy men and women [11–13]. ATP III advises limiting egg yolks to no more than two per week to keep dietary cholesterol under 200 mg/day [2].

Monounsaturated fat

Epidemiologic data shows that the Mediterranean diet, which is rich in MUFA, is associated with a lower incidence of CHD [14]. This hypothesis has now been corroborated by a secondary prevention clinical trial, the Lyon Diet Heart Study [15]. In this study the participants who consumed a Mediterranean-style diet supplemented with canola oil based margarine, high in alpha-linolenic acid (ALA), had a 70% reduced risk of total and CVD mortality and non-fatal myocardial infarction (MI). The Mediterranean diet contains less meat than the Western-style diet and more fish, fruits, vegetables and alcohol. This diet is also low in saturated fat and rich in antioxidants and phytochemicals, and may beneficially affect LDL oxidation and thrombus formation independent of effects on lipoprotein levels.

Oleic acid is the most common dietary form of MUFA and when substituted for saturated fat, reduces LDL cholesterol levels [5]. A diet high in MUFA, lowers LDL cholesterol and serum triglycerides without lowering HDL cholesterol levels [2]. Thus, providing calories from MUFA that might otherwise be provided from PUFA or carbohydrate, can lower LDL without lowering HDL or raising triglyceride levels.

Monounsaturated fat is the preferred type of dietary fat for patients with metabolic syndrome who present with an atherogenic dyslipidemia characterized by elevated apolipoprotein B and triglyceride levels, low HDL levels, and small dense LDL particles. Increasing MUFA by as much as 20% as recommended by the TLC diet plan is likely to benefit patients whose hypertriglyceridemia worsens with high carbohydrate, low-fat diets. However, since all fats are calorically dense, (i.e.1 tablespoon of oil contains 15 g of fat and approximately 135 calories), liberal use of fat can lead to weight gain, and adversely affect triglyceride and HDL levels. Dietary sources of MUFA include: canola and olive oil, olives, peanuts and pecans, tahini paste (used as an ingredient in hummus) and avocado.

Polyunsaturated fat

The two major categories of PUFA are omega-3 and omega-6 fatty acids (FA). Vegetable or seed oils such as corn, sunflower, safflower, sesame, and cottonseed contain omega-6 FA. The major omega-6 FA is linoleic acid, an essential fatty acid required in the diet. Linoleic acid is converted to arachidonic acid, the precursor for the synthesis of prostaglandins [5]. The Institute of Medicine's Food and Nutrition Board set recommended intakes for linoleic acid at 17 g/day for men and 12 g/day for women [16].

Overall, Americans have greater intakes of omega-6 FA compared to omega-3 FA as they are contained in commonly used foods such as margarines, commercial salad dressings, and mayonnaise. The ratio of omega-6: omega-3 FA intake is estimated to be 20 : 1 in the typical Western diet [17]. Substitution of PUFA for saturated fat in the diet lowers LDL levels and reduces risk for CHD, however, TLC sets an upper limit of 10% of total calories from PUFA [2].

Omega-3 FA include long chain marine fats, such as eciosapentanoic acid (EPA) and docosahexenoic acid (DHA) and the plant-based essential fatty acid, ALA. Current intake of omega-3 FA in the US is 1.6 g/day [18]. Food sources of ALA are soybean and canola oil, tofu, walnuts, and flaxseed. EPA and DHA are contained in fatty fish such as salmon, mackerel, tuna, herring, and sardines. Growing evidence indicates that omega-3 FA are cardioprotective beyond their effects on lipoprotein levels [19]. The GISSI-Prevenzione trial was the largest randomized controlled clinical trial demonstrating the effect of supplemental

EPA plus DHA on secondary prevention of CHD. After a period of 3.5 years those individuals receiving 850 mg of concentrated EPA and DHA experienced a 15% reduction in stroke and nonfatal myocardial infarction (MI) and a 45% reduction in sudden cardiac death compared to the control group [20]. Omega-3 FA have also been associated with decreased risk of arrhythmia, lower plasma triglyceride levels, reduced platelet aggregation, and lower risk of nonfatal MI [18,20].

The American Heart Association (AHA) has updated its recommendations for secondary prevention of CVD to include 1 g/day of EPA plus DHA which amounts to approximately 7 ounces of fish or several over-the-counter fish oil capsules per day. In primary prevention, the AHA recommends eating fish at least twice per week. Higher doses of fish oil (6–9 capsules) may be used in treating patients with severe hypertriglyceridemia (>1000 mg/dL). A prescription brand of fish oil is now approved by the FDA Omacor®; (Reliant Pharmaceuticals), it provides approximately 840 mg EPA/DHA per capsule. In addition to its possible cardioprotective effects, fish is generally low in total and saturated fat.

Plant sources of ALA can be increased in the diet as they can be converted to EPA and DHA in humans. The recommendations for ALA are 1.6 and 1.1 g/day for men and women respectively [16]. This amount can be obtained in 1 tbsp canola or walnut oil, ½ tbsp ground flax seed or <1 tsp flaxseed oil.

Soluble fiber

Epidemiologic evidence strongly supports an inverse association between fiber intake and CVD [7]. Inclusion of soluble fiber in the diet can decrease LDL levels. Based on evidence from a meta-analysis of over 50 clinical trials, ATP III recommends the inclusion of at least 5–10 g/day of viscous fiber daily into a low saturated, low trans fat diet. This amount of soluble fiber has been shown to reduce LDL levels by about 5% [2]. The hypocholesterolemic effect of soluble fiber results from its ability to form a gel-like substance in the gut, which binds and removes bile acids from the body through the stool before they are reabsorbed. Compensatory hepatic conversion of cholesterol into new bile acids reduces serum cholesterol. Soluble fiber can also substitute for foods that are high in saturated fat. Some of the best dietary sources that provide 2–4 g of viscous fiber per serving include dried beans (lima, pinto, kidney), oatmeal, oat bran, citrus fruits, pears and brussel sprouts [21]. Unfortunately fewer than 25% of Americans eat five or more daily servings of fruits and vegetables per day according to data from the Behavioral Risk Factor Surveillance System and Centers for Disease Control.

The current *US Dietary Guidelines* recommend that individuals consume at least three servings of whole grains daily [22]. Examples of whole-grain foods and flours include amaranth, barley, brown rice, buckwheat, bulgur, corn, farro, millet, oatmeal and whole oats, popcorn, quinoa, sorghum, spelt, teff, whole rye, whole or cracked wheat and wild rice and wheat berries. Whole grains are high in protein and fiber and low in fat. Numerous studies have supported the role of whole grains in reducing the risk of heart disease, stroke and type 2 diabetes [23–27]. More and more whole grain foods are entering supermarkets daily in the form of pasta products, breads, cookies, cereals and frozen dinners, which, while positive, is adding to the confusion of food shoppers. Counsel patients to look for the word "whole" in front of the type of grain and ideally this should be the first or second ingredient listed on the food label. The Whole Grains Council has also developed an official Whole Grain stamp to help consumers identify whole grain products more easily.

Plant stanols/sterols

Plant stanols/sterols are natural components of plants which compete with dietary and biliary cholesterol for absorption in the intestinal lumen. They are found naturally in vegetable oils and nuts. As cholesterol absorption is reduced, the liver increases cholesterol synthesis and LDL receptor activity, which results in a reduction in serum LDL levels. Plant sterols are very poorly absorbed by the human body [28]. They differ from plant stanols in that they contain a double bond in their sterol ring structure.

In 1995, a landmark trial demonstrated that 24 g of a plant stanol ester spread that provided 2.6 g/day of plant stanols reduced total cholesterol levels by 10% and LDL cholesterol levels by 14% in a mildly hypercholesterolemic northern European population [29]. A minimum range of 0.8–1.0 g/day of sterols and stanols is required to produce a clinically significant reduction of LDL cholesterol. A dose–response relationship has been demonstrated at doses up to 2 g/day, leading health and government agencies to recommend intakes of 2 g/day [21].

Other studies have reported additive effects of plant stanol and sterol esters and bile acid sequestrants [31] and statins [32]. In one study, LDL cholesterol was reduced by an additional 17% (vs. 7% for placebo) when 3 g/day of plant stanol in ester form was added to the diet of patients on a stable statin dose [32].

The NCEP and the AHA recommend intake of 2–3 g/day of sterols or stanols as an adjunct to LDL cholesterol-lowering strategies for cardiovascular risk reduction [2]. There are currently two cholesterol-lowering margarines on the market in the US, Benecol® which contains sitostanol and is derived from wood pulp and Take Control® which contains sitosterol from soybean oil. Both come in regular and light variations, which can be used in place of margarine or butter in most applications. The full-fat version of both products are formulated so that they can be used in cooking, frying, and baking, in addition to their use as traditional spreads. The "light" versions contain water and therefore cannot be used in cooking. Plant stanols and sterols show benefits after two weeks of consuming 2–3 servings/day with meals. Manufacturers of functional foods are also exploring ways to incorporate plant stanol and sterol esters into beverages and other foods such as orange juice, yogurt, and granola bars.

Few adverse effects related to either the short- or long-term use of plant stanol/sterol ester-containing products have been reported. However, there have been some concerns that the addition of plant stanols and sterols to the diet may affect the absorption of fat-soluble vitamins [28].

The "portfolio" diet

The traditional Mediterranean diet is low in saturated fat, high in MUFAs from nuts and olive oil, and high in fiber from fruits and vegetables. Jenkins *et al.* tested a combination dietary approach on a smaller, more controlled scale using a "portfolio" diet [33]. In this study, 46 hyperlipidemic adults were randomized to a low-saturated fat diet group (control), a low-saturated fat diet plus lovastatin (20 mg/day) group, or the "portfolio" diet group. The "portfolio" diet was low in fat and contained 1 g plant sterols in an enriched margarine; 21.4 g soy protein; 9.8 g viscous fibers from oats, barley, and psyllium; and 14 g (0.5 ounce) of whole almonds per 1000 kcal. Decreases in LDL cholesterol were 8%, 30.9%, and 28.6% for each group, respectively, with no significant difference between the statin and dietary "portfolio" group. High-sensitivity C-reactive protein was also reduced by 28% and 33% in the diet and statin groups, respectively, without any changes in the control group. This study provides strong evidence that a dietary approach incorporating the TLC diet and other functional foods can significantly reduce LDL cholesterol levels and, thus, can be expected to reduce CHD risk.

Recently Jenkins *et al.* looked at the effectiveness of the portfolio diet under "real-world" conditions in the same participants who had undergone metabolic studies comparing the same dietary portfolio with the effects of a statin medication. More than 30% of the participants who ate the portfolio diet in everyday life had LDL reductions of >20% after 1 year which was not significantly different from what was observed with the response to a metabolically controlled diet or first generation statin therapy [34].

Hypertension

Definition and prevalence

Hypertension is an independent risk factor for both CHD and stroke. This relationship is both continuous and consistent [35]. Hypertension is traditionally defined in patients with persistent systolic blood pressure (SBP) of 140 mmHg or greater and/or diastolic blood pressure (DBP) of 90 mmHg or greater, or taking antihypertensive medication. Hypertension frequently coexists with other cardiovascular risk factors, including obesity, dyslipidemia, insulin resistance, and glucose intolerance. The risk of CVD doubles with each incremental elevation in blood pressure (BP) of 20/10 mmHg starting at 115/75 mmHg [35].

Antihypertensive therapy has been associated with mean reductions of 35–40% in stroke incidence; 20–25% in MI; and more than 50% in heart failure in clinical trials [35]. Therefore, hypertension management is a critical component of preventive therapies for reducing morbidity and mortality from CVD.

According to the most recent NHANES III data (1999–2000) 65 million, or 1 out of every 3, Americans are hypertension [36]. This represents a 30% increase in the total number of adults with hypertension over the last decade. Individuals who are normotensive at age 55 years have a 90% chance of developing hypertension at some point in their lifetime. There is substantial evidence that dietary modifications effectively lower BP [37]. This information should compel primary care clinicians and other health care professionals to focus their efforts on improving the lifestyle practices of their patients. The importance of these efforts is highlighted by the fact that the prevalence of obesity and hypertension in children and adolescents 8–17 years of age has also risen [37].

Medical Nutrition Therapy for Hypertension

The National High Blood Pressure Education Program for the Prevention, Detection, Evaluation, and Treatment of High Blood Pressure released the Seventh Report of the Joint National Committee (JNC 7) sponsored by the Department of Health and Human Services and the National Institutes of Health, National Heart, Lung, and Blood Institute in 2003 [35]. According to the JNC 7 report, diet and lifestyle changes should be the first line of therapy for hypertension. Lifestyle modification may not completely obviate the need for antihypertensive medications, but it can dramatically reduce the amount of antihypertensive medication required to reach target blood pressure goals. The recent guidelines of the National High Blood Pressure Education Program estimate that a reduction in SBP of as little as 2 mmHg could save more that 70,000 lives in the US each year [35]. Table 7.3 outlines the specific diet

Table 7.3 Lifestyle modifications to manage hypertension. (JNC 7)

Modification	Recommendations	Approximate systolic BP reduction
Weight reduction	Maintain normal body weigh (BMI 18.5–24.9)	5–20 mmHg for each 10 kg weight loss
Adopt DASH eating plan	Consume diet rich in fruits, vegetables, low-fat dairy foods and low saturated fat	8–14 mmHg
Dietary sodium reduction	Reduce sodium to no more than 2.4 g/day or 6 g/day NaCl	2–8 mmHg
Increase physical activity	Engage in regular aerobic activity such as walking (30 min/day on most days)	4–9 mmHg
Moderate alcohol consumption	Limit alcohol to no more than 2 drinks/day for men and 1 drink/day for women	2–4 mmHg

Source: [35].

and lifestyle interventions as recommended by JNC 7 to manage high blood pressure and the approximate reductions in SBP that can be achieved.

Several key questions asked during a focused diet history will enable the clinician to develop a nutrition plan for the patient with hypertension.

Do you use the salt shaker at the table or in cooking?

Evidence from clinical trials has demonstrated that a moderate reduction in sodium intake is associated with a reduction in BP levels in both hypertensive and normotensive individuals. In addition, clinical trials have documented that a reduced sodium intake can prevent hypertension (with or without weight loss) and lower BP in patients on antihypertensive medications [37]. Observational studies have shown the age-related rise in SBP can be diminished by limiting sodium intake [37]. Thus, recommendations to limit dietary sodium directed at all Americans are essential for the primary prevention of hypertension in the US population. The Institute of Medicine has set an acceptable intake level of sodium at 1.5 g/day (65 mEq), which is probably unachievable for most Americans [37]. Data from NHANES between 1974 and 1994 suggest an increasing trend in sodium intake, which is not surprising considering the increasing consumption of commercially prepared foods and foods eaten outside the home [38]. Current daily consumption of sodium in the US is estimated to be between 140–150 mEq (approximately 3.5 g sodium or 8–9 g salt/sodium chloride) [39].

Foods that contribute the most sodium to the diet are canned, smoked, and processed foods, including frozen and prepared dinners, deli meats, and fast food. Condiments and snack foods also contain significant amounts of sodium. Because foods prepared outside of the home often contain added salt, more home preparation of food and care in food selection when dining in restaurants is advised. Primary care clinicians should recommend that patients with high–normal BP (135/85 mmHg) limit their sodium intake to 2000–3000 mg/day of sodium, which is equivalent to about 5–7.5 g/day of salt (1–1.5 tsp/day) (See Appendix I).

In practice, this means not adding table salt to foods during preparation or at meals. Encourage patients to substitute fresh herbs, pepper, or salt substitutes made from potassium chloride (such as Mrs. Dash® and NuSalt®) for table salt. In some products, potassium chloride may be substituted for sodium chloride. This additional potassium may be contraindicated in certain conditions, such as renal insufficiency. Potassium supplements should also be avoided when taking certain medications, such as angiotensin-converting enzyme (ACE) inhibitors and potassium-sparing diuretics, because of the possibility of drug–nutrient interactions.

Do you read labels for sodium content?

Since the Nutrition Labeling and Education Act of 1990 (NLEA), most processed foods display the Nutrition Facts panel, which provides sodium content to help monitor intake. During the last several decades, many lower sodium products have become available, offering greater variety to individuals who wish to maintain a low-sodium diet. The NLEA regulates nutrient-content claims used on food packages to describe the amount of nutrients per serving. Labeling claims for the sodium content of foods and beverages include the following.

• Low: ≤140 mg sodium per serving; products labeled "no added salt" are usually low in sodium but are not sodium-free because they contain naturally occurring sodium.

• Reduced or less: at least 25% less sodium compared to the amount typically present in that food.

• Light or lite: at least 50% less sodium per reference amount. A "lightly salted" product has 50% less added sodium than is normally added to the food; label must declare "not a low sodium food" if the product does not contain 140 mg sodium or less.

How many servings of fruits, vegetables and dairy foods do you eat everyday?

Aside from the benefits of sodium restriction and weight loss, investigators for the original Dietary Approaches to Stop Hypertension (DASH) trial found that a diet consisting of 8–10 servings of fruits and vegetables (four of each), two servings of low-fat dairy foods and low in saturated fat was optimal for lowering BP (See Appendix R) [40]. Among mildly hypertensive subjects SBP was reduced by 11 mmHg and DBP are reduced by 5.5 mmHg in response to the DASH diet. In the follow-up DASH-sodium trial, investigators demonstrated a synergistic effect between sodium restriction (3300 mg/day, 2400 mg/day, and 1500 mg/day) and the DASH diet in reducing BP [41].

On average, how many alcoholic beverages do you drink each week?

A large number of epidemiologic studies have established a relationship between alcohol consumption and BP [42]. Chronic excess consumption of alcohol can adversely affect BP as well as BP responsiveness to antihypertensive medications [43]. In the Atherosclerosis Risk in Communities Study, one in five cases of hypertension were estimated to be attributed to a daily intake of alcohol greater than or equal to 30 g (approximately 2 drinks) [44]. Several potential mechanisms have been identified in an attempt to explain the relationship between alcohol and elevated blood pressure, including hormonal and catecholaminergic effects, increased vascular tone, and abdominal obesity. Although an immediate effect of alcohol intake is vasodilation, sustained chronic alcohol intake is associated with increased formation of the vasoconstrictor, thromboxane [43].

It appears that the relationship between alcohol and BP is dependent on the amount, and not the type, of alcohol ingested. Furthermore, the relationship is independent of the effects of obesity, smoking, and a high sodium intake

[45]. A standard drink in the US is defined as 14 g of alcohol. This amount of alcohol is in 12 ounces of beer, 5 ounces of table wine, and 1.5 ounces of 80 proof (40% alcohol) liquor. Both the epidemiologic and randomized controlled trials provide strong evidence that in persons who drink three or more alcoholic drinks per day, a reduction in alcohol consumption can effectively lower BP [43,44].

In addition to its effects on blood pressure, increased alcohol consumption is associated with an increased risk of cardiomyopathy, hemorrhagic and ischemic strokes, certain cancers, cirrhosis, pancreatitis, gastritis, suicides, and accidents [44,46]. Conversely moderate alcohol consumption is associated with a lower incidence of atherosclerotic CVD. The cardioprotective effects associated with alcohol intake may be related to increases in high-density lipoprotein and apolipoproteins A-I and A-II, antioxidant polyphenols (quercetin, resveratrol, catechin), and reduced platelet aggregation [44,46,47]. Therefore, the current public health recommendation is moderation in alcohol consumption, defined as two drinks per day for men and one drink per day for women [48]. Alcohol provides 7 calories per gram and therefore contributes "empty calories" (nutrient-poor) to the diet which may displace more nutrient-dense foods. In patients where weight reduction is indicated, abstaining from alcohol can aid in weight management. During clinical encounters, all hypertensive patients should be questioned about their current drinking habits, including quantity and frequency of alcohol intake, in addition to their diet and exercise behaviors.

Metabolic syndrome

Definition, prevalence and diagnosis

Metabolic syndrome (MES) has been identified as an independent risk factor for CVD by ATP III and a secondary target of therapy in hypercholesterolemic patients after LDL reduction. With growing awareness that the metabolic syndrome, in which altered serum lipid levels, insulin resistance, elevated BP, and abdominal obesity greatly increase risk of diabetes and CVD morbidity and mortality, the importance of lifestyle modification has been heightened. Recent estimates indicate that 24% of US adults meet current NCEP criteria for metabolic syndrome contributing to the burgeoning epidemics of diabetes and CVD [49]. Physicians must be able to recognize patients with metabolic syndrome, make them aware of their increased risk of developing type 2 diabetes and CVD, and provide brief, but effective counseling on lifestyle changes specifically directed at achieving lipid and non-lipid goals.

Metabolic syndrome (**called dysmetabolic syndrome on ICD9 codes**), represents a cluster of metabolic abnormalities associated with abdominal obesity. Obesity frequently leads to insulin resistance, which in turn may lead to hypertension, atherogenic dyslipidemia, and impaired fasting glucose levels [50–51]. Research has also shown that other factors, such as a tendency toward

Table 7.4 Diagnostic criteria for metabolic syndrome according to the ATP III/AHA guidelines.

Component	ATP III/AHA diagnostic criteria (three of the following)
Abdominal/central obesity	Waist circumference ≥102 cm (≥40 in) in men ≥8 cm (≥35 in) in women
Elevated triglycerides	≥150 mg/dL (1.7 mmol/L) *Or* on drug treatment for elevated triglycerides
Low HDL-cholesterol	<40 mg/dL (<1.03 mMol/L) for men <50 mg/dL (<1.3 mMol/L) for women *Or* on drug treatment for reduced HDL-cholesterol
High blood pressure	≥130/85 mmHg or documented use of antihypertensive therapy
High fasting glucose	≥100 mg/dL (≥6.1 mMol/L) or on drug treatment for elevated glucose

Source: [52].

a prothrombotic and proinflammatory state, also contribute to this syndrome [50]. According to the NCEP, the criterion for metabolic syndrome includes at least three of the five clinical factors listed in Table 7.4.

The diagnosis of metabolic syndrome can serve as a starting point for discussing lifestyle modification. The five clinical criteria for metabolic syndrome can be established by means of a focused history, a brief physical exam, and fasting laboratory tests. Clinicians should add waist circumference measurement to their clinical exam or assign clinical support staff to obtain this along with the patient's BP prior to the clinician's evaluation. Waist circumference is an important marker of visceral fat which is more prognostic of metabolic syndrome than body mass index (BMI) [53]. Waist circumferences should be measured as self-reported pants size will almost always be smaller than the patient's true girth. To get the correct waist measurement, wrap a tape measure around the smallest area below the rib cage and above the umbilicus. Accuracy is important, especially for patients at risk, because abdominal obesity is a crucial pathophysiologic link to other features of metabolic syndrome, particularly insulin resistance. A waist circumference of greater than 40 inches for men and greater than 35 inches for women defines significant abdominal obesity. According to the International Diabetes Federation, waist circumference norms are smaller in populations of Asian, East Indian, and European decent (www.idf.org).

As suggested by the NCEP and the American Diabetes Association (ADA), a complete fasting lipid panel (total cholesterol, HDL-cholesterol (HDL-C), LDL-cholesterol (LDL-C), and triglyceride levels) should be performed, along with a 12-hour fasting serum glucose level in patients with identified cardiac risk. Laboratory measures of insulin resistance may provide additional value in assessing CVD risk when added to the NCEP definition of metabolic syndrome [54–55]. Insulin resistance can be identified by various methods such as the homeostasis model assessment (HOMA) index and the euglycemic insulin clamp technique [56]. However, lack of standardized assays and significant physiological variation in plasma insulin levels, even in the fasting state, make these techniques less applicable in clinical practice.

Medical Nutrition Therapy for Metabolic Syndrome

According to the NCEP, the initial and most effective strategies to treat metabolic syndrome are weight reduction and increased physical activity. Once the discussion has been initiated, the clinician can make a number of basic suggestions to help patients address this important medical condition. Getting patients to make lifestyle changes can be difficult. They are often more motivated by a possible diagnosis of diabetes rather than the threat of CVD, so using the ADA term *pre-diabetes* may be one way to stimulate interest (See Chapter 15 on Behavior Change). If lifestyle changes alone do not achieve NCEP lipid targets, drug therapy should be considered, preferably with either niacin or fish oil, to address disorders of the HDL–TG (triglyceride) axis that are characteristic of metabolic syndrome. However, if the LDL-C level has not reached the NCEP goal, this lipid abnormality should be addressed first, usually by prescribing a statin [51]. ATP III guidelines for the treatment of metabolic syndrome are summarized in Table 7.5.

Taking a diet and physical activity history

Since dietitians may be readily available in the busy primary care setting, getting a patient started on therapy requires a focused dietary and physical activity

Table 7.5 ATP III guidelines for treatment of metabolic syndrome.

Targeted area	Goal
Treat LDL-C first	
CHD and CHD risk equivalent (10-year risk for CHD >20%)	<100 mg/dL
Multiple (2+) risk factors and 10-year risk ≤20%	<130 mg/dL
Prescribe weight control	10% from baseline
Prescribe physical activity	30–40 min/day for 3–5 days/week
Monitor treatment of hypertension	<130/85 mmHg
Treat elevated triglycerides and low HDL-C	
Goal of non-HDL-C for patients with triglyceride ≥200 mg/dL and ≤499 mg/dL	High CHD risk: <130 mg/dL Intermediate CHD risk: <160 mg/dL Low CHD risk: <190 mg/dL

Non-HDL defined as VLDL + LDL
Source: [57].

assessment. Medical nutrition therapy in patients with metabolic syndrome is intended to:
• reduce weight by reducing total calories and increasing physical activity;
• replace calories from saturated fat and simple carbohydrates with monounsaturated fatty acids and omega-3 FAs.

Several key questions asked during a focused diet history will enable the clinician and the patient to develop a nutrition plan to achieve these goals. Since patients with metabolic syndrome will benefit from dietary changes related to specific nutrients and to overall total calories, reviewing every question at an initial visit may take up too much time. So specific issues should be discussed over the course of several visits, depending on time availability and a patient's motivation level. Prioritize issues depending on diagnosis and laboratory results. Improvements in nutritional status – as indicated by weight, BMI, waist circumference, BP, and lipid and glucose levels – should be documented. Patients who require complex dietary changes and those who are highly motivated and have many specific questions would benefit from a referral to a registered dietitian.

The activity assessment should focus on identifying how frequently the patient is involved in moderate to vigorous activity followed by suggesting increasing daily functional physical activity. One method of initiating an exercise regimen is by writing a prescription that specifies the frequency for a regular walking program, and suggest other ways to increase daily physical activity in everyday life.

Assessing carbohydrate intake: simple vs. complex

While the NCEP recommends that carbohydrates be the major source of calories (50–60% of total calories), patients need to be aware that both the quantity and quality of their carbohydrate intake influences their risk for metabolic syndrome and can increase body weight [51]. Excess consumption of simple sugars can increase TG levels while depressing HDL-C levels [56,58]. In the last decade, nutritionists and physicians have recommended low-fat diets for CVD prevention. The message was misinterpreted as sanctioning an increase in the consumption of fat-free, carbohydrate-rich processed foods. This worrisome trend, coupled with decreased physical activity, is believed to be associated with the epidemic of obesity and diabetes in this country and an increase in the prevalence of metabolic syndrome. Consequently a number of high-protein, low-carbohydrate diets, such as the Atkins and Zone diets, became very popular despite the lack of rigorous scientific investigation [59,60]. While these diets result in weight loss, their effects on lipids, bone metabolism, renal function, and cardiovascular risk are still unknown.

One of the major misconceptions about these diets is the notion that all carbohydrates are created equal. This ignores the important distinction between the two major subtypes of carbohydrates–simple and complex, which affect blood glucose and lipid metabolism very differently. Several epidemiologic studies have found that diets rich in whole grains are associated with a lower risk of CVD, type 2 diabetes and stroke [27,56,61,62]. According to the AHA and the NCEP, the intake of simple carbohydrates should be minimized, while the intake of complex sources of carbohydrates, which are higher in fiber, should be increased [48]. This emphasis of complex over refined carbohydrates is embodied in the glycemic index (GI) concept, in which complex sources of carbohydrates (low GI) are preferred to refined products (high GI) [63]. The GI ranks foods according to their ability to raise postprandial blood glucose levels compared with 50 g glucose or equivalent carbohydrate load as white bread. Diets tailored to lower the GI have been shown in small studies to reduce TG levels and raise HDL-C levels [63]. In a recent cross-sectional study among participants of the Framingham Offspring Study, consumption of whole grain foods and low GI diets were inversely associated with insulin resistance and risk of metabolic syndrome [64]. Whether GI-tailored diets will be effective, acceptable, and understandable to patients over the long-term remains to be seen.

Simple or refined carbohydrates are foods that have a high concentration of disaccharides such as sucrose (sugar), fructose (found in fruits), and lactose (found in milk). The primary offender is sugar, which has been associated with reductions in HDL-C levels and increases in TG levels. It has also been linked in some, but not all, epidemiologic studies to CVD and obesity [58]. The major sources of sugar in the American diet are table sugar, naturally sweetened beverages such as regular soda and fruit juices, or foods such as sweetened cereals, candy, dried fruit, and baked and frozen desserts. Based on epidemiologic data, the average American consumed 150 lb of sugar in 1995, up from 120 lb in 1970 [58]. Complex carbohydrates are primarily represented by fresh fruits, vegetables, whole grains and legumes and serve as natural sources of dietary fiber.

The NCEP recommends the inclusion of 20–30 g/day of dietary fiber, 10 g/day of which should come from soluble or viscous fiber. In the US the average adult fiber intake is only 16 g/day. Soluble fiber alone has no effect on the HDL-TG axis, but it does have a modest effect on reducing LDL-C levels and has been shown in epidemiologic studies to reduce the risk of CVD [7]. Oatmeal, beans, citrus fruits, split peas, and broccoli are some of the best sources of soluble fiber, with approximately 2–4 g per serving (See Appendix O). In addition, foods that contain dietary fiber often take longer to eat and may increase satiety by delaying gastric emptying, which assists in glucose handling and weight management. Carbohydrate consumption can easily be assessed by asking patients the following four simple questions.

What do you like to drink during the day?
Regular soda, sugar-sweetened iced tea, soft drinks, sports drinks (such as Gatorade) and fruit juices contribute a significant amount of calories and simple carbohydrates, both of which can affect body weight and TG levels. By quantifying patients' beverage intake and suggesting that they substitute plain or seltzer water with meals and snacks, you can help them save

hundreds of calories per day. If they are able to make only one dietary change, this may be the most realistic and effective one. In addition, alcohol intake should always be quantified. Although alcohol has been shown to be cardio-protective in certain patients, it contributes a significant amount of calories and can raise TG levels. For example, 6 oz red wine has approximately 120 calories, and 12 oz of regular beer has 150 calories, equivalent to a 12 oz can of regular soda. Alcohol also weakens the patient's resolve not to overeat and can thus contribute to many collateral calories. Limit alcohol in all patients with metabolic syndrome to one drink per day or seven per week.

How much bread, pasta, and potatoes do you generally eat?
In our culture, people tend to eat far too much of these foods, leading to ex-cessive carbohydrate and calorie consumption. Ask specifically about white bread, dinner rolls, bagels, soft pretzels, white pasta, white rice, and mashed or fried potatoes. Unless fortified, these foods tend to be low in nutrient value and high in calories. Suggest that patients eat whole grains such as wheat, rye, or pumpernickel breads, whole wheat pasta, brown rice, or baked pota-toes with the skin instead. Advise them to try one substitution every 2 weeks as a way of introducing new foods. This approach will increase fiber intake, delaying glucose absorption and improving the HDL-TG axis.

What type of snacks and desserts do you eat?
Snacks and desserts such as cookies, crackers, pretzels, candy bars, cakes, pies, and ice cream contain high amounts of simple carbohydrates as well as satu-rated and trans fats and calories, which could contribute to weight gain and increased TG levels in patients with metabolic syndrome. Remind patients to check the labels of snack foods for hidden sugars in the guise of ingredients such as brown sugar, molasses, honey, high fructose corn syrup, sorbitol, and juice concentrate. Substituting fresh fruit for desserts will also help reduce to-tal fat and calories, but patients should also be advised to skip the snack and share the dessert. If patients cannot give up snacking, suggest a piece of fruit or small handful of walnuts, pecans, almonds or unsalted dry roasted peanuts. A serving of nuts will help increase MUFA and fiber intake, which can improve the dyslipidemia associated with the metabolic syndrome.

How often do you eat fruits and vegetables?
Increasing fruit and vegetable intake will address both the glucose and BP abnormalities in patients with the metabolic syndrome. You can help your patient reach the goal of 7–9 servings a day by suggesting that they add fruit to their morning cereal; snack on fresh fruit, celery, or carrot sticks; or even drink a glass of a low-sodium vegetable beverage (such as V8 vegetable juice).

Key diet history questions for patients

Several key questions will help the clinician focus on specific nutritional recommendations for the individual patient.

Questions for all patients
- How many meals do you eat outside the home?
- How many servings of fruits and vegetables do you eat everyday?
- How many servings of dairy foods do you eat everyday?
- On average how many alcoholic beverages do you drink weekly?
- How often do you exercise, including walking?

For the patient with hypercholesterolemia
- What type of oil do you use in cooking?
- Do you use butter or margarine (Soft tub or stick)?
- Do you eat full-fat cheese, whole milk, and ice cream?
- How often do you eat fatty meats (bacon, sausage, hot dogs, spare ribs)
- How often do you eat fried foods?

For the patient with hypertension
- Do you use a salt shaker at the table or in cooking?
- Do you read labels for sodium content?
- How often do you eat canned, processed, or salted foods?

For the patient with metabolic syndrome
- What do you like to drink during the day?
- How many servings of bread, pasta, and potatoes do you eat daily?
- What type of snacks and desserts do you eat?

Source: [65].

Physical activity and cardiovascular risk factors

Physical activity may prevent and treat many of the established risk factors for CVD including high BP, insulin resistance and impaired glucose tolerance, high triglyceride levels, low HDL-C levels, and obesity [66]. In addition, sustained physical activity is beneficial to prevent weight regain and improve fitness [67]. According to the CDC, more than 60% of US adults do not get the recommended amount of physical activity and approximately 25% are not active at all [68]. Both observational and intervention studies suggest that brisk walking for 30 minutes per day on most days of the week can reduce the risk of CVD and type 2 diabetes by at least 30% [69]. The recently published Diabetes Prevention Program study reinforced the exercise approach by showing that incorporating 150 minutes per week of at least moderate physical activity could reduce the risk of developing type 2 diabetes by 58% [70]. This level of physical activity can be achieved simply by increasing levels of physical

Table 7.6 Common examples of moderate and vigorous physical activity.

Moderate activity	Vigorous activity
Walking 3–4.5 mph	Race walking 5 mph or greater or jogging
Bicycling 5–9 mph on level terrain	Bicycling more than 10 mph or on a steep uphill terrain
Water aerobics	Step aerobics
Yoga	Performing jumping jacks
Ballroom dancing	Karate, judo, tae kwon do
Tennis-doubles	Tennis-singles
Golf, wheeling or carrying clubs	Squash, racquetball
Weight training using free weights	Circuit weight training
Hand washing and waxing a car	Cross-country and downhill skiing
Gardening and yard work: raking leaves, weeding, light snow shoveling, stacking wood, pushing a power lawn mower	Gardening and yard work: pushing a non-motorized lawn mower, heavy snow shoveling (more than 10 lbs per minute), hand-splitting firewood
Moderate housework: scrubbing bathroom, washing windows, vacuuming	Heavy housework: moving or pushing heavy furniture
Sailing, recreational swimming, treading water	Swimming: steady paced laps

Source: Adapted from [71].

activity in daily life. Routine daily activities include actions such as taking the stairs instead of the elevator at work or parking farther away from one's destination and then walking [70]. Clinicians can assess activity levels in their patient by asking, "Do you exercise regularly, including walking?" This question can initiate the physical activity discussion. Several common activities that constitute at least moderate physical activity are listed in Table 7.6. Other simple tips for increasing physical activity include:
• exercising with a partner;
• taking multiple 5-minute walks throughout the day; and
• wearing a step counter (pedometer) to keep track of the number of steps taken throughout the day: the goal should be at least 5000 steps per day.

By assessing baseline physical activity and providing patients with an exercise prescription, health care professionals can start the process of getting sedentary patients with metabolic syndrome to be more physically active.

Conclusion

In conclusion, if primary care clinicians spend time focusing on these lifestyle recommendations, the burden of cardiovascular disease may be reduced in the years to come. Table 7.7 provides a summary of the dietary and physical activity interventions for hyperlipidemia, hypertension, and metabolic syndrome as outlined in this chapter.

Table 7.7 Medical Nutrition Therapy targeting specific abnormalities.

Abnormality	Diet and physical activity interventions	Practical advice
Abdominal obesity	Weight reduction Increase physical activity	Reduce portion sizes to cut calories 30 minutes of moderate intensity exercise daily
Hypercholesterolemia	Limit saturated and trans fats Weight reduction Increase soluble fiber Include plant stanol/sterols Increase physical activity	Replace saturated and trans fats (butter, cheese, bacon, french fries) with PUFAs (soybean oil) or MUFAs (nuts, canola oil or olive oil) Replace refined carbohydrates (bagels, bread, soft pretzels, white rice and pasta) with brown rice, oatmeal, fresh fruits and vegetables Replace stick margarine with soft tub margarine, Benecol or Take Control spreads 30 minutes of moderate intensity exercise daily
Hypertriglyceridemia	Weight reduction Increase physical activity Reduce total carbohydrates Increase low GI foods Increase omega-3 fatty acids Limit alcohol	Replace refined carbohydrates (white bread, potatoes, pasta) with MUFAs (nuts, avocado, canola oil or olive oil) Replace soda and juices with water, seltzer and diet beverages Eat fish at least once a week Limit alcohol to no more than 2 drinks/ day for men and 1 drink/day for women Limit intake of sweets and baked desserts
Low HDL-C	Weight reduction Increase physical activity Replace carbohydrates with monounsaturated fat Quit smoking	Reduce portion sizes to cut calories 30 minutes of moderate intensity exercise daily Eat fish, nuts, avocado. Use olive or canola oils in salad dressing and for cooking Join a smoking cessation program
Hypertension	Weight reduction Increase physical activity Reduce sodium intake Reduce saturated fat intake Increase fruits and vegetables Increase low-fat dairy products Moderate alcohol consumption	Reduce portion sizes to cut calories 30 minutes of moderate intensity exercise daily Reduce salt intake to no more than 2.4 g/day or 6 g/day NaCl by using more herbs in cooking Read labels for sodium content Skip the salt shaker Consume at least 5 servings of fruits and vegetables every day 3 servings of low-fat dairy/day Limit alcohol to no more than 2 drinks/day for men and 1 drink/day for women

(Continued)

Table 7.7 (*Continued*)

Abnormality	Diet and physical activity interventions	Practical advice
High fasting glucose	Weight reduction Increase physical activity Reduce total carbohydrates Replace carbohydrates with MUFAs Increase low GI foods Increase dietary fiber (>30 g/day)	Reduce portion sizes to cut calories 30 minutes of moderate intensity exercise daily Replace refined grains with whole grains, such as oatmeal, brown rice, whole wheat bread and MUFAs (nuts, avocado, canola oil or olive oil) Add legumes and beans for soluble fiber

Source: Darwin Deen, MD, Albert Einstein College of Medicine, Lisa Hark, PhD, RD, and Frances Burke, MS, RD, University of Pennsylvania School of Medicine. 2007. Used with permission.

References

1 Thom T, Haase N, Rosamond W *et al.* Heart Disease and Stroke Statistics–2006 Update: A Report From the American Heart Association Statistics Committee and Stroke Statistics Subcommittee. *Circulation* 2006;113(6): e85–e151.

2 National Heart, Lung, and Blood Institute *Third Report of the National Cholesterol Education Program Expert Panel on Detection, Evaluation, and Treatment of High Blood Cholesterol in Adults (Adult Treatment Panel III). Executive Summary.* Bethesda, MD: National Institutes of Health; 2001. NIH publication 01-3670.

3 Grundy SM, Cleeman JI, Merz NB *et al.*, for the Coordinating Committee of the National Cholesterol Education Program. Implications of recent clinical trials for the National Cholesterol Education Program Adult Treatment Panel III guidelines. *Circulation* 2004;110:227–39.

4 Olendzki B, Speed C, Domino FJ. Nutritional assessment and counseling for prevention and treatment of cardiovascular disease. *American Family Physician* 2006;73:257–264.

5 Schaefer EJ. Lipoproteins, nutrition, and heart disease. *Am J Clin Nutr* 2002;75:191–212.

6 Fletcher B, Berra K, Ades P *et al.* AHA Scientific Statement. Managing abnormal blood lipids, a collaborative approach. *Circulation* 2005;112:3184–209.

7 Hu FB, Willett WC. Optimal diets for prevention of coronary heart disease. *JAMA* 2002;288:2569–78.

8 Lichtenstein AH, Ausman LM, Jalbert SM, Schaefer EJ. Effects of different forms of dietary hydrogenated fats on serum lipoprotein cholesterol levels. *N Engl J Med* 1999;340:1933–40.

9 US Food and Drug Administration. Department of Health and Human Services. Revealing Trans Fats. *FDA Consumer*. September–October 2003. Pub No. FDA04–1329C.

10 Turley SD. Cholesterol metabolism and therapeutic targets: rationale for targeting multiple metabolic pathways. *Clin Cardiol* 2004;6(Suppl 3):III16–21.

11 Hu FB, Stampfer MJ, Rimm EB *et al.* A prospective study of egg consumption and risk of cardiovascular disease in men and women. *JAMA* 1999;281:1387–94.

12 Kritchevsky SB. A review of scientific research and recommendations regarding eggs. *J Am Coll of Nutr* 2004;23:596S–600S.

13 AHA Dietary Guidelines Revision 2000: A Statement for Healthcare Professionals from the Nutrition Committee of the American Heart Association. *Circulation* 2000; 102:2284–2299.

14 Parikh P, McDaniel MC, Ashen MD *et al.* Diets and cardiovascular disease. *J Am Coll Cardiol* 2005;45:1379–87.

15 de Lorgeril M, Renaud S, Mamelle N *et al.* Mediterranean alpha-linolenic acid-rich diet in secondary prevention of coronary heart disease. *Lancet* 1994;343:1454–9.

16 Food and Nutrition Board, Institute of Medicine, National Academy of Sciences. *Dietary Reference Intakes for Energy, Carbohydrate, Fiber, Fat, Fatty Acids, Cholesterol, Protien, and Amino Acids*, National Academy of Medicine. National Academies Press. Washington, DC, 2002.

17 DeFilippis AP, Sperling LS. Understanding omega 3's. *Am Heart J* 2006;151:564–70.

18 Harper CR, Jacobson TA. The fats of life: the role of omega-3 fatty acids in the prevention of coronary heart disease. *Arch Intern Med* 2001;161:2185–92.

19 Oh R. Practical Applications of fish oil in primary care. *J Am Board Fam Pract* 2005;18:28–36.

20 Kris-Etherton PM, Harris WS, Appel LJ. AHA Nutrition Committee. Fish consumption, fish oil, omega-3 fatty acids, and cardiovascular disease. *Circulation* 2002;106:2747–57.

21 Marlett JA, McBurney MI, Slavin JL. Position of the American Dietetic Association: health implications of dietary fiber. *J Am Diet Assoc* 2002;102:993–1000.

22 US Department of Agriculture Dietary Guidelines. http://www.healthierus.gov /dietaryguidelines/

23 Jensen MK, Koh-Banerjee P, Hu FB, Franz M, Sampson L, Gronbaek M, Rimm EB. Intakes of whole grains, bran, and germ and the risk of coronary heart disease in men. *Am J Clin Nutr* 2004;80:1492–9.

24 Jacobs, Jr DR, Meyer KA, Kushi LH, Folsom AR. Is whole grain intake associated with reduced total and cause-specific death rates in older women? The Iowa Women's Health Study. *Am J Public Health* 1999;89:322–9.

25 Anderson JW, Hanna TH, Peng X, Kryscio RJ. Whole grain foods and heart disease risk. *J Am Coll Nutr* 2000;19:291S–299S.

26 Liu S, Manson JE, Stampfer MJ *et al.* Whole grain consumption and risk of ischemic stroke in women: A prosective study. *JAMA* 2000;284:1534–40.

27 Bazzano LA, Serdula M, Liu S. Prevention of type 2 diabetes by diet and lifestyle modification. *J Am Coll Nutr* 2005;24:310–19.

28 Lichtenstein AH, Deckelbaum RJ for the American Heart Association Nutrition Committee. AHA Science Advisory. Stanol/sterol ester-containing foods and blood cholesterol levels. A statement for healthcare professionals from the Nutrition Committee of the Council on Nutrition, Physical Activity, and Metabolism of the American Heart Association. *Circulation* 2001;103(8):1177–9.

29 Miettinen TA, Puska P, Gylling H, Vanhanen H, Vartiainen E. Reduction of serum cholesterol with sitonstanol-ester margarine in a mildly hypercholesterolemic population. *N Engl J Med* 1995;333:1308–12.

30 Hallikainen MA, Sarkkinen ES, Uusitupa MI. Plant stanol esters affect serum cholesterol concentrations of hypercholesterolemic men and women in a dose-dependent manner. *J Nutr* 2000;130:767–76.

31 Gylling H, Miettinen TA. LDL cholesterol lowering by bile acid malabsorption during inhibited synthesis and absorption of cholesterol in hypercholesterolemic coronary subjects. *Nutr Metab Cardiovasc Dis* 2002;12:19–23.

32 Blair SN, Capuzzi DM, Gottlieb SO, Nguyen T, Morgan JM, Cater NB. Incremental reduction of serum total cholesterol and low-density lipoprotein cholesterol with the addition of plant stanol ester-containing spread to statin therapy. *Am J Cardiol* 2000;86:46–52.

33 Jenkins DJ, Kendall CW, Marchie A *et al*. Effects of a dietary portfolio of cholesterol-lowering foods vs lovastatin on serum lipids and C-reactive protein. *JAMA* 2003;290:502–10.

34 Jenkins DJ, Kendall CW, Faulkner DA *et al*. Assessment of the longer-term effects of a dietary portfolio of cholesterol-lowering foods in hypercholesterolemia. *Am J Clin Nutr* 2006;83:582–91.

35 National High Blood Pressure Education Program Coordinating Committee. The seventh report of the Joint National Committee on Prevention, Detection, Evaluation and Treatment of High Blood Pressure. The JNC 7 Report. *JAMA* 2003;289:2560–72.

36 Fields LE, Burt VL, Cutler JA, Hughes J, Roccella EJ, Sorlie P. The burden of adult hypertension in the United States 1999 to 2000: a rising tide. *Hypertension* 2004 Oct;44:398–404.

37 Appel LJ, Brands MW, Daniels SR, Karanja N, Elmer PJ, Sacks FM. Dietary approaches to prevent and treat hypertension. A Scientific Statement from the American Heart Association. *Hypertension*. 2006;47:296–308.

38 Loria CM, Obarzanek E, Ernst ND. Choose and prepare foods with less salt: dietary advice for all Americans. *J Nutrition* 2001;131:536S–551S.

39 Elliot P. Salt and Blood Pressure. In: Izzo JL Jr, Black HR eds. *Hypertension Primer: The Essentials of High Blood Pressure*. 3rd ed. Dallas, Texas: American Heart Association; 2003;277–9.

40 Appel LJ, Moore TJ, Obarzanek E *et al*. A clinical trial of the effects of dietary patterns on blood pressure. *N Engl J Med* 1997;336:1117–24.

41 Sacks FM, Svetkey LP, Vollmer WM *et al*., for the DASH-Sodium Collaborative Research Group. Effects on blood pressure of reduced dietary sodium and the Dietary Approaches to Stop Hypertension (DASH) diet. *N Engl J Med* 2001;344:3–10.

42 Xin X, He J, Frontini MG, Ogsen LG. Motsamai OI, Whelton PK. Effects of alcohol reduction on blood pressure: a meta-analysis of randomized controlled trials. *Hypertension* 2001;38:1112–17.

43 Cushman WC. Alcohol use and blood pressure. In: Izzo JL Jr, Black HR eds. *Hypertension Primer: The Essentials of High Blood Pressure*. 3rd ed. Dallas, Texas: American Heart Association; 2003;290–4.

44 Fuchs FD, Chambless LE, Whelton PK, Nieto FJ, Heiss G. Alcohol consumption and the incidence of hypertension. The Atherosclerosis Risk in Communities Study. *Hypertension* 2001;37:1242–50.

45 Klatsky AL. Alcohol and hypertension. *Clin Chim Acta* 1996;246:91–105.

46 Goldberg IJ, Mosca L, Piano MR, Fisher EA. AHA Science Advisory. Wine and your heart: A science advisory for healthcare professionals from the Nutrition Committee, Council on Epidemiology and Prevention, and Council on Cardiovascular Nursing of the American Heart Association. *Stroke* 2001 Feb;32(2):591–4.

47 De Oliveira e Silva ER, Foster D, McGee Harper M *et al*. Alcohol consumption raises HDL cholesterol levels by increasing the transport rate of apolipoproteins A-I and A-II. *Circulation* 2000;102:2347–52.

48 Krauss RM, Eckel RH, Howard B *et al*. AHA Dietary Guidelines: revision 2000: a statement for healthcare professionals from the Nutrition Committee of the American Heart Association. *Circulation* 2000;102:2284–99.

49 Ford E, Giles W, Dietz W. Prevalence of the metabolic syndrome among US adults. *JAMA* 2002;287:356–9.

50 Reaven G. Metabolic syndrome:pathophysiology and implications for management of cardiovascular disease. *Circulation* 2002;106:286–8.

51 Szapary PO, Hark LA, Burke FM. The metabolic syndrome: a new focus for lifestyle modification. *Patient Care* 2002;36:75–88.

52 Grundy SM, Cleeman JI, Daniels SR *et al*. Diagnosis and management of the metabolic syndrome: an American Heart Association/National Heart, Lung, and Blood Institute Scientific Statement. *Circulation* 2005;112(17):2735–52.

53 Rexrode KM, Carey VJ, Hennekens CH *et al*. Abdominal adiposity and coronary heart disease in woman. *JAMA* 1998;280:1843–8.

54 Reilly MP, Wolfe M, Rhodes T, Girman C, Mehta N, Rader DJ. Measures of insulin resistance add incremental value to the clinical diagnosis of metabolic syndrome in association with coronary atherosclerosis. *Circulation* 2004;110:803–9.

55 Sierra-Johnson J, Johnson BD, Allison TG, Bailey KR, Schwartz GL, Turner ST. Correspondence between the Adult Treatment Panel III criteria for metabolic syndrome and insulin resistance. *Diabetes Care* 2006;29:668–72.

56 Deen D. Metabolic syndrome: a practical guide for clinicians. *Am Fam Physician* 2004, 69(12): 2875–82.

57 Vega LG. Obesity, the metabolic syndrome, and cardiovascular disease. *Am Heart J* 2001;142:1108–16.

58 Howard BV, Wylie-Rosett J. Sugar and cardiovascular disease: a statement for healthcare professionals from the Committee on Nutrition of the Council on Nutrition, Physical Activity, and Metabolism of the American Heart Association. *Circulation* 2002;106: 523–7.

59 Freedman MR, King J, Kennedy E. Popular diets: a scientific review. *Obesity Research* 2001; 9(Suppl 1):1S–40S.

60 St. Jeor ST, Howard BV, Prewitt TE, Bovee V, Bazzarre T, Eckel RH. Dietary protein and weight reduction: a statement for healthcare professionals from the Nutrition Committee of the Council on Nutrition, Physical Activity, and Metabolism of the American Heart Association. *Circulation* 2001;104:1869–74.

61 Liu S. Intake of refined carbohydrates and whole grains in relation to risk of type 2 diabetes mellitus and coronary heart disease. *J Am Coll Nutr* 2002;21:298–306.

62 Meyer KA, Kushi LH, Jacobs DR Jr, Slavin J, Sellers TA, Folsom AR. Carbohydrates, dietary fiber, and incident type 2 diabetes in older women. *Am J Clin Nutr* 2000;71:921–30.

63 Ludwig DS. The glycemic index: physiological mechanisms relating to obesity, diabetes, and cardiovascular disease. *JAMA* 2002;287:2414–23.

64 McKeown NM, Meigs JB, Lui S, Saltzmann E, Wilson PWF, Jacques P. Carbohydrate nutrition, insulin resistance, and the prevalence of the metabolic syndrome in the Framingham Offspring Cohort. *Diabetes Care* 2004;27:538–46.

65 Hark L and Morrison G (eds). *Medical Nutrition and Disease, 3rd edition*. Blackwell Publishing, Malden, MA. 2003.

66 Thompson PD, Buchner D, Pina IL, *et al*; American Heart Association Council on Clinical Cardiology Subcommittee on Exercise, Rehabilitation, and Prevention; American Heart Association Council on Nutrition, Physical Activity, and Metabolism Subcommittee on Physical Activity. Exercise and physical activity in the prevention and treatment of atherosclerotic cardiovascular disease: a statement from the Council on Clinical Cardiology (Subcommittee on Exercise, Rehabilitation, and Prevention) and the Council on Nutrition, Physical Activity, and Metabolism (Subcommittee on Physical Activity). *Circulation* 2003;107(24):3109–3116.

67 Stone NJ, Saxon D. Approach to the treatment of the patient with metabolic syndrome: lifestyle therapy. *Am J Cardiol* 2005;96(suppl): 15E–21E.

68 *Physical Activity and Health: A Report of the Surgeon General*. Atlanta, GA: US Dept of Health and Human Services. Centers for Disease Control and Prevention, National Center for Chronic Disease Prevention and Health Promotion; 1996.

69 Chakravarthy MV, Joyner MJ, Booth FW. An obligation for primary care physicians to prescribe physical activity to sedentary patients to reduce the risk of chronic health conditions. *Mayo Clin Proc* 2002;77:165–73.

70 Knowler WC, Barrett-Connor E, Fowler SE *et al*. Reduction in the incidence of type 2 diabetes with lifestyle intervention or metformin. *N Engl J Med* 2002;346:393–403.

71 Ainsworth BE, Haskell WL, Leon AS *et al*. Compendium of physical activities: classification of energy costs of human physical activities. *Medicine and Science in Sports and Exercise.* 1993;25:71–80. www.gov/ncdcccdphp/dnpa/physical/pdf/PA_Intensity_table_2_1.pdf

CHAPTER 8

Diabetes, Pre-diabetes and Hypoglycemia

Marion J Franz and Richard Wender

Introduction to medical nutritional therapy

There have been major changes in nutrition recommendations and therapy over the past decade. Medical nutrition therapy (MNT) remains essential for effective diabetes management and successful nutrition therapy is an ongoing process. When prioritizing nutrition recommendations, the focus is first on the interventions that are likely to have the most positive effect on metabolic outcomes. Using effective teaching and counseling skills helps to develop relationships of trust and mutual respect. Outcomes must be measured and effective nutrition therapy is a process of problem solving, adjustment and readjustment.

It is essential that primary care clinicians understand nutrition issues and guide the patient's efforts. This can be accomplished by reinforcing basic and important messages, by referring patients with a new diagnosis of prediabetes or diabetes for nutrition therapy, by promoting the importance of lifestyle modifications, and by providing support for the lifestyle intervention process.

Medical nutrition therapy for diabetes is guided by evidence-based recommendations that require using the best available scientific evidence while taking into account individual circumstances, cultural and ethnic concerns, and involving the patient in decision making. Understanding the expected outcomes from nutrition therapy as well as evaluating the best implementation approach can assist the primary care clinician in the clinical decision making process. If treatment goals are not being achieved by lifestyle interventions (nutrition therapy and physical activity), changes in medication(s) are required. Table 8.1 outlines appropriate therapeutic goals, established by the American Diabetes Association [1].

It is essential that primary care clinicians express support for lifestyle changes and diabetes education. Referring patients with diabetes or pre-diabetes to registered dietitians (RDs) for MNT and diabetes self-management training (DSMT) is an important first step. Although MNT has the greatest impact at initial diagnosis, it continues to be effective throughout the disease process. However, one counseling session is not enough – continuing education and follow-up is beneficial. The results of nutrition interventions, regardless of

Table 8.1 Glucose, lipids, and blood pressure recommendations for adults with diabetes.

Glycemic control	
A1C	<7.0%*
Preprandial plasma glucose	90–130 mg/dL (5.0–7.2 mMol/L)
Postprandial plasma glucose	<180 mg/dL (<10.0 mMol/l)
Blood pressure	<130/80 mmHg
Lipids	
LDL cholesterol	<100 mg/dL (<2.6 mMol/L)
Triglycerides	<150 mg/dL (<1.7 mMol/L)
HDL cholesterol	>40 mg/dL (>1.1 mMol/L)[†]

*Referenced to a nondiabetic range of 4.0–6.0% using a Diabetes Control and Complications Trial (DCCT) based assay.
[†]For women, it has been suggested that the HDL goal be increased by 10 mg/dL.
Source: [1].

whether the clinical outcomes have improved, stayed the same, or worsened, must be shared with the primary care clinician and the diabetes education team. Failure to achieve therapeutic goals often results from progression of diabetes as opposed to dietary noncompliance. Helping patients understand the natural progression of diabetes is a responsibility of the care team.

This chapter reviews expected outcomes from diabetes MNT, prioritizes evidence-based lifestyle recommendations for type 1 and type 2 diabetes and pre-diabetes and summarizes strategies that primary care clinicians can use to be supportive of lifestyle interventions and education.

Medical Nutrition Therapy outcomes for diabetes

Primary care clinicians need to be knowledgeable about both expected outcomes from an intervention and when to re-evaluate these outcomes. Individuals should be referred for MNT at diagnosis and outcomes should be assessed at 6 weeks to 3 months. However, ongoing support for lifestyle interventions and six month to one year assessments and review of MNT are important. Randomized controlled clinical trials and outcomes research support MNT provided by RDs as effective in reaching treatment goals. In persons with newly diagnosed type 2 diabetes, decreases in hemoglobin A1c (A1C) of approximately 2 units and in persons with an average duration of type 2 diabetes of 4 years, decreases of 1 unit (a 12–24% decrease in A1C) can be expected [2]. These outcomes are similar to those from oral glucose lowering medications. In persons with type 1 diabetes who were taught to adjust their insulin doses based on planned carbohydrate intake [3] or with newly diagnosed type 1 diabetes [2], A1C may decrease by approximately 1 unit. The outcomes of the initial intervention can be seen by 3 months. If goals have not been met, medication(s) need to be added or adjusted. However, attention to lifestyle

Table 8.2 Effectiveness of medical nutrition therapy.

Endpoint	Expected outcome	When to evaluate
Glycemic control		
A1C	1–2 unit (15–22%) decrease	6 weeks to 3 months
Plasma fasting	50–100 mg/dL (2.78–5.56	
Glucose	mMol/L) decrease	
Lipids		
Total cholesterol	24–32 mg/dL [0.62–0.82 mmol/l] (10–16%) decrease	6 weeks; if goals are not achieved, intensify nutrition therapy and evaluate again in 6 weeks
LDL cholesterol	19–25 mg/L (0.46–0.65 mmol/L) (12–16%) decrease	
Triglycerides	15–17 mg/dL (0.17–0.19 mmol/L) (8%) decrease	
HDL cholesterol	With no exercise: 7% decrease With exercise: No decrease	
Blood pressure (in hypertensive patients)	5 mmHg decrease in systolic and 2 mmHg decrease in diastolic	Measure at every visit

Source: Adapted with permission from [2].

continues to be important as medications are more effective when attention is also given to food intake and physical activity. Table 8.2 is a summary of the mean expected outcomes from MNT on glucose, lipids, and / or blood pressure.

Diabetes nutrition recommendations

Primary care clinicians should be knowledgeable about evidence-based diabetes nutrition recommendations. Prior to 1994, diabetes nutrition recommendations attempted to define an ideal nutrition prescription that would apply to all persons with diabetes and which identified calorie levels and ideal percentages of carbohydrate, protein, and fat. Although individualization was recommended, this approach did not allow for much, if any, real individualization. In 1994, the American Diabetes Association (ADA) recommended that instead of a rigid nutrition prescription, the nutrition prescription should be based on treatment goals, the patient's metabolic profile, known strategies that would assist the patient to meet treatment goals, and most importantly, on changes the patient is willing and able to make. Some changes could include those listed below [4].

1) Reducing energy intake: eating smaller food portions reduces caloric intake and is associated with improvements in glycemic control.

2) Consistently eating three meals a day, especially breakfast: it is important to make time in schedules for eating and to not skip meals.

3) Gradually increasing physical activity: the goal is to accumulate 30 minutes a day or at least 150 min/week.

This more flexible and realistic approach continues with the current ADA nutrition recommendations [5,6]. In addition, the technical review and position statement grade the recommendations (A, B, C, and expert consensus) based on the level of available evidence. The grading of nutrition recommendations can also be used to prioritize care. Table 8.3 is a summary of nutrition-related recommendations for diabetes.

Table 8.3 Nutrition-related recommendations for diabetes.

Nutrient	Recommendations
Carbohydrate	A dietary pattern that includes carbohydrate from fruits, vegetables, whole grains, legumes, and low-fat milk is encouraged for good health (Grade B)
	Monitoring carbohydrate, whether by carbohydrate counting, exchanges, or experience based estimation remains a a key strategy in achieving glycemic control (Grade A)
	Sucrose-containing foods can be substituted for other carbohydrates in the meal plan or, if added to the meal plan, covered with insulin or other glucose lowering medications; care should be taken to avoid excess energy intake (Grade A)
	Non-nutritive sweeteners and sugar alcohols are safe when consumed within the daily intake levels established by the Food and Drug Administration (Grade A)
	As for the general population, people with diabetes are encouraged to consume a variety of fiber-containing foods; however, evidence is lacking to recommend a higher fiber intake for people with diabetes than for the population as a whole (Grade B)
	The use of the glycemic index and load provides a modest additional benefit over that observed when total carbohydrate is considered alone (Grade B)
	Low carbohydrate diets, restricting total carbohydrate to <130 g/day, are not recommended in the management of diabetes (Expert Consensus)
	All persons with diabetes can benefit from basic information about carbohydrates: what foods contain carbohydrate (starches, fruits, starchy vegetables, milk, sweets), average 15 g portion sizes, and how many servings to select for meals (and snacks, if desired)
Protein	For individuals with diabetes and normal renal function, there is insufficient evidence to suggest that usual protein intake (15–20% of energy) should be modified (Expert Consensus)
	In persons with diabetes, ingested protein does not increase plasma glucose concentrations but does increase serum insulin responses (Grade A)
	Reduction of protein intake to 0.8–1.0 g/kg/day in individuals with diabetes and the earlier stages of chronic kidney disease (CKD) and to 0.8 g/kg/day in the later stages of CKD may improve measures of renal function, such as urine albumin excretion rate and glomerular filtration rate (Grade B)
	Protein does not slow the absorption of carbohydrate or affect peak glucose response. There is no evidence that adding protein to bedtime snacks is helpful nor that adding protein to the treatment of hypoglycemia improves treatment or prevents subsequent hypoglycemia

(Continued)

Table 8.3 Nutrition-related recommendations for diabetes. (*Continued*)

Fat	The cardiovascular risk of individuals with diabetes is considered to be equivalent to that of nondiabetic individuals with pre-existing cardiovascular disease; therefore, individuals with diabetes may benefit from lowering saturated fatty acids to <7% of total calories (Grade A)
	Intake of *trans* fat should be minimized (Expert Consensus)
	Individuals with diabetes may benefit from lowering dietary cholesterol to <200 mg/day (Expert Consensus)
	Saturated or *trans* fats can be reduced if weight loss is desirable or replaced with either poly- or monounsaturated fat if weight loss is not a goal
Micronutrients	There is no evidence of benefit from vitamin or mineral supplementation in persons with diabetes who do not have underlying deficiencies. Exceptions include folate for the prevention of birth defects (Grade A)
	Although difficult to ascertain, if deficiencies of vitamins and minerals are identified, supplementation may be beneficial (Expert Consensus)
	Routine supplementation with antioxidants, such as vitamin E and C and carotene, is not advised because of lack of efficacy and concern related to long-term safety (Grade A)
	Benefit from chromium supplementation in persons with diabetes or obesity has not been clearly demonstrated and therefore can not be recommended (Expert Consensus)
	In both normotensive and hypertensive persons, a reduced sodium intake (e.g., 2300 mg/day) with a diet high in fruits, vegetables and low-fat dairy products lowers blood pressure (Grade A)
Alcohol	If adults with diabetes choose to drink alcohol, daily intake should be limited to 1 drink or less for women and 2 drinks or less for men (Expert Consensus)
	One drink is defined as 12 oz beer, 5 oz wine, or 1.5 oz of distilled spirits, each of which contains ~15 g alcohol
	In individuals with diabetes, moderate alcohol consumption when ingested with food has minimal, if any, effect on glucose and insulin levels. For individuals using insulin or insulin secretagogues, alcohol should be consumed with food to reduce the risk of hypoglycemia (Grade B)
	Studies suggest a U or J-shaped association with moderate consumption of alcohol (~15–45 g/day) and decreased risk of type 2 diabetes and diabetes-related coronary heart disease
	Heavy and chronic consumption of alcohol is associated with an increased incidence of diabetes and deterioration in glucose control in people with diabetes
Energy balance	Structured programs that emphasize lifestyle changes including education, reduced energy and fat intake, regular physical activity, and regular participant contact, can produce long-term weight loss on the order of 5–7% of starting weight (Grade A)
	Physical activity and behavior modification are important components of weight loss programs and are most helpful in maintenance of weight loss (Grade B)
	Weight loss medications may be useful in the treatment of overweight and obese individuals with type 2 diabetes and can help achieve a 5–10% weight loss when combined with lifestyle modification (Grade B)
	Bariatric surgery is appropriate for some individuals with type 2 diabetes and a BMI $\geq$35 kg/m^2 and can result in marked improvements in glycemia. The long-term benefits and risks of bariatric surgery in individuals with prediabetes or diabetes continue to be studied. (Grade B)

(Continued)

Table 8.3 Nutrition-related recommendations for diabetes. (*Continued*)

Children and adolescents with diabetes	For youths with type 1 diabetes, individualized food/meal plans and physiological insulin regimens can provide flexibility to accommodate irregular meal times and schedules, varying appetite, and varying activity levels (Expert Consensus)
	Increased physical activity, reduced energy and fat intake, and improved eating habits is strongly encouraged for youth with type 2 diabetes and their family members (Expert Consensus)
Pregnancy and lactation	Nutrition requirements during pregnancy and lactation are similar for women with and without diabetes. (Expert Consensus)
	MNT for gestational diabetes focuses on food choices for appropriate weight gain, normoglycemia, and absence of ketones. (Expert Consensus)
Older adults	Obese older adults with diabetes may benefit from modest energy restriction and an increase in physical activity; energy requirement may be less than for a younger individual of a similar weight. (Expert Consensus)

Source: [5,6].

Prioritizing nutrition interventions for type 1 diabetes and other insulin users

For persons requiring insulin therapy, the first nutrition-related priority for primary care clinicians is to integrate an insulin regimen into the patient's lifestyle. With the many insulin regimens now available, an insulin regimen can usually be developed which will conform to the individual's preferred food choices and meal routine. The food/meal plan is developed first and is based on the individual's appetite, preferred foods and usual schedule of meals and physical activity. After the registered dietitian works with the individual with diabetes to develop a food plan, this information is shared with the health care provider who determines the insulin regimen. Insulin therapy can then be integrated into food and physical activity schedules. Table 8.4 lists the types of insulin currently available, their onset of action, peak effects, usual effective duration, and when to evaluate their effect.

Insulin administered via the pulmonary route (inhaled insulin) has also been approved by the FDA and also may be used as bolus insulin. Exubra, involving a spray-dried insulin powder contained in a blister packet and a simple inhalation device, is currently approved, but other inhaled insulin systems are under development.

Physiological insulin therapy consists of a basal (background) insulin and bolus (meal, rapid-acting) insulin or insulin pump therapy. Normal-weight persons require approximately 0.5 unit and persons with type 2 diabetes 1–1.5 units of insulin per kg of body weight with approximately half of this being for basal insulin and the reminder covering meal insulin needs. The half of the total insulin dose that is to be used to cover meals can be divided into thirds: one-third for each meal. These doses can then be adjusted based on blood glucose monitoring.

Table 8.4 Insulin therapy.

Type of insulin	Onset of action	Peak action	Usual effective duration	Monitor effect after
Bolus insulin (mealtime)				
Rapid-acting	<15 min	1–2 h	3–4 h	2 h
Insulin lispro (Humalog)				
Insulin aspart (Novolog)				
Insulin glulisine (Apidra)				
Short-acting	0.5–1 h	2–3 h	3–6 h	4 h (next meal)
Regular				
Basal insulin (background)				
Long-acting				
Insulin glargine (Lantus)	~1 h	Peakless	20–24 h	10–12 h
Insulin determir (Levemir)	1–2 h	5–14 h	14–23 h	10–12 h
Intermediate-acting				
NPH	2–4 h	6–10 h	10–16 h	8–12 h
Mixtures				
70/30 (70% NPH, 30% regular)	0.5–1 h	Dual	10–16 h	
Humalog Mix 75/25 (75% neutral protamine lispro [NPL], 25% lispro)	<15 min	Dual	10–16 h	
Novolog Mix 70/30 (70% neutral protamine aspart [NPA], 30% aspart)	<15 min	Dual	10–16 h	

Source: Adapted from [7].

The total carbohydrate content of meals is the major determinant of the meal-rapid-acting insulin dose and the postprandial glucose response. After determining the basic dose of insulin needed to cover the usual meal carbohydrate, individuals can be taught how to adjust meal insulin doses based on the amount of carbohydrate they plan to eat (insulin : carbohydrate ratios). Approximately 1.5 units of insulin at breakfast and 1 unit at lunch and dinner are usually needed for every 10 g carbohydrate eaten. In a trial using this ratio, the postprandial glucose response remained constant over a wide range of ingested carbohydrates and was not affected by the glycemic index, fiber, calorie or fat content of the meals [8]. This approach was further confirmed in the dose adjustment for normal eating randomized controlled trial [3].

The insulin : carbohydrate ratios can also be used to determine the bolus insulin doses. In order to determine the proper ratio, an individual must be consistent in their carbohydrate intake and the bolus insulin adjusted to cover that amount of carbohydrate. The servings, or grams, of carbohydrate per meal are then divided by the bolus insulin dose to determine how many units of insulin are needed to cover the servings, or grams, of carbohydrate. For example, if an individual usually eats five servings (75 g) of carbohydrate for dinner and the postmeal glucose is within target range by taking 5 units of rapid-acting insulin at meals, the insulin : carbohydrate ratio is 1:15 g (1 serving) [75 ÷ 5, which equals 1 unit of insulin per 15 g of carbohydrate]. Individuals can then adjust their bolus insulin based on the carbohydrate they plan to eat.

Patients with type 2 diabetes who initially may be reluctant to do basal–bolus insulin management often make the transition to multiple daily insulin injection regimens after gaining confidence in their ability to safely and effectively use insulin through less intensive regimens. Common regimens used may be once-daily glargine and once- or twice-daily premixed insulins. Conventional or fixed insulin therapy consisting of rapid-acting (or regular), and intermediate-acting insulins given before breakfast and the evening meal is another common insulin regimen. Sometimes the intermediate-acting insulin, instead of being given at the evening meal, is given at bedtime. For this particular time of insulin therapy, consistency in the day-to-day carbohydrate content as well as the timing of meals is important [9].

Prioritizing nutrition interventions over the continuum of type 2 diabetes

In order to prioritize nutrition therapy for type 2 diabetes, it should be recognized that the progressive nature of type 2 diabetes demands progressive changes in both medication(s) and nutrition therapy. The two primary metabolic abnormalities in type 2 diabetes are insulin resistance (deficient response to insulin) and beta-cell failure (impairment in insulin secretion). Over time, beta-cell function steadily declines. This progressive decline in beta-cell function requires that medical therapy progresses from MNT as monotherapy to MNT in combination with glucose-lowering medications and/or insulin.

Type 2 diabetes results from coexisting defects at multiple organ sites: resistance to insulin action in muscle, defective pancreatic insulin secretion, and unrestrained hepatic glucose production. These defects are all worsened by increased lipolysis in adipose tissues releasing free fatty acids which contribute to defective insulin action (lipotoxicity). A major goal of therapy is to achieve euglycemia in order to slow beta-cell exhaustion (glucotoxicity). To achieve adequate glycemic control, eventually medications need to be added. Glucose-lowering medications are usually first-line therapy and can be very effective in patients with a short duration of diabetes and, thus, relatively adequate beta-cell function. However, due to the progressive nature of type 2 diabetes that leads to insulin deficiency, many patients with type 2 diabetes will eventually need insulin [10]. The United Kingdom Prospective Study (UKPDS) showed that more than half of the patient population required insulin at the end of the 10-year study and the investigators predicted that most of the patients would need insulin during their lifetimes [11].

Classes of oral medications target the mechanisms underlying insulin resistance and insulin deficiency. Administered as monotherapy each of the classes of medications (except alpha glucosidase inhibitors) in controlled clinical trials resulted in an approximate 1–2 unit reduction in A1C compared to placebo [12]. Because the various drug classes have different mechanisms of action, they can be used in combination to provide additive glycemic benefits. Two new injectable medications have also been approved for use in diabetes. Incretin mimetics have the same glucose-lowering effects as the body's natural incretin hormones. Exenatide is only approved for people who take either metformin, a sulfonylurea, or both. An amylinominetic is a form of amylin, a hormone co-secreted with insulin by the beta cells of the pancreas. Pramlintide is approved as adjunct therapy to insulin in people with type 2 and type 1 diabetes. Table 8.5 lists classes of oral glucose lowering agents, common drugs in each class, and their mechanism of action.

A new class of oral drugs—dipeptidyl peptidase-4 (DPP-4) inhibitors–which prevent or slow down incretin degradation, are being approved for use in type 2 diabetes. Examples are sitagliptin (Januvia) and vildagliptin (Galvus).

Just as medical management of type 2 diabetes changes as the disease progresses, the nutrition care process also changes. MNT for patients with type 2 diabetes differs in several aspects from the strategies for prevention or delay

Table 8.5 Glucose lowering medications for type 2 diabetes.

Class and generic names	Mechanism of action
Sulfonylureas (Second generation) Glipizide (Glucotrol) Glipizide, long-acting (Glucotrol XL) Glyburide, micronized (Glynase Prestabs) Glimepiride (Amaryl)	Stimulates insulin secretion from the beta cells
Meglitinide Repaglinide (Prandin), Nateglinide (Starlix)	Stimulates insulin secretion from beta cells
Biguanide Metformin (Glucophage) Metformin Extended Release (Glucophage XR) Metformin, liquid (Riomet)	Decreases hepatic glucose production
Thiazolidinediones Pioglitazone (Actos) Rosiglitazone (Avandia)	Improves peripheral insulin sensitivity
Alpha Glucosidase Inhibitors Acarbose (Precose), Miglitol (Glyset)	Delays carbohydrate absorption
Incretin Mimetics Exenatide (Byetta)	Enhances glucose-dependent insulin secretion and suppresses glucagon secretion
Amylinominetic Pramlintide (Smylin)	Decreases glucagon production which decreases mealtime hepatic glucose release and prevents postprandial hyperglycemia
Combination Drugs Metformin/glyburide (Glucovance) Metformin/rosiglitazone (Avandamet) Metformin/glipizide (Metaglip) Rosigliatazone/glimepiride (Avandaryl)	Combined action of each medication

Source: Adapted from [7].

of type 2 diabetes. The goal of MNT progresses from prevention of obesity or weight gain to improving insulin resistance to contributing to improved metabolic control. However, basic throughout the process is the recommendation that individuals achieve optimal nutrition through healthy food choices and a physically active lifestyle. Healthy food choices include substantial intakes of whole grain foods, fruits, vegetables and legumes. A literature review [13] concluded that these foods are also associated with an improvement in insulin sensitivity and other indicators of carbohydrate metabolism including improved glycemic control in people with diabetes.

MNT treatment guidelines for type 2 diabetes are often first based on the goal of glycemic control, as lifestyle modifications have an immediate impact on glucose concentrations, but of equal concern are optimal lipid levels and blood pressure goals. As individuals move from being insulin resistant to insulin deficient, the goal of MNT shifts from weight loss to control of glucose, lipid, and blood pressure. Although moderate weight loss may be beneficial for some individuals, primarily those who are still insulin resistant, for many it is too late for weight loss to improve hyperglycemia [14]. Furthermore, often when medications – including insulin – need to be combined with nutrition therapy, preventing an expected weight gain becomes a key consideration. However, glycemic control must still take precedence over concerns about weight.

Teaching individuals how to make appropriate food choices (usually by means of carbohydrate counting) and using data from blood-glucose monitoring to evaluate short-term effectiveness are important components of successful MNT for type 2 diabetes. Carbohydrate counting is useful in the management of all types of diabetes. However, instead of grouping foods into six lists as in the exchange system, it groups foods into three categories: carbohydrate, meat and meat substitutes, and fat. The carbohydrate list is composed of starches, starchy vegetables, fruits, milk, and sweets; one serving is the amount of food that contains 15 grams of carbohydrate. Table 8.6 lists some examples of a carbohydrate serving.

Table 8.6 Carbohydrate servings.*

Starch	Milk
1 slice of bread (1 oz)	1 cup skim/reduced-fat milk
1/3 cup cooked rice or pasta	2/3 cup fat-free fruited yogurt sweetened with
3/4 cup dry cereal	non-nutritive sweetener or fructose (6 oz)
4–6 crackers	
1/2 large baked potato with skin (3 oz)	
3/4 oz pretzels, potato, or tortilla chips	
Fruit	**Sweets and desserts**
1 small fresh fruit (4 oz)	2 small cookies
1/2 cup fruit juice	1 tablespoon jam, honey, syrup, table sugar
1/4 cup dried fruit	1/2 cup ice cream, frozen yogurt, or sherbet

*One serving contains 15 g of carbohydrate.
Source: Marion Franz, MS, RD, CDE, Nutrition concepts by Franz, Inc. 2007. Used with permission.

Women with type 2 diabetes often do well with three-to-four carbohydrate servings per meal and one-to-two for a snack. Men with type 2 diabetes, because they generally require more calories than women, may need four-to-five carbohydrate servings per meal and one-to-two for a snack. Food records, along with blood glucose monitoring data, can then be used to evaluate if treatment goals are being met, or if there is a need for additional lifestyle and/or medication changes. When insulin is required, consistency in timing of meals and of their carbohydrate content becomes important.

Learning how to use Nutrient Facts on food labels is also useful. First, individuals should take note of the serving size and the total amount (grams) of carbohydrate. The total grams of carbohydrate are then divided by 15 to determine the number of carbohydrate servings in the serving size.

Carbohydrate counting does not mean that meat and fat portions can be ignored. Individuals with diabetes must also know the approximate number of meat and fat servings they should select for meals and snacks. Weight control is important as is the maintenance of a healthy balance of food choices.

Clinicians should give greater attention to counseling for increasing physical activity and improving fitness, primarily for the benefits associated with enhanced cardiorespiratory fitness that are independent of weight. Fitness, independent of body mass index and body fatness, is related to a decrease in all-cause death rates in men with diabetes [15]. Lower cardiorespiratory fitness, as opposed to being overweight and obese, is also an important predictor of all-cause mortality in women with diabetes [16].

Many individuals with type 2 diabetes also have dyslipidemia and hypertension, so decreasing intakes of saturated fat, cholesterol, and sodium should also be a priority. Lifestyle strategies should be implemented as soon as diabetes is diagnosed in order to prevent the chronic complications of the disorder.

Pre-Diabetes

Primary care clinicians have an important role in the prevention of diabetes. For individuals who have progressed to pre-diabetes, the benefits of lifestyle modifications were conclusively documented in the Finnish Prevention Study [17] and the Diabetes Prevention Program (DPP) [18]. Both studies emphasized a low-calorie, low-fat diet and increased physical activity. A sustained, moderate weight loss of 5–7% of body weight and a goal to achieve 150 minutes a week of physical activity, reduced the overall risk of diabetes by 58% in the intervention group; an outcome attributed specifically to changes in participants' lifestyles. Structured programs that emphasize regular contact with study participants were necessary to accomplish the study objectives.

Based on these findings, the American Diabetes Association and the National Institute of Diabetes, Digestive, and Kidney Disease recommend that lifestyle modification – modest weight loss (5–10% of body weight) and modest physical activity (30 min daily) – is the first line of defense to prevent or delay the onset of type 2 diabetes [19]. People with pre-diabetes are also at high risk for cardiovascular disease (CVD) and have a marked increase in the number and severity of cardiovascular disease (CVD) risk factors. In the DPP, the intensive lifestyle intervention also improved CVD risk factor status – reduced blood pressure levels and elevated HDL cholesterol levels – compared with placebo and metformin therapy [20]. At 3 years of follow-up, the intensive lifestyle group was 27–28% less likely to be using medication for hypertension and 25% less likely to be using medication for hyperlipidemia compared with the placebo and metformin groups.

Several studies have documented evidence for reduced risk of diabetes with increased intake of whole grains and dietary fiber [21,22]. Whole grain-containing foods have been associated with improved insulin sensitivity, independent of body weight and dietary fiber with improved insulin sensitivity and improved ability to secrete insulin. Although some studies have demonstrated an association between glycemic index/glycemic load and risk for diabetes, other studies have not [6].

Hypoglycemia of non-diabetic origin

Primary care clinicians are often asked about hypoglycemia of non-diabetic origin which is defined as a clinical syndrome with diverse causes in which low levels of plasma glucose eventually lead to neuroglycopenia. Symptoms, such as sweating, shaking, weakness, hunger, headaches, and irritability, can develop if the brain and nervous system are deprived of the glucose they need to function. Hypoglycemia can be difficult to diagnose because these typical symptoms can be caused by many different health problems besides hypoglycemia. Hypoglycemia can best be defined by the presence of three features known as Whipple's triad:

1) a low plasma or blood glucose level;

2) symptoms of hypoglycemia present at the same time as the low blood glucose values; and

3) amelioration of the symptoms by correction of the hypoglycemia.

Hypoglycemic syndromes are classically divided into fasting (food-deprived) hypoglycemia or postprandial (reactive) hypoglycemia, which occurs in response to food.

The management of hypoglycemic disorders involves two distinct components: the relief of neuroglycopenic symptoms with restoration of blood glucose concentrations to the normal range, and the correction of the underlying cause. The immediate treatment is to eat foods or beverages containing carbohydrate. If an underlying problem is causing hypoglycemia, appropriate treatment of this disease or disorder is essential.

Almost no research has been done to determine what type of food-related treatment is best for the prevention of hypoglycemia. Traditional advice has been to avoid foods containing sugars and to eat protein- and fat-containing foods. However, recent research on the glycemic index and sugars has raised questions about the appropriateness of restricting only sugars, as these foods have been reported to have a lower glycemic index than many of the starches which were encouraged in the past. There is no evidence that ingestion of protein or fat is helpful. Evidence-based recommendations cannot be made for hypoglycemia of non-diabetic origin as minimal research is available; however, recommendations from clinical practice experience are summarized.

The goal of treatment is to adopt eating habits that will keep blood glucose levels as static as possible. Patients with hypoglycemia may also benefit from learning carbohydrate counting and limiting carbohydrate servings (15 g of carbohydrate per serving) to 2–4 for meals and 1–2 for snacks. Foods containing lean protein that are low in total fat can be eaten at meals or with snacks. These foods would be expected to have minimal effect on blood glucose levels and can promote satiety and provide calories. However, because protein, as well as carbohydrate, stimulates insulin release, a moderate intake may be advisable.

The following guidelines can be used for avoiding hypoglycemic symptoms:

Guidelines for avoiding hypoglycemic symptoms

1) Eat small meals, with snacks interspersed between meals and at bedtime. This means eating five to six small meals rather than two to three large meals to steady the release of glucose into the bloodstream.

2) Spread the intake of carbohydrate foods throughout the day. Most individual can eat 2 to 4 servings of carbohydrate foods at each meal and 1 to 2 servings at each snack. Furthermore, if carbohydrate is removed from the diet, the body loses its ability to handle carbohydrate properly. Carbohydrate foods include starches, fruits and fruit juices, milk and yogurt, and foods containing sugars.

3) Avoid foods that contain large amounts of carbohydrate. Examples of such foods are regular soft drinks, syrups, candy, regular fruited yogurts, pies, cookies and cakes.

4) Avoid beverages and foods containing caffeine. Caffeine can cause the same symptoms as hypoglycemia and make the individual feel worse.

5) Limit or avoid alcoholic beverages. Drinking alcohol on an empty stomach and without food can lower blood glucose levels by interfering with the liver's ability to release stored glucose (gluconeogenesis). If an individual chooses to drink alcohol, it should be done in moderation and food should always be eaten along with the alcoholic beverage.

6) Decrease fat intake. A high-fat diet, especially saturated fats, has been shown to affect the body's ability to use insulin (insulin resistance). Decreasing fat intake can also help with weight loss, if weight is a problem. Excess weight also interferes with the body's ability to use insulin.

Source: adapted from [23].

Role of primary care clinicians

Primary care clinicians often have a very limited amount of time to discuss lifestyle interventions with patients at risk for or with diabetes. Far too often well-intended but scientifically unfounded nutrition advice is given to these patients, occasionally accompanied by a simplistic dietary instruction sheet.

Primary care clinicians can begin the process of education by emphasizing to patients with type 1 diabetes the need for a physiological insulin regimen or alerting patients with type 2 diabetes to the natural progression of the disease. Patients, as well as health care providers, are often reluctant to begin insulin therapy when needed. Changing the educational message at diagnosis of type 2 diabetes may help patients anticipate and accept insulin therapy later. Insulin should not be considered a last resort but instead a very effective treatment of diabetes. Insulin should not be seen as a punishment for inadequate compliance with lifestyle behavior change. The need for insulin arises from the decline in beta-cell function rather than failure of diet or the arrival of a grim and unmanageable stage of diabetes. This simply reflects the natural progression of the disease, and patients need to be reassured that it is not their fault.

Interventions that can be used, depending on the individual's stage of change

• Individuals in **precontemplation** may be unaware that they have a problem – or are simply not motivated to change. **Personalizing the individual's risk factors** can help them become aware of a problem. Helping them perceive a greater number of benefits from lifestyle changes increases motivation to change.

• Individuals in **contemplation** are aware that they have a problem and are seriously thinking about change. **Encourage individuals to think about the personal benefits of change**. Discuss barriers to change and come up with some practical strategies to overcome them. Written material, websites, and phone resources can all help contemplators.

• Individuals in **preparation** are at the stage of decision making. At this point, **designing a specific action plan with a start date and providing some simple guidelines** can facilitate small behavioral changes the individual is trying to make.

• Individuals in **action** are making overt efforts to change. **Counseling strategies** such as stressing the importance of self-monitoring by recording food intake and physical activity, assisting in changing thinking patterns from unrealistic goals to realistic and achievable goals, and advice to eat at specific times and to set aside time and a place for physical activity can help the individual focus their efforts.

• Individuals in **maintenance** are working to stabilize their behavior change. **Continued support** is important; help in identifying individuals in their family or systems in the community that can provide the needed support is essential.

Secondly, primary care clinicians can identify the patient's stage of change and take appropriate action based on the patient's readiness to make behavior changes. Different intervention strategies are needed for individuals at different stages of the change process – precontemplation, contemplation, preparation, action, and maintenance [24] (see Chapter 15).

The following brief interventions can be used depending on the individual's stage of change.

As individuals are in the process of making and maintaining lifestyle changes, the primary care provider can also be supportive by:

• Asking about food, physical activity, and stress. The act of asking places importance on these issues and provides credibility to the counseling provided by registered dietitians and other diabetes educators.

• Writing down and setting one or two lifestyle change goals – not weight loss goals – based on patient's assessment of what they need to do.

• Promoting realistic expectations.

• At office follow-up ask, for food and physical activity records.

• Changes in two food habits can have a major impact on improved metabolic control: discontinuing drinking regular soft drinks [25] and eating breakfast and other meals at consistent times [26,27]. If individuals have already made these changes clinicians should be complementary and supportive.

• Encourage a goal of 150 minutes of accumulated physical activity per week. Recommend starting with small goals – 5 minutes every day. Using monitoring tools such as a pedometer to identify total steps per day provides reinforcement.

Finally, primary care clinicians can facilitate and identify systems in the community for follow-up and support. Support from family and friends must be provided in the right balance. Some support is important in promoting adherence, but more than the desired amount negatively affects these behaviors. And just as support from family and friends is important, continuing education and support from health care providers is also essential and can enhance the patient's problem-solving skills and decision-making strategies.

References

1 American Diabetes Association. Standards of medical care in diabetes – 2006 (Position Statement). *Diabetes Care* 2006;29(suppl 1):S4–S42.
2 Pastors JG, Franz MJ, Warshaw H, Daly A, Arnold M. How effective is medical nutrition therapy in diabetes care? *J Am Diet Assoc* 2003;103:827–31.
3 DAFNE Study Group. Training in flexible, intensive insulin management to enable dietary freedom in people with type 1 diabetes: dose adjustment for normal eating (DAFNE) randomized trial. *BMJ* 2002;325:746–52.

4 Savoca MR, Miller CK, Ludwig DA. Food habits are related to glycemic control among people with type 2 diabetes mellitus. *J Am Diet Assoc* 2004;104:560–66.

5 Franz MJ, Bantle JP, Beebe CA, *et al.* Evidence-based nutrition principles and recommendations for the treatment and prevention of diabetes and related complications (Technical Review). *Diabetes Care* 2002;25:148–98.

6 American Diabetes Association. Nutrition recommendations and interventions for diabetes: a position statement of the American Diabetes Association. *Diabetes Care* 2006;29:2140–57.

7 Franz MJ, Reader D, Monk A. *Implementing Group and Individual Medical Nutrition Therapy for Diabetes*. Alexandria, VA, American Diabetes Association, 2002.

8 Rabasa-Lhoret R, Garon J, Langlier H, Poisson D, Chiasson J-L. Effects of meal carbohydrate on insulin requirements in type 1 diabetic patients treated intensively with the basal-bolus (ultralente-regular) insulin regimen. *Diabetes Care* 1999;22:667–73.

9 Wolever TMS, Hamad S, Chiasson J-L, *et al.* Day-to-day consistency in amount and source of carbohydrate intake associated with improved glucose control in type 1 diabetes. *J Amer Coll Nutr* 1999;18:242–7.

10 DeWitt DE, Hirsch IB. Outpatient insulin therapy in type 1 and type 2 diabetes mellitus. *JAMA* 2003;289:2254–64.

11 Wright A, Burden AC, Paisey RB, Cull CA, Holman RR. Sulfonylurea inadequacy: efficacy of addition of insulin over 6 years in patients with type 2 diabetes in the U.K. Prospective Diabetes Study (UKPDS 57). *Diabetes Care* 2002;25:330–6.

12 Inzucchi SE. Oral antihyperglycemic therapy for type 2 diabetes. Scientific review. *JAMA* 2002;287:360–72.

13 Venn BJ, Mann JI. Cereal grains, legumes and diabetes. *Eur J Clin Nutr* 2004;58:1443–61.

14 Wolf AM, Conaway MR, Crowther JQ, *et al.* Translating lifestyle intervention to practice in obese patients with type 2 diabetes. *Diabetes Care* 2004;27:1570–6.

15 Church TS, Cheng YJ, Earnest CP, *et al.* Exercise capacity and body composition as predictors of mortality among men with diabetes. *Diabetes Care* 2004;27:83–8.

16 Farrell SW, Braun LA, Barlow CE, Cheng YJ, Blair SN. The relation of body mass index, cardiorespiratory fitness, and all-cause mortality in women. *Obesity Research* 2002;10: 417–23.

17 Tuomilehto J, Lindstrom J, Eriksson JG, *et al.* for the Finnish Diabetes Prevention Study Group. Prevention of type 2 diabetes mellitus by changes in lifestyle among subjects with impaired glucose tolerance. *N Engl J Med* 2001;344:1343–50.

18 Diabetes Prevention Program Research Group. Reduction in the incidence of type 2 diabetes with lifestyle intervention or metformin. *N Engl J Med* 2002;346:393–403.

19 American Diabetes Association and National Institute of Diabetes and Digestive and Kidney Diseases. The prevention or delay of type 2 diabetes. *Diabetes Care* 2003;26(suppl 1):S62–S69.

20 The Diabetes Prevention Program Research Group. Impact of intensive lifestyle and metformin therapy on cardiovascular disease risk factors in the Diabetes Prevention Program. *Diabetes Care* 2005; 28:888–94.

21 Liese AD, Schulz M, Fang F, Wolever TMS, D'Agostino RB Jr, Sparks KC, Mayer-Davis EJ. Dietary glycemic index and glycemic load, carbohydrate and fiber intake, and measures of insulin sensitivity, secretion, and adiposity in the Insulin Resistance Atherosclerosis Study. *Diabetes Care* 2005;28:2832–38.

22 McKeown NM, Meigs JB, Liu S, Wilson PW, Jacques PF. Whole-grain intake is favorably associated with metabolic risk factors for type 2 diabetes and cardiovascular disease in the Framingham Offspring Study. *Am J Clin Nutr* 2002;76:390–8.

23 International Diabetes Center, *Reactive and Fasting Hypoglycemia,* Minneapolis, MN: International Diabetes Center, Park Nicollet Institute; 2004.

24 Prochaska JO, Velicer WF. The Transtheoretical model of health behavior change. *Am J Health Promotion* 1997;12:38–48.

25 Teff KL, Elliott SS, Tschöp M, *et al.* Dietary fructose reduces circulating insulin and leptin, attenuates postprandial suppression of ghrelin, and increases triglycerides in women. *J Clin Endocrinol Metab* 2004;89:2963–72.

26 Farshchi HR, Taylor MA, Macdonald IA. Deleterious effect of omitting breakfast on insulin sensitivity and fasting lipid profiles in healthy lean women. *Am J Clin Nutr* 2005;81:388–96.

27 Farshchi HR, Taylor MA, Macdonald IA. Beneficial metabolic effects of regular meal frequency on dietary thermogenesis, insulin sensitivity, and fasting lipid profiles in healthy obese women. *Am A Clin Nutr* 2005;81:16–24.

CHAPTER 9

Gastrointestinal disorders

Marianne Aloupis and Thomas Faust

Gastrointestinal (GI) complaints, even seemingly mild, can negatively impact quality of life. Primary care physicians are often the gateway between the evaluation and treatment of digestive disorders. Patients seek care for various symptoms from food intolerances to chronic digestive diseases. Symptoms such as abdominal pain, nausea, and altered bowel habits may be caused by dietary intolerance, underlying GI pathology or anxiety. The role of a primary care physician is to differentiate between mild complaints and potentially life-threatening medical conditions. Once a diagnosis is found, the physician becomes a partner in the management of GI complaints. Management of these disorders frequently includes some degree of dietary manipulation. Some dietary guidelines, such as a diet rich in whole grain foods, can be useful across the spectrum of most GI symptoms whereas certain disorders require specific nutritional modifications. A physician with a strong understanding of the role of nutrition in GI illnesses will be better suited to optimize disease management and improve the patient's quality of life.

Digestion and absorption

Nutrient digestion requires a controlled process of mechanical and chemical breakdown, with subsequent enzymatic and secretory responses that facilitate nutrient absorption. Carbohydrate digestion requires adequate amylase to convert starches into disaccharides, which then undergo further hydrolysis into monosaccharides. Monosaccharides are absorbed through a process of either diffusion or active transport. Dietary fats require a complex series of lipase secretion resulting in the hydrolysis of free fatty acids from the triglyceride backbone. Once hydrolyzed, monoglycerides, glycerol and fatty acids, as well as fat-soluble vitamins, undergo emulsification by bile acids in order to promote diffusion across the cell membrane of the enterocyte. Protein digestion requires adequate gastric acidity which activates pepsin and other proteases allowing breakdown of proteins into amino acids and di- and tri-peptides [1]. Defects in any of the mechanical, chemical, or secretory processes involved in digestion can result in nutrient maldigestion and malabsorption.

Malabsorption

Inadequate nutrient absorption can occur as a result of many diseases of the digestive system. In order to effectively treat the symptoms of malabsorption, one must first identify the cause. Once the underlying cause has been identified, appropriate treatment can be implemented. The management of disorders of carbohydrate, protein, and fat malabsorption can be improved with appropriate nutrition therapy.

Carbohydrate malabsorption

Lactose malabsorption is the most common form of carbohydrate malabsorption and is usually caused by suboptimal activity of the enzyme lactase. Lactase is necessary for hydrolysis of lactose into glucose and galactose for uptake by the intestinal absorptive cells. Characteristic symptoms of lactose intolerance include bloating, abdominal pain, flatulence, nausea, or diarrhea after consumption of dairy products. These symptoms are caused by the passage of undigested lactose into the colon where it is metabolized by colonic bacteria, producing excess fluid and gas in the bowel.

The diagnosis of lactose intolerance can often be made by symptomatic improvement after temporary avoidance of dairy products. It is best to confirm the diagnosis with a lactose tolerance test or a breath hydrogen test as many other GI disorders, such as irritable bowel syndrome (IBS), inflammatory bowel disease (IBD), or celiac sprue can mimic the symptoms of lactose intolerance [2].

Lactose malabsorption is often caused by a genetically determined decline in lactase production. The prevalence of lactase deficiency is approximately 5–20% of Caucasians, but may be as high as 50–80% of Latinos, 60–80% of African Americans and Ashkenazi Jews, and nearly 100% of Asians and American Indians [3]. Thus while lactase deficiency may be pathological in infants, it is normal in most teens and adults. Secondary lactase deficiency can occur as a result of other intestinal disorders including bacterial overgrowth, mucosal injury, or IBDs. Effective treatment of underlying disorders may improve lactose tolerance [4]. Research suggests that lactose malabsorption may increase with age, although older persons who develop lactase deficiency may be asymptomatic [5].

Despite the high prevalence of lactose malabsorption, dietary manipulation can allow individuals with lactose intolerance to consume adequate dietary calcium from dairy products [6]. The severity of symptoms is often related to the quantity of lactose consumed. With recent research identifying the health benefits of a diet high in calcium, all individuals, regardless of lactose malabsorption, should be encouraged to include low-fat dairy products in their diet (dietary guidelines recommend three servings of dairy per day). Lactose hydrolyzed products can be well tolerated, as can yogurt and other fermented dairy products [7]. Ongoing research examining the use of probiotics is attempting to determine if modification of colonic bacteria can improve symptoms of lactose intolerance.

Table 9.1 Nutritional management of lactose intolerance.

Dairy products and foods that contain dairy products are high in lactose. Many people do not produce enough lactase which is the enzyme necessary for the digestion of the milk sugar, lactose. Symptoms of lactose intolerance vary among individuals but may include cramps, bloating, diarrhea, gas, or nausea after consuming dairy products. The following tips may help you to better tolerate dairy foods:

• Continue to include yogurt and dairy foods as tolerated.
• Drink milk with a meal or other foods.
• Substitute lactose-reduced dairy foods for regular dairy foods.
• Try hard cheeses, such as cheddar or Swiss, that are low in lactose.
• Take lactase enzyme tablets before eating dairy products.
• Add lactase enzyme drops to regular milk.

Although dairy products contain the highest amounts of lactose in our diets, other foods may contain significant amounts of lactose. If you continue to have symptoms of lactose intolerance after making the changes listed above, you may need to look for "hidden sources" of lactose in foods. The following ingredients may not be well tolerated by persons with lactose intolerance:

• Whey or lactose.
• Non-fat milk solids, buttermilk, or malted milk.
• Margarine or sweet or sour cream.

Other foods that may contain small amounts of lactose include some breads, baked goods, dry cereals, breakfast drinks, milk chocolate, instant potato, pancake, biscuit or cookie mixes, and non-kosher luncheon meats.

Source: Adapted from [9].

Appropriate nutrition therapy for patients suffering from lactose malabsorption or intolerance is outlined in Table 9.1. Lactose intolerant patients who are unable to tolerate adequate intake of dairy products should be encouraged to consume calcium-fortified foods or to include a daily calcium supplement to ensure intake of 1000–1200 mg calcium per day [8,11]. Table 9.2 identifies the Dietary Reference Intake (DRI) of calcium by age group. Calcium contents of commonly consumed foods are listed in Appendices G and H [12].

Protein malabsorption

Celiac disease, also termed gluten intolerance, is a disorder of small bowel absorption characterized by chronic inflammation of small bowel mucosa, villous

Table 9.2 Dietary Reference Intake (DRI) for calcium.

Age group	DRI
Children age 1–3 years	500 mg/day
Children age 4–8 years	800 mg/day
Females and males age 9–18 years	1300 mg/day
Females and males age 19–50 years	1000 mg/day
Females and males age 51–70 years	1200 mg/day
Females and males > 70 years	1200 mg/day

Source: [10].

atrophy, and crypt hyperplasia. It is caused by an intolerance to gliadin, the protein fraction of wheat, in genetically predisposed individuals [13]. Disease presentation is variable and can occur at any age. Presenting symptoms of celiac disease can be GI in nature (diarrhea, weight loss, vomiting, abdominal pain, bloating, distension, anorexia and constipation) or may be less specific and include iron deficiency anemia, folic acid or vitamin B_{12} deficiency, osteoporosis or osteomalacia, infertility, or elevated transaminases [13]. In recent years, "silent" celiac disease has been described and may present with symptoms similar to IBS [14].

Testing for celiac disease should be pursued in patients with persistent GI symptoms, such as chronic diarrhea, malabsorption, weight loss, or abdominal distension. Testing should also be considered in patients with unexplained iron deficiency anemia, vitamin deficiencies, infertility or elevated transaminases [13]. Recent research suggests a higher prevalence of celiac disease among patients with osteoporosis [15], but conflicting data have been presented. High-risk populations for celiac disease include patients with autoimmune endocrinopathies especially type 1 diabetes mellitus, first- and second-degree relatives of persons with celiac disease, and Turner syndrome [13]. The diagnostic evaluation of celiac disease should occur while the patient is on a gluten-containing diet and should include serologic testing followed by small bowel biopsy if serologic testing is positive. The NIH consensus statement on celiac disease recommends the IgA antihuman tissue transglutaminase (TTG) and IgA endomysial antibody immunofluorescence (EMA) tests. Positive results warrant small bowel biopsies. Once a definitive diagnosis is made, treatment of celiac disease should include the following elements:

- Consultation with an experienced dietitian.
- Education about the disease.
- Lifelong adherence to a gluten-free diet.
- Identification and treatment of nutritional deficiencies.
- Access to an advocacy group.
- Continuous follow-up by a multidisciplinary team.

Clinical evaluation should include an assessment of vitamin and mineral deficiencies. Initial blood work should include liver function tests, serum iron or ferritin, folate or red blood cell folate, and vitamin B_{12}. A DEXA (dual energy x-ray absorptiometry) scan should also be performed to assess bone density and fracture risk. Identified deficiencies should be repleted, but long-term supplementation is likely not required once the disease is under control. Annual evaluation of vitamin status should be done as deficiencies of folate and vitamin B_6 have been documented in patients on long-term gluten free diets [16].

The gluten-free diet excludes all foods containing wheat, rye, and barley. Recent evidence suggests that patients can safely consume small amounts of oat-containing foods [17], however, questions about safety remain with an oats-containing gluten-free diet. Some patients report worsened GI symptoms when including oats in the diet, although mucosal integrity is maintained [17]. In the United States, there is concern for gluten contamination of oats [18].

Table 9.3 Gluten-free diet guidelines.

Celiac disease, sometimes called gluten intolerance, is a disorder that prevents wheat products from being properly digested. Gluten is found in most grain products, including wheat, barley, and rye. The list below provides basic guidelines for a gluten-free diet. It is important to get additional education from a nutrition professional who specializes in celiac disease. To find a registered dietitian, contact your local hospital or the American Dietetic Association (www.eatright.org or 1-800-877-1600).

Allowed foods
• Allowed grains/flours: rice, corn, soy, potato, tapioca, beans, garfava, sorghum, quinoa, millet, buckwheat, arrowroot, amaranth, teff, and nut flours.
• Plain meat, chicken, fish, fruits and vegetables do not contain gluten.

Foods NOT ALLOWED
• Grains/flours: Wheat (including durum, semolina, kamut, spelt), rye, barley, farro and triticale in any form. Oats are not recommended.
• Foods that often contain gluten: breading and coating mixes, broth or soup bases, communion wafers, croutons, imitation bacon or seafood, marinades or sauces, processed meats, self-basting poultry, soy sauce, stuffings, thickeners.

Read ingredient lists on all food labels The following list includes ingredients which may contain gluten: brown rice syrup, caramel color, dextrin, flour or cereal products, malt or malt flavoring, malt vinegar, modified food starch, soy sauce or soy sauce solids.

Check with your pharmacist about the gluten content of medications or products like mouthwash.

Source: Adapted from the Celiac Disease Foundation, the Gluten Intolerance Group [19].

Patients should be encouraged to avoid oats unless their disease is mild or in remission. If oats are incorporated into the diet, patients should be aware of the risk for increased intestinal symptoms. Table 9.3 describes the principles of a gluten-free diet.

After diagnosis, patients should be referred to a dietitian for education on a gluten-free diet. In addition, information on patient resources and support groups should be provided. See Table 9.4 for patient resources.

Table 9.4 Patient resources for celiac disease.

Celiac Sprue Association: www.csaceliacs.org or 1-877-CSA-4CSA
Nonprofit organization providing patient advocacy, gluten free diet education, and links to national and local chapters/support groups

Celiac Disease Foundation: www.celiac.org or 1-800-990-2354
Nonprofit organization focusing on awareness, education, and advocacy about celiac disease

Gluten Intolerance Group of North America: www.gluten.net or 206-246-6652
Provides up-to-date information, education and support for patients and health care professionals

American Dietetic Association: www.eatright.org or 1-800-877-1600
National organization of registered dietitians and nutrition professionals

Celiac.com: www.celiac.com
Patient information website; includes gluten free on-line store

Whole grains that can be safely included in a gluten-free diet include rice, corn, buckwheat, millet, amaranth, and quinoa [14]. A recent study examining the nutritional quality of gluten-free diets demonstrated that despite adherence to dietary restrictions, diet quality was poor. The majority of females in the study consumed suboptimal intakes of whole grain foods, fiber, calcium, and iron. While males were more likely to consume adequate amounts of fiber and iron, diet choices remained low in calcium and whole grain foods [20]. To improve diet quality, individuals with celiac disease should be encouraged to consume 6–11 servings of whole grain or enriched gluten-free grains and three servings of gluten-free dairy products per day. The primary care physician should reinforce the need for life-long diet adherence, particularly after symptom resolution.

Fat malabsorption

Fat malabsorption is a common finding in many GI disorders and may be characterized by complaints of steatorrhea. Fat malabsorption occurs in cases of impaired luminal transport of products of digestion, and is often seen in disorders causing widespread mucosal injury, such as celiac disease, IBD, and bacterial overgrowth. Treatment of the underlying mucosal disorder may allow for resolution of fat malabsorption. Conversely, steatorrhea can also be caused by maldigestion of fats, as seen in chronic pancreatitis, cystic fibrosis, and bile salt deficiencies [21]. Untreated fat malabsorption may result in weight loss, failure to thrive, osteomalacia, bone pain, infertility, dysmenorrhea, and amenorrhea [1]. In addition, deficiencies of the fat-soluble vitamins may occur.

Adoption of a low-fat diet may aid in symptom management. See Table 9.5 for low-fat diet guidelines. Patients following a low-fat diet may have difficulty consuming adequate calories to maintain weight. Additional calories can be added to the diet with the use of medium chain triglyceride (MCT) oil, which provides 115 calories per tablespoon (available through Novartis Medical Nutrition). MCT oil is rapidly hydrolyzed and does not require bile salts or micelle formation for digestion. Factors limiting the use of MCT oil include poor palability and possible side effects of nausea and vomiting, therefore patients are typically unable to consume more than 3–4 tablespoons per day. Oral nutrition supplements with added MCT oil (i.e., Optimental®, Peptinex®, or Peptamen®) are commercially available and may provide some benefit.

In patients with pancreatic exocrine insufficiency, supplemental pancreatic enzymes may be necessary, whereas in patients with a history of ileal resection, conjugated bile acids may allow resolution of fat malabsorption. Recent evidence suggests that patients with chronic pancreatitis may benefit from early screening for fat malabsorption, even in the absence of clinically significant steatorrhea. Patients may present with pain after meals resulting in reduced caloric intake but not suffer from overt steatorrhea [23].

Table 9.5 Low fat diet.

A low fat diet is sometimes recommended for patients with GI disorders that cause fat malabsorption. Reducing the amount of fat in your diet may help to reduce symptoms such as nausea, abdominal pain, cramping, or diarrhea.

Basic guidelines of a low-fat diet

Avoid adding fats to your foods (butter, margarine, mayonnaise, salad dressings, oils).

Read food labels to determine fat content. Low-fat foods contain less than 3 g fat per 100 calories.

Increase intake of foods that do not contain fat to ensure adequate calories in your diet.

Low fat food choices	High fat food choices
Bread, cereal, and grains	
Breads (whole wheat, white, or rye bread), English muffins, bagels, most cooked or cold cereals, rice, pasta, noodles, potatoes	Cheese bread, quick breads, egg bagels, biscuits, pancakes, snack crackers, peanut butter or cheese crackers, cereals containing nuts or granola, fried potatoes, potatoes, rice, pasta, or noodles prepared with cheese or cream sauces
Meat, Poultry, Fish, Beans, Nuts	
Lean cuts of beef, pork, veal, or lamb (chuck, sirloin, round, 95% lean ground beef; tenderloin cuts) Ham, Canadian bacon Poultry (without skin) Canned fish packed in water Low-fat luncheon meats (turkey, ham) Legumes cooked without added fats Egg whites, egg substitute Egg yolk (1/day)	Fried or breaded meats, poultry, or fish Fatty cuts of meat, including ribs, roasts, ground beef (<95% lean), corned beef, sausage, duck or goose Canned fish packed in oil High fat luncheon meats (bologna, salami, frankfurters, etc.) Dried beans or peas prepared with added fat or high-fat meat Nuts and peanut butter
Milk, yogurt, and cheese	
Nonfat or low-fat milk, fat-free or low-fat cheeses, low-fat or non-fat yogurt or cottage cheese	Whole milk, buttermilk, chocolate milk, cream, regular or processed cheeses, cream cheese, sour cream
Fruits and vegetables	
Fresh, frozen, or canned fruits and vegetables	Avocado Vegetables prepared with added fat, cream sauces or cheese sauces
Snacks, condiments, beverages	
Fat-free broth or soups Sherbet, fruit ice, angel food cake, graham crackers, nonfat frozen desserts Honey, jams, jellies, syrups, hard candy, jelly beans Coffee, tea, soda, non-fat dairy products Baked snack chips, plain crackers (ex. saltines)	Cream or cheese sauces, gravies Cakes, cookies, pies, ice cream Coconut, chocolate High fat snack foods such as chips, crackers, buttered popcorn

Source: Adapted from [22].

Fat malabsorption places patients at risk for vitamin and mineral deficiencies, specifically fat-soluble vitamins: A, D, E, K. Monitoring for fat-soluble vitamin deficiencies should occur on an annual basis, with aggressive repletion as needed. Provision of fat-soluble vitamins in a water-miscible form may allow patients to have better vitamin absorption. Deficiencies of calcium, magnesium, zinc and iron may also be present due to impaired absorption and increased intestinal losses and should be aggressively repleted.

Inflammatory bowel diseases

Crohn's disease and ulcerative colitis are chronic, inflammatory conditions of the GI tract. There is a high prevalence of malnutrition in patients suffering from both disorders. It is estimated that more than 50% of patients with Crohn's disease and 18–60% of patients with ulcerative colitis have some type of nutritional deficiencies [24,25]. The pathogenesis of malnutrition in this set of diseases is multifactorial. One of the primary causative agents is suboptimal oral intake. Patients frequently limit their dietary intake due to anorexia, which may be caused by elevated levels of tumor necrosis factor-alpha and other cytokines [26]. Fear of symptom exacerbation may cause patients to significantly limit their food choices. Taste changes may occur as a result of antibiotics or zinc deficiency. Other causes of malnutrition in this population are malabsorption and maldigestion, particularly in patients suffering from Crohn's disease.

The assessment of patients with IBD should include an emphasis on nutritional status. Recent weight loss, dietary changes, and symptom exacerbation should be reviewed. To prevent micronutrient deficiencies, patients who are following highly restricted diets should be encouraged to increase dietary variety as digestive tolerance permits to prevent micronutrient deficiencies. Iron deficiency is quite common in ulcerative colitis and appropriate supplementation should be provided. Although ulcerative colitis does not result in malabsorption, patients remain at risk for nutrient deficiencies due to poor dietary intake as a result of GI symptoms associated with eating. Deficiencies of fat-soluble vitamins, folate, and vitamin B_{12} have been documented. Metabolic bone disease is a frequent finding in patients with IBD and deficiencies of vitamin D and calcium should be corrected to prevent further bone loss. Folate supplementation should be recommended in patients taking sulfasalazine.

Medical nutrition therapy for IBD

Nutritional recommendations vary depending on disease activity. Although there is no specific diet for IBD, modification of dietary intake may prevent exacerbation of abdominal pain, cramping, and diarrhea. A low-residue, low-lactose, low-fat diet, as well as small frequent meals may improve food tolerance. Particularly in patients with Crohn's disease, foods that are high in insoluble fiber should be avoided to decrease the risk of obstruction in strictured or inflamed sections of the small bowel. Symptoms of lactose intolerance and fat malabsorption may occur during disease exacerbations. As inflammation resolves, dietary restrictions should be reduced based on patient tolerance.

Although a low-fiber diet has often been recommended in IBD, recent evidence suggests that soluble fiber can be beneficial. Soluble fiber is found in oats, legumes, barley, and some fruits, as well as in guar gum and psyllium. Soluble fiber sources are fermented by the colonic bacteria and produce short chain fatty acids such as butyrate, which is a preferred energy source for the colonocyte. The various benefits associated with short chain fatty acids include a trophic effect on intestinal mucosa, increased water and sodium resorption, and promotion of mucosal restitution. Butyrate may also have an anti-inflammatory effect on intestinal mucosa by inhibition of nuclear factor-κB activation of pro-inflammatory mediators [27]. Some research demonstrates that diets high in soluble fiber may prevent disease remission. Until further research is available, soluble fiber should be encouraged as tolerated to potentially alleviate symptoms of IBD.

Probiotics are another area of ongoing research in IBD. It appears that consumption of probiotics may act to beneficially impact the intestinal microflora and improve GI symptoms. Although it is too early to recommend probiotic supplements for routine treatment in IBD, incorporating probiotics in the diet with active culture yogurt may be beneficial.

Patients with ileal disease or ileal resection are at an increased risk of developing oxalate stones. Due to impaired small bowel reabsorption of bile salts, available free fatty acids bind calcium, leaving oxalate free to be absorbed. The risk of oxalate stones can be reduced in patients with bile salt malabsorption by adhering to a low oxalate diet, ensuring adequate hydration, and consuming oral calcium supplements which bind to oxalate and prevent colonic absorption [1]. Foods and beverages high in oxalate include dark, leafy greens, green beans, sweet potatoes, Rhubarb, berries, cocoa, chocolate, peanut butter, tea and beer. For a complete list, see Appendix N.

Gastric disorders

Gastroesophageal reflux disease

Gastroesophageal reflux disease (GERD), characterized by symptoms of acid reflux and heartburn, has been reported to effect as much as 20% of the population [29]. As many as one in seven persons may suffer from daily symptoms of heartburn [30], which can decrease quality of life and may increase risk for development of esophageal adenocarcinoma. Although the underlying causes of GERD are not known, the pathogenesis has been related to decreases in lower esophageal sphincter pressure.

Weight may be a significant risk factor for development of GERD, with increasing body mass index (BMI) having a strong correlation with reflux symptoms [30]. The impact of dietary factors has been evaluated as a causative agent for reflux disease. Although limited data is available, fatty foods, chocolate, alcohol and caffeine (coffee, tea, cola) have been frequently associated with GER

Table 9.6 Medical nutrition therapy for GERD.

In order to reduce symptoms associated with GERD, it may be necessary to modify your diet. The following tips may help decrease discomfort associated with meals and heartburn.

- Limit intake of high fat, high calorie meals
- Eat smaller meals more frequently during the day
- Drink most fluids between meals rather than with meals
- Increase intake of high fiber foods, such as fruits and vegetables, and whole grains
- Sit up or take a walk after eating. Lying down after a meal can worsen symptoms
- Limit foods that worsen symptoms, such as alcohol, chocolate, coffee, or caffeine-containing beverages, mints, citrus fruits, tomato products, spicy foods, or carbonated beverages

---

Source: [19].

symptoms. High fat intake, particularly saturated fat, has recently been found to increase risk of GERD [31]. Although fatty foods are thought to decrease the competence of the lower esophageal sphincter, excessive calorie consumption at one meal may be more of a risk factor than fat content, per se [32]. There is some evidence that increasing dietary fiber may have a protective effect against reflux [33].

Nutrition therapy for patients with GERD should be focused at minimizing exacerbation of reflux symptoms. Patients may have varying degrees of sensitivity to different high-risk foods. The goals of therapy should be to prevent relaxation of the lower esophageal sphincter, reduce volume of gastric acid, and prevent esophageal irritation. In addition, encouraging patients to gradually increase their intake of whole grain foods may reduce their reflux symptoms. Table 9.6 identifies medical nutrition therapy for patients with GERD.

Peptic ulcer disease

The management of peptic ulcer disease (PUD) has changed significantly in recent decades. Early treatment of PUD included a bland diet as a mainstay of treatment. It is now understood that most gastric and duodenal ulcers are caused by damage to the gastric mucosa, and the most common causative agents are *Helicobacter pylori* and non-steroidal anti-inflammatory drugs (NSAIDS) [34]. Treatment of the underlying cause of PUD may allow for resolution of symptoms.

Although gastric acid is not responsible for ulcer development, reduction in gastric acid may facilitate healing and decrease abdominal discomfort. Gastric acid secretion occurs as a result of vagal stimulation of the parietal cells by the sight or taste of food. Certain foods are potent gastric acid secretagogues, including coffee, tea, colas, and alcohol [35]. No difference has been found in randomized controlled trials that compared restricted to unrestricted diets in the resolution of ulcers. The focus of nutrition therapy should be based on individual tolerance and patients should be encouraged to avoid their individual triggers. Foods that are often poorly tolerated include coffee, orange juice, fried

Table 9.7 Medical nutrition therapy for peptic ulcer disease.

Limit intake of caffeine containing beverages and foods including coffee, tea, iced tea, colas, and chocolate

Avoid alcohol, especially on an empty stomach

Eat three small meals per day

Don't skip meals

Avoid eating spicy foods, fried foods, and citrus fruits as these foods may worsen symptoms

Avoid other foods or drinks that cause discomfort

foods, spicy foods and fruits. After treatment of *H. pylori,* improved tolerance of these trigger foods has been demonstrated [36]. Table 9.7 outlines medical nutrition therapy for symptom management of PUD.

Colonic disorders

Diarrhea

Diarrhea is characterized by increased frequency of watery stools, and may be acute or chronic in nature. Acute diarrhea often resolves on its own, whereas chronic diarrhea lasts for more than 4 weeks. Up to 5% of the population may suffer from chronic diarrhea [37]. Diarrhea occurs in many underlying GI illnesses, and therefore appropriate evaluation of symptoms is vital. Malabsorptive disorders, such as lactose intolerance, celiac disease, or IBD may result in chronic diarrhea. Assessment should identify the frequency of stools, duration of symptoms, and potential weight loss. Stool characteristics (i.e., watery, inflammatory, or fatty) can aid in the further evaluation of the pathogenesis of diarrhea. Secretory diarrhea occurs as a result of a disruption in electrolyte transport within the epithelium with resultant diarrhea. It may be caused by enterotoxins, intestinal resections or mucosal disease, or mesenteric atherorsclerosis. Osmotic diarrhea occurs after ingestion of poorly absorbed cations and anions, such as sorbitol or sugar alcohols, magnesium, sulfate, or phosphate, or may be related to deficiencies of disaccharidases, as in lactase deficiency [38].

Particularly in chronic diarrhea, a comprehensive evaluation is necessary to determine the underlying cause. Management of diarrhea to prevent electrolyte abnormalities and potential weight loss is vital. Adequate fluids are also necessary to prevent dehydration and oral, rehydration solutions are beneficial in compensating for electrolyte losses. While diarrhea may be worsened by the intake of insoluble fibers, soluble fibers may aid in improvement as they form a gel within the intestinal lumen, thus slowing intestinal transit. Table 9.8 reviews sources of soluble and insoluble dietary fiber. After diarrhea resolves, patients may tolerate gradual reintroduction of insoluble fiber, such as whole grain breads and cereals, in their diet. Other foods that may worsen diarrhea, such as lactose-containing foods or high-fat foods, should be avoided

Table 9.8 Food sources of soluble and insoluble fiber.

Soluble fiber	Insoluble fiber
Apples	Whole-wheat flour
Citrus fruits	Bran
Strawberries	Vegetables
Carrots	Whole grains
Oats	Wheat
Beans	Fruits with edible seeds (strawberries,
Legumes	blueberries, etc)
Barley	
Fiber supplements:	
Psyllium (Metamucil®)	
Guar gum (Benefiber®)	

Source: Adapted from [39].

until diarrhea begins to resolve. Eating yogurt with adequate colonies of active cultures may promote restoration of normal gut flora.

A thorough medication history can identify potential drugs that may exacerbate diarrhea. Sorbitol or lactose-containing medications should be adjusted if possible. Significant amounts of sorbitol and other sugar alcohols found in low carbohydrate or sugar-free foods can also play a role. Patients should be encouraged to eliminate these foods temporarily and assess for symptom resolution.

Constipation

Constipation is a common complaint with prevalence estimates of 12–19% in North America. Risk factors for constipation include advancing age and female gender, with females being twice as likely as males to report symptoms [40]. Constipation is defined as less than 2–3 bowel movements per week [41] and is caused by disordered movement of stool in the colon. The causes of constipation are varied and may be a side effect of multiple diseases or prescribed medications. It is important to rule out structural causes of constipation as well as organic disease.

Nutrition therapy for constipation focuses on increasing fluid intake, gradually increasing fiber intake, and increasing physical activity. It is important that patients are instructed to make gradual dietary changes, as rapid fluctuations in dietary fiber can worsen symptoms of constipation and abdominal discomfort. Dietary fiber intake should be increased as tolerated to approximately 20–35 g/day by including fruits, vegetables, whole grains, legumes, and nuts in the diet. The Dietary Guidelines for Americans recommend at least 2 cups or 3–4 servings of fruits and 2 ½ cups or 4–5 servings of vegetables every day. A recent population-based study demonstrated that women who are physically active on a daily basis and consumed approximately 20 g fiber per day had a three-fold lower prevalence of constipation [42]. See Table 9.9 for recommendations for a high fiber diet. See appendix O for food sources of dietary fiber.

Table 9.9 High fiber food choices.

Increasing the amount of dietary fiber can help manage symptoms of constipation. Dietary fiber should be increased gradually to prevent excessive gas, abdominal cramping and bloating. Over several weeks, fiber intake should be increased to 20–35 g/day (as tolerated). It is important to drink additional fluid as fiber intake is increased. Aim for at least 6–8 glasses of water or liquids per day. Daily physical activity is also beneficial in the management of constipation

Grains (bread, cereal, rice, pasta)	Pumpernickel, rye or whole-wheat bread Whole wheat bagel, matzo, or pasta Bran cereals, Bran Flakes, shredded wheat, oatmeal Cooked barley, bulgur, or brown rice Rye and whole grain crackers, graham wafers Dried beans, peas, or legumes (cooked), potatoes (cooked) with skin Popcorn, air-popped Bran muffin
Fruits (the listed fruits contain higher amounts of fiber. Fruits not listed typically contain less than 2 g fiber per serving, but can still be included in a healthy diet)	High fiber (5+ g/serving): apple (with skin), blackberries, blueberries, figs/dates, kiwi fruit, mango, pears, prunes, raspberries Medium fiber (2–4 g/serving): apple (no skin), oranges, raisins, rhubarb (cooked/stewed), strawberries, tangerine
Vegetables (the listed vegetables contain higher amounts of fiber. Vegetables not listed typically contain less than 2 g fiber per serving, but can still be included in a healthy diet)	High fiber (5+ g/serving): green peas, snowpeas, swiss chard Medium fiber (2–4 g/serving): bean sprouts, string beans, broccoli, Brussels sprouts, carrots, eggplant, parsnips, turnips
Nuts and seeds	Almonds, peanuts, peanut butter, sunflower seeds, sesame seeds

Source: Adapted from [62].

Irritable bowel syndrome

IBS is a functional GI disorder characterized by abdominal pain, altered bowel motility, and bloating or abdominal distension. The pathogenesis of irritable bowel syndrome is not well understood, but researchers have suggested abnormal GI motility, visceral hypersensitivity, dietary intolerances, and psychological or emotional dysfunction as potential causes.

The abdominal pain associated with IBS is variable, and can be described as mild to severe. Diarrhea and constipation may occur in varying degrees [38]. An evaluation for organic causes of GI symptoms is indicated. Recent evidence has suggested that carbohydrate malabsorption may precipitate symptoms of IBS [43,44]. Testing for lactose or fructose malabsorption should be considered in patients with symptoms consistent with IBS. If IBS is diagnosed, treatment focuses on management of symptoms.

The nutritional therapy of IBS is variable, as many patients have specific food intolerances. Following a lactose-restricted diet may improve symptoms of IBS. In addition, reducing the amount of dietary fructose, found in fruits, fruit juices, and foods prepared with high fructose corn syrup may be beneficial. A high fiber diet is often recommended, as it aids in water absorption, promotes bulking of the stool and can improve intestinal transit. Although many studies have examined the role of fiber supplements in the treatment of irritable bowel symptoms, randomized controlled trials have failed to consistently show an improvement when fiber supplements were compared to placebo [45,46]. However, some patients report symptomatic improvement. Dietary fiber, primarily insoluble, was recently determined to be well tolerated in patients with both constipation-predominant- and diarrhea-predominant-IBS, although relief of symptoms was similar to that found in a control group on a low fiber diet, suggesting a placebo effect [47]. Researchers have demonstrated that guar gum causes less bloating than wheat bran, but both forms of fiber resulted in symptomatic improvement [48]. The authors noted that patients reported better tolerance to guar gum [48], which may result in better treatment adherence. Research examining a role for probiotics, such as lactobacillus or bifidobacteria, in IBS is ongoing. It is thought that restoration of normal gut flora may allow for better utilization of butyrate. Additional research is needed to determine the ideal balance between diet, fiber supplements and probiotics in the management of IBS.

Because symptoms are variable, encouraging patients to keep a food diary may allow them to determine specific dietary triggers for their IBS. Foods identified as triggers should be limited. In addition, a trial of a high-fiber diet may produce symptomatic improvement in some patients. Table 9.11 outlines high-fiber choices. Patients should be instructed to increase fiber intake gradually, and to increase fluid intake as fiber intake increases. Avoidance of lactose or fructose containing foods, as well as gas-producing foods, may reduce complaints of bloating and abdominal pain. Table 9.10 provides a list of

Table 9.10 Tips to decrease gas and bloating.

Certain foods can produce excess gas during digestion and may worsen symptoms of abdominal pain or bloating. Various foods effect people in different ways; avoid these foods only if they cause discomfort. The following diet tips may improve symptoms.

Foods that may cause gas:
Beans, cabbage, cauliflower, brussel sprouts, broccoli, asparagus, peppers, cucumbers, onions, garlic, radishes, sauerkraut
Raw apples, avocado, melon
Eggs, fried and fatty foods, spicy foods, carbonated beverages

Swallowing air may also cause excess gas. *To prevent this:*
Eat slowly
Avoid chewing gum, carbonated beverages, and smoking

Source: Adapted from [49].

dietary tips to reduce gas and bloating. Patients who avoid dairy products due to symptoms of lactose intolerance should be encouraged to consume other calcium-rich foods or calcium supplements to meet the RDI of calcium.

Diverticulosis

Diverticulosis is a disorder of the colon, most often the sigmoid colon, caused by multiple potential factors including age-related changes in the colonic wall, abnormal increases in colonic intraluminal pressure, motor dysfunction, or inadequate fiber intake. The incidence of diverticulosis increases with age and suboptimal dietary fiber intake. The prevalence of diverticular disease has been reported at 10% of the population, most often occurring after age 40. It has been estimated that more than 50% of patients over age 60 have evidence of diverticulosis [38].

Treatment of diverticulosis is focused on increasing dietary fiber intake via whole grain foods, fruits, and vegetables. Patients should aim to consume 25–30 g fiber per day [50]. Table 9.9 and Appendix O lists high-fiber food choices. It may be necessary to increase fiber intake with the use of fiber supplements, such as psyllium or guar gum. Early recommendations for diverticular disease encouraged the elimination of foods containing nuts and seeds due to concerns that these items could become lodged within the diverticuli. No evidence is available to support this claim, and these recommendations have been questioned. Increasing fluid intake is vital as fiber intake is increased. Although no evidence is available to provide an exact recommendation for fluid intake, encouraging at least 64 ounces of fluids daily is reasonable.

Diverticulitis

Diverticulitis occurs when there is inflammation or perforations at the site of diverticuli. Management focuses on resolution of inflammation. Bowel rest is often indicated with gradual diet advancement. In the acute phase, patients should maintain a low fiber intake until the inflammation is resolved. The diet should be advanced slowly as tolerance permits, and fiber intake should be gradually increased. Eventual return to a high-fiber diet should be encouraged, as well as consumption of adequate fluids.

Liver disease

Fatty liver

The development of fatty liver can occur as a result of chronic alcohol use or as a side effect of many medications. Recently, much emphasis has been focused on the development of non-alcoholic fatty liver disease (NAFLD). As the prevalence of obesity increases, so does the risk of NAFLD. Histologic changes seen in NAFLD are often macrovesicular hepatic steatosis [51]. Patients at risk for NAFLD are patients who demonstrate symptoms consistent with the metabolic syndrome, including obesity, hypertension, and insulin resistance.

In patients who experience fatty liver as a result of alcohol use, abstinence from alcohol should be encouraged. Medical nutrition therapy of NAFLD should be aimed at promotion of gradual weight loss of 1–2 pounds per week. The ideal dietary composition for patients with NAFLD is unclear [52], but reduction in total calorie and fat intake and increased dietary fiber intake will likely aid in weight loss and improve other symptoms associated with metabolic syndrome. Increased physical activity will aid the patient in weight loss maintenance. Patients may benefit from referral to a registered dietitian or weight loss programs that offer a support component, either through local clinics, hospitals or commercial programs.

Medical nutrition therapy for cirrhosis

Malnutrition and vitamin deficiencies are extremely prevalent in cirrhosis, affecting anywhere between 10–100% of patients. Compensated cirrhotics are at much lower nutritional risk. Severity of malnutrition worsens as disease severity increases, and profound muscle wasting is often seen. The causes of malnutrition in this population are variable. There is impaired nutrient metabolism, causing patients to move more rapidly from a fed state to a fasting state. Malabsorption may occur as a result of diminished bile acid production. Calorie requirements may be increased acutely during complications of ascites or spontaneous bacterial peritonitis. GI symptoms, such as anorexia, nausea and early satiety may impact the intake of adequate nutrients [53]. In addition, many patients with cirrhosis are often placed on highly restricted diets, further worsening their nutrient and vitamin intake.

Risk factors for development of cirrhosis include alcohol-related liver disease, hepatitis, NAFLD or non-alcoholic steatohepatitis (NASH), and cholestatic diseases. The nutrition therapy is variable depending on the cause of cirrhosis and the degree of decompensation.

To prevent worsening of cirrhosis, patients who consume alcohol should be encouraged to abstain. Nutrient deficiencies, particularly the B vitamins (thiamin, folate, B_{12}), are often seen in patients with alcoholic cirrhosis and it is usually necessary to provide additional vitamin supplementation. The macronutrient content of the diet in cirrhosis is difficult to generalize. Patients may suffer from insulin resistance, in which case intake of carbohydrates may need to be modified. Patients should be encouraged to limit their intake of refined carbohydrates and increase consumption of whole grains. Fat intake should be adjusted based on symptoms of intolerance, particularly in cholestatic diseases. In patients with significant malnutrition and anorexia, increasing calorie intake by way of higher fat, energy dense food choices may be helpful. Individuals with persistently inadequate oral intake may benefit from oral nutrition supplements, such as Ensure® or Boost®, to increase calorie and protein intake. Oral supplements high in branched-chain amino acids are available; however, due to limited data demonstrating benefits use of these supplements is limited.

Protein restrictions have frequently been recommended in cirrhosis, especially with accompanying encephalopathy, often at levels of 40 g/day. However, there is significant research demonstrating that excessive protein restriction can worsen outcomes in cirrhosis [54]. Protein restrictions should be limited to periods of acute encephalopathy, with gradual increases in protein intake after the resolution of encephalopathy. Cirrhosis is a catabolic illness, and evidence suggests that patients will benefit from protein intake in a range of 1.0–1.5 g protein/kilogram/day [55]. Protein requirements should be based on the estimated dry weight. Patients may have better tolerance to certain forms of dietary protein, such as vegetable and dairy proteins [56], as these foods are higher in branched chain amino acids. In addition, the increased fiber content of vegetable protein sources may facilitate nitrogenous losses in the stool. Avoidance of raw seafood and shellfish should be encouraged due to the risk of *vibrio vulnificus* infections [57].

Many patients with cirrhosis will develop ascites, and therefore a low-sodium diet is also indicated. Restriction of sodium to 2000 mg/day is often recommended. Further restrictions in sodium worsen the palatability of the diet and increase the risk of inadequate nutrient intake. Fluid restriction may also be indicated. See Appendix I for foods high in sodium.

Multiple vitamin deficiencies have been described in patients with cirrhosis as a result of inadequate nutrient intake, malabsorption, and altered metabolism. A daily multivitamin with mineral supplement should be recommended. In patients with significant steatorrhea, it may be necessary to provide additional supplementation of the fat-soluble vitamins, preferably in a water-soluble form.

Gallbladder disease

Cholelithiasis

Cholelithiasis is caused by a combination of lithogenic bile, cholesterol crystallization, and gallbladder stasis. The majority of cases of gallstone disease are related to cholesterol stones. Female gender, pregnancy, age, obesity, and certain ethnic backgrounds are associated with an increased risk of cholelithiasis. Rapid weight loss, family history, and certain medications may also increase the risk of disease development.

Although there are no specific diet recommendations for the management of gallstone disease, dietary factors may play a role in gallstone development. Excess energy intake as well as diets high in saturated fats and refined sugars have been identified as risk factors [59]. The combination of dietary factors that predispose one to weight gain and obesity also predispose persons to gallstone disease. Recent evidence from long-term population studies suggests that high fiber diets may reduce risk. In addition, there has been a correlation between diets that include frequent consumption of nuts and reduced risk of cholelithiasis in both men and women [60,61].

Patients who are at risk for development of gallstone disease should be encouraged to adopt healthy lifestyle habits, including a diet low in saturated fats and refined sugars and high in dietary fiber. Increased consumption of whole grain breads and cereals, fruits and vegetables will increase dietary fiber intake and potentially reduce risk. If weight loss is indicated, patients should be encouraged to make gradual changes to support weight loss of 1–2 pounds per week. Rapid weight loss has been associated with gallstone formation.

In patients with current gallstone disease, a diet that restricts fat to 25–30% of calories is indicated. Further restriction of fat should be avoided as it may prevent adequate stimulation of gallbladder contraction. Food intolerances may be reported, specifically with foods that cause gas and bloating. Avoiding these foods may aid in symptom control. If overweight or obese, gradual weight loss should be encouraged. If steatorrhea is reported, supplementation of fat soluble vitamins may be indicated.

Summary

Digestive disorders are often complex illnesses requiring a multi-faceted approach. Rarely is there one solution that will work for all patients. In addition to medical treatment of the underlying disease, nutritional therapy may be needed to improve GI symptoms. The impact of dietary manipulations, such as dietary fiber in irritable bowel syndrome or a gluten-free diet in celiac disease, demonstrates the intricate role that nutrition therapy plays in the management of chronic digestive disorders. Further research is needed to provide additional evidence on the ideal diet modifications for various GI disorders such as IBD and NAFLD. Based on the available data, it is clear that a well-balanced diet which includes adequate amounts of whole grains, fruits and vegetables can aid in the maintenance of GI well-being. In the setting of chronic GI diseases, referral to a dietitian for in-depth nutritional counseling may be necessary. Understanding the rationale for various therapeutic diets will allow the primary care physician to promote diet compliance. A primary care physician who incorporates current nutrition guidelines into daily practice will empower patients to better manage their digestive health.

References

1 Compher C, Lichenstein GR, Gastrointestinal Disease. In Hark, L, Morrison G. *Medical Nutrition & Disease: A Case-Based Approach* (3rd edition). Blackwell Publishing: Malden MA. 2003: 232–3.

2 Srinivasan R, Minocha A. When to suspect lactose intolerance. Symptomatic, ethnic, and laboratory clues. *Postgrad Med* 1998;104:109–11;115–16;122–3.

3 Sahi T. Genetics and epidemiology of adult-type hypolactasia. *Scand J Gastroenterol* 1994;29 Suppl 202:7–20.

4 Swagerty DL, Walling AD, Klein RM. Lactose intolerance. *Am Fam Physician* 2002;65:1845–50;1855–6.

5 DiStefano M, Veneto G, Malservisi S, Stocchi A, Corazza GR. Lactose malabsorption and intolerance in the elderly. *Scand J Gastroenterol* 2001;36:1274–8.

6 Suarez FL, Adshead J, Furne JK, Levitt MD. Lactose maldigestion is not an impediment to the intake of 1500 mg calcium daily as dairy products. *Am J Clin Nutr* 1998;68:1118–22.

7 Rizkalla SW, Luo J, Kabir M, Chevalier A, Pacher N, Slama G. Chronic consumption of fresh but not heated yogurt improves breath-hydrogen status and short-chain fatty acid profiles: a controlled study in healthy men with or without lactose maldigestion. *Am J Clin Nutr* 2000;72:1474–9.

8 Food and Nutrition Board, National Academy of Sciences Institute of Medicine. Dietary Reference Intakes for Calcium, Phosphorus, Magnesium, Vitamin D, and Fluoride. Standing Committee on the Scientific Evaluation of Dietary Reference Intakes. National Academy Press: Washington DC. 1997.

9 The American Dietetic Association. Lactose-Controlled Diet. In: *Manual of Clinical Dietetic* (6th edition). 2000: pp. 212–13.

10 Food and Nutrition Board. Institute of Medicine. *Dietary Reference Intakes for Calcium, Phosphorous, Magnesium, Vitamin D and Fluoride.* National Academy of Sciences. National Academies Press. Washington, D.C. 1997.

11 Office of Dietary Supplements, NIH Clinical Center, Dietary Factsheet: Calcium. 2004. http://ods.od.nih.gov.

12 Nutrient Data Laboratory, US Dept. of Agriculture. Calcium contrent of selected foods. USDA, 2005. www.nal.usda.gov.

13 National Institutes of Health Consensus Development Conference Statement. Celiac Disease 2003. http://consensus.nih.gov.

14 Chand, N. Mihas AA. Celiac disease: current concepts in diagnosis and treatment. *Clin Gastroenterology.* 2006;40(1):3–14.

15 Stenson WF, Newberry R, Lorenz R, Baldus C, Civitelli R. Increased prevalence of celiac disease and need for routine screening among patients with osteoporosis. *Arch Intern Med* 2005;165:393–9.

16 Hallert C, Grant C, Grehn S *et al.* Evidence of poor vitamin status in celiac patients on a gluten-free diet for 10 years. *Aliment Pharmacol Ther* 2002;16:1333–9.

17 Peraaho M, Kaukinen K, Mustalahti K *et al.* Effect of an oats-containing gluten-free diet on symptoms and quality of life in celiac disease. A randomized study. *Scand J Gastroenterol* 2004;39:27–31.

18 Thompson T. Gluten contamination of commercial oat products in the United States. *N Engl J Med* 2004;351:2021–22.

19 Compher C, Lichenstein GR, Gastrointestinal disease. In Hark L, Morrison G, *Medical Nutrition and Disease: A Case-Based Approach* (3rd edition). Blackwell Publishing: Malden MA. 2003, pp. 238–9.

20 Thompson T, Dennis M, Higgins LA, Lee AR, Sharrett MK. Gluten-free diet survery: are Americans with celiac diease consuming recommended amounts of fiber, iron, calcium and grain foods? *J Hum Nutr Diet* 2005;18(3):163–9.

21 Feldman M, Friedman L, Sleisinger M. *Sleisinger and Fordtran's Gastrointestinal and Liver Disease* (7th edition). Elsevier: Philadelphia PA. 2002, p. 144.

22 The American Dietetic Association. Fat-Restricted Diet. In: *Manual of Clinical Dietetic* (6th edition). 2000: pp. 697–702.

23 Dumasy V, Delhaye M, Cotton F, Deviere J. Fat malabsorption screening in chronic pancreatitis. *Am J Gastroenterol* 2004;99(7):1350–4.

24 O'Keefe SJ. Nutrition and gastrointestinal disease. *Scand J Gastroenterol Suppl* 1996; 220:52.

25 Burke A, Lichtenstein GR, Rombeau JL. Nutrition and ulcerative colitis. *Baillieres Clin Gastroenterol* 1997;11:153.

26 Jeejeebhoy KN. Clinical nutrition:6. Management of nutritional problems of patients with crohn's disease. *CMAJ* 2002;166(7):913–18.

27 Goh J, O'Morain C.A. Review article: nutrition and adult inflammatory bowel disease. *Aliment Pharmacol Ther* 2003;17:307–20.

28 The American Dietetic Association. High Oxalate Foods. In: *Manual of Clinical Dietetic* (6th edition). 2000: p. 485.

29 Locke GR III, Talley NJ, Fett SL, Zinsmeister AR, Melton LJ III. Prevalence and clinical spectrum of gastroesophageal reflux: a population-based study in Olmsted County, Minnesota. *Gastroenterology* 1997;112:1448–56.

30 Nandurkur S, Locke GR III, Fett S, Zinsmeister AR, Cameron AJ, Talley NJ. Relationship between body mass index, diet, exercise and gastro-oesophageal reflux symptoms in a community. *Aliment Pharmacol Ther* 2004;20:497–505.

31 El-Serag HB, Satia JA, Rabeneck L. Dietary intake and the risk of gastro-oesophageal reflux disease: a cross-sectional study in volunteers. *Gut* 2005;54:11–17.

32 Colombo P, Mangano M, Bianchi PA, Penagini R. Effect of calories and fat on postprandial gastro-oesophageal reflux. *Scand J Gastroenerol* 2002;37:3–5.

33 Nilsson M, Johnsen R, Ye W, Hveem K, Lagergren J. Lifestyle related risk factors in the aetiology of gastro-oesophageal reflux. *Gut* 2004;53:1730–5.

34 Sontag SJ. Guilty as charged: bugs and drugs in gastric ulcer. *Am J Gastroenterol* 1997;92(8):1255–61.

35 McArthur K, Hogan D, Igenberg JI. Relative stimulatory effects of commonly ingested beverages on gastric acid secretion in humans. *Gastroenterology* 1982;83:199–203.

36 Olafsson S, Berstad A. Changes in food tolerance and lifestyle after eradication of *Helicobacter pylori*. *Scand J Gastroenterol* 2003;38(3):268–76.

37 Fine KD, Schiller LR. AGA technical review on the evaluation and management of chronic diarrhea. *Gastroenterology* 1999;116:1464.

38 Feldman M, Friedman L, Sleisinger M. *Sleisinger and Fordtran's Gastrointestinal and Liver Disease* (7th edition). Elsevier: Philadelphia PA. 2002, p. 131.

39 Ettinger S, Macronutrition: Carbohydrates, Proteins and lipids. In Mahan LK, Escott-Stump S, *Krause's Food, Nutrition, and Diet Therapy* (11th edition). Saunders: Philadelphia PA. 2004, p. 47.

40 Higgins PD, Johanson JF. Epidemiology of constipation in North America: a systematic review. *Am J Gastroenterol* 2004;99(4):750–9.

41 Locke, GR III, Pemberton, JH, Phillips, SF. AGA technical review on constipation. *Gastroenterology* 2000;119:1766.

42 Dukas L, Willet WC, Giovannucci EL. Association between physical activity, fiber intake, and other lifestyle variables and constipation in a study of women. *Am J Gastroenterol* 2003;98(9):1790–6.

43 Vesa TH, Seppo LM, Marteau, PR, Sahi T, Korpela R. Role of irritable bowel syndrome in subjective lactose intolerance. *Am J Clin Nutr* 1998;67:710–15.

44 Choi YK, Johlin FC Jr, Summers RW, Jackson M, Rao SS. Fructose intolerance: an under-recognized problem. *Am J Gastroenterol* 2003;98:1348–53.

45 Snook J, Shepard HS. Bran supplementation in the treatment of irritable bowel syndrome. *Aliment Pharmacol Ther* 1994;8:511–14.

46 Lucey MR, Clark ML, Lowndes J, Dawson AM. Is bran efficcious in irritable bowel syndrome? A double-blind, placebo-controlled crossover study. *Gut* 1978;28:221–5.

47 Aller R, de Luis DA, Izaola O *et al*. Effects of a high-fiber diet on symptoms of irritable bowel syndrome: a randomized clinical trial. *Nutrition* 2004;20:735–7.

48 Parisi GC, Zill M, Miani MP *et al*. High-fiber diet supplementation in patients with irritable bowel syndrome (IBS). A multicenter, randomized, open trial comparison between wheat bran diet and partially hydrolyzed guar gum (PHGG). *Dig Dis Sci* 2002;47(8):1697–1704.

49 Beyer PL, Medical nutrition therapy for lower gastrointestinal tract disorders. In Mahan LK, Escott-Stump S, *Krause's Food, Nutrition, and Diet Therapy* (11th edition). Saunders: Philadelphia PA. 2004, p. 707.

50 Marlett, JA, McBUrney MI, Slavin JL. Health implications of dietary fiber. *J Am Diet Assoc* 2001;102:993–1000.

51 Sanyal AJ. American Gastroenterological Association. AGA technical review on nonalcoholic fatty liver disease. *Gastroenterology* 2002;123(5):1705–25.

52 Solga S, Alkhuraishe AR, Clark JM *et al*. Dietary composition and nonalcoholic fatty liver disease. *Dig Dis Sci* 2004;49(10):1578–84.

53 A.S.P.E.N. Board of Directors and The Clinical Guidelines Task Force. Guidelines for the use of parenteral and enteral nutrition in adult and pediatric patients: liver disease. *JPEN* 2002;26(1)Suppl:65SA–67SA.

54 Merli M, Riggio O, Dally L. Does malnutrition affect survival in cirrhosis? *PINC Hepatol* 1997;25:672–7.

55 Plauth M, Merli M, Kondrup J, Weimann A, Ferenci P, Muller MJ. ESPEN guidelines for nutrition in liver disease and transplantation. *Clin Nutr* 1997;16:43–55.

56 Bianci GP, Marchesini G, Fabbri A *et al*. Vegetable versus animal protein diet in cirrhotic patients with chronic encephalopathy. A randomized cross-over comparison. *J Intern Med* 1993;233:385–92.

57 Chen Y, Satoh T, Tokunya O. Vibrio vulnificus infection in patients with liver disease: reports of five autopsy cases. *Virchows Archiv* 2002;44(1):88–92.

58 Brown L, Hill P, Klaver S, Sodium Restricted Diet. In: *Manual of Clinical Dietetic* (6th edition). The American Dietetic Association. 2000: pp. 770–4.

59 Cuevas A, Miquel JF, Reyes MS, Zanlungo S, Nervi F. Diet as a risk factor for cholesterol gallstone disease. *J Amer Coll Nutr* 2004;23(3):187–96.

60 Tsai CJ, Leitzman MF, Hu FB, Willett WC, Giovannucci EL. Frequent nut consumption and decreased risk of cholecystectomy in women. *Am J Clin Nutr* 2004;80(1):76–81.

61 Tsai CJ, Leitzman MF, Hu FB, Willett WC, Giovannucci EL. A prospective cohort study of nut consumption and the risk of gallstone disease in men. *Am J Epid* 2004;160(10):961–8.

62 The American Dietetic Association. High-Fiber Diet. In: *Manual of Clinical Dietetic* (6th edition). 2000: pp. 710–11.

Further reading

Hebden JM, Blackshaw E, D'Amato M, Perkins AC, Spiller RC. Abnormalities of GI transit in bloated irritable bowel syndrome: effect of bran on transit and symptoms. *Am J Gastroenterol* 2002;97:2315–20.

Suarez FL, Savaiano DA, Levitt MD. A comparison of symptoms after the consumption of milk or lactose-hydrolyzed milk by people with self-reported severe lactose intolerance. *N Engl J Med* 1995;333:1–4.

CHAPTER 10

Everything else

Marion Vetter and Katherine Chauncey

The quality of food intake is important to all medical conditions. A healthy diet can lower an individual's susceptibility to disease and boost immune response. Assessment of current dietary intake is always recommended as a part of a preventive medical visit. Following are specific dietary and nutritional recommendations for medical problems commonly seen in the primary care setting.

Urinary tract infections

Urinary tract infections (UTIs) account for more than 11 million physician visits annually in the United States and have become increasingly resistant to first-line antibiotic therapy [1]. Women are more susceptible to UTIs than men.

Urinary tract infections are ascending infections that are commonly caused by coliform bacteria. *Escherichia coli* (*E. coli*) is the most frequent pathogen. Dietary factors which can affect the bacterial flora include cranberry juice, yogurt with lactobacillus and adequate fluid intake.

Cranberry juice
Cranberry juice has long been purported to reduce the incidence of UTIs. Early research focused on the acidification of the urine as the mechanism through which cranberry juice exerted its bacteriostatic effect, but this was not substantiated. Recent evidence indicates that cranberry proanthocyanidins (condensed tannins) may inhibit P-fimbriated *E. coli* from adhering to uroepithelial cells, the initial step in development of UTIs [2]. There is now good evidence that certain components in cranberry juice (tannins and fructose) can bind to type 1 fimbriated *E. coli* to reduce their ability to adhere to uroepithelial cells. Additional compounds, including the flavonol epicatechin, have also been found to inhibit adhesion to the genitourinary lining [3]. The anti-adhesion effect of cranberry juice can last up to 10 hours [2]; therefore, ingestion of two 8 oz servings of cranberry juice, 10 hours apart, may be beneficial in UTI-susceptible individuals. Cranberry juice cocktail can contain 30 g sugar and 120 calories per 8 oz serving. Patients with diabetes or glucose intolerance should consume the light versions sweetened with artificial sweetener which contain two-thirds less calories and sugar than the regular versions. Cranberry capsules are also available and have been shown to be equally effective.

Probiotics

Probiotics are live beneficial microorganisms administered in adequate amounts to confer a positive health effect to the host. Probiotics are important in maintaining the balance of microbes to favor beneficial bacteria over the potentially harmful ones. *Lactobacillus* and bifidobacteria are the most commonly used probiotics and are often found in fermented dairy foods such as yogurt. Multiple studies have examined the role of probiotics in preventing recurrent UTIs. *Lactobacillus* colonizes the gut lumen, replacing potentially pathogenic coliform bacteria and decreasing the risk of recurrent UTIs [4]. Additionally, *lactobacillus* restores rather than destroys the normal urogenital flora. This helps to prevent vaginal candidiasis, a common problem following antimicrobial therapy [5]. Yogurt products in the supermarket containing the beneficial bacteria will carry a symbol from the National Yogurt Association and the designation *"Meets National Yogurt Association Criteria for Live and Active Culture Yogurt."* Products without this designation cannot be depended upon to carry the beneficial bacteria. Generally, the recommendation for consumption of yogurt to help prevent UTI is 6–8 oz per day.

Fluids

Clear evidence about the benefit of increased fluid intake is still somewhat lacking. Several studies suggest that copious intake of fluids can actually dilute antibacterial factors present in the urine (such as Tamm–Horsfall glycoprotein) and may increase the risk of infection [5]. However, fluid intake remains a controversial issue and no clear recommendations have been established [4]. Checking that the patient is consuming adequate fluid of 8 cups per day is reasonable. Recommendations beyond that is a matter of clinical judgment.

Nutritional recommendations for UTI

1) Maintain adequate fluid intake of 8 cups of water, juice, milk, or other beverages. Tea and coffee can be considered part of fluid intake.

2) Recommend two 8 oz glasses of cranberry juice cocktail per day; 10–12 hours apart for UTI-susceptible individuals. For others, one glass 3–4 times per week is satisfactory. "Sugar-Free" juice for diabetes and overweight patients.

3) Increase intake of dairy products, such as yogurt, that contain live and active cultures as specified by the National Yogurt Association. Patients should look for the association's symbol on the product.

4) Improve overall quality of food intake by increasing fruits, vegetables, whole grains, fish, poultry, olive or canola oil, and nuts. Decrease intake of soda, candy, and processed foods.

Source: Marion Vetter, MD, RD and Katherine Chauncey, PhD, RD, FADA. 2007. Used with permission.

Table 10.1 Dietary triggers for migraine headaches.

Offending food or behavior	Chemical trigger
Cheese	Tyramine
Chocolate	Phenylethylamine, theobromine
Citrus fruits	Phenolic amines, octopamine
Hot dogs, ham, cured meats	Nitrites, nitric oxide
Dairy foods	Allergenic proteins (casein, etc)
Fatty and fried foods	Linoleic and oleic fatty acids
Food dyes, additives	Tartrazine, sulfites
Artificial sweetener	Aspartame
Wine, beer	Histamine, tyramine, sulfites
Caffeineated beverages	Caffeine withdrawal
Fasting, skipping meals	Hypoglycemia, stress hormone release
Inadequate sleep	Sleep dept

Source: [6].

Migraine headache

Migraines typically begin with the depolarization of cortical neurons and sensitization of the trigeminal nerve ganglia. A secondary phase involving vasoconstriction, vasodilatation, and vascular inflammation is mediated by neurotransmitters, most notably serotonin. Dietary triggers may play some role in the pathogenesis of migraines by modulating either the release of neurotransmitters or by stimulating neuroreceptors. Commonly implicated foods include chocolate, cheese, fruits, caffeine and alcohol. Food sensitivities that are immunologically mediated are very rare causes of migraines. Clinical studies vary widely in the percentage of patients who report food-triggered migraines, from as few as 7% to as many as 44% [6]. Several commonly implicated food components are described below and a comprehensive list of triggers for migraine are provided in Table 10.1.

Biogenic amines and migraines

Biogenic amines are organic bases that are formed by the decarboxylation of free amino acids. They have potent vasoconstrictive properties and include tyramine, histamine, and phenylethylamine. Specifically, tyramine is thought to stimulate the release of norepinephrine from sympathetic nerve endings with subsequent cerebral vasoconstriction [7]. Biogenic amines can occur naturally in many foods or may be produced as a byproduct of fermentation or decay. Foods containing significant amounts of biogenic amines include fermented products such as cheese, sauerkraut, processed meats, alcoholic beverages, chocolate, and yeast extracts. Cheese typically contains large amounts of tyramine, while chocolate contains notable quantities of phenylethylamine. Biogenic amines were first implicated as potential precipitants of migraines when it was noted that patients taking monoamine-oxidase inhibitors often developed headaches when consuming tyramine-rich foods

[8]. Similarly, patients with diet-triggered migraines may also have impaired tyramine metabolism secondary to either a deficiency of monoamine-oxidase or a defect in one of the enzymes involved in the conjugation of tyramine [6]. Consequently, levels remain high and cerebral vasoconstriction ensues. Low-tyramine diets for migraine prophylaxis remains controversial. Jansen *et al.* [8] reviewed the evidence for diet-triggered migraines and found no relation between the ingestion of amines and food intolerance reactions. However, other studies have suggested a strong correlation between amine-rich foods and headaches.

Caffeine and caffeine-withdrawal migraines

Given the popularity of soft drinks, teas, and coffee, large quantities of caffeine may be consumed on a daily basis. An eight-ounce cup of coffee has roughly 300 mg of caffeine, compared to 35 mg in a 12-ounce can of cola. Abrupt cessation of caffeinated beverages can precipitate a migraine, most typically within 24–48 hours. Although caffeine intake initially causes cerebral vasoconstriction, a rebound vasodilatation and increased blood flow occurs when caffeine is discontinued [6].

Alcohol and migraines

Alcohol, most frequently red wine, is often implicated as a migraine trigger. Compounds found in alcoholic beverages including histamine, tyramine, sulfites, and phenolic flavinoids are thought to mediate several different pathways in the pathogenesis of migraines. Tyramine releases norepinephrine causing vasoconstriction, while the flavinoids have been associated with increased serotonin levels. Red wine is a particularly potent trigger in food-sensitive patients, as it has higher levels of phenolic flavinoids and histamine [6].

Monosodium glutamate triggered migraines

Monosodium glutamate (MSG) is most commonly associated with Asian foods. However, it is a flavor enhancer that is incorporated into many other food items including snack foods, frozen foods, sauces, salad dressings, and canned soups, and may be purchased by consumers as a flavor enhancer or meat tenderizer. MSG is a potent vasoconstrictor, which can result in headache, palpitations, sweating, and flushing shortly after ingestion. Although many patients may report intolerance to MSG, it is estimated that only 1.8% of patients have a true reaction after consuming large amounts [6].

Medical Nutrition Therapy for headaches

Elimination diets are used to help patients identify their individual dietary triggers, if any. Elimination diets have two phases: the first phase, where foods are eliminated and symptoms will be reduced (if successful); and the second phase, where foods are gradually reintroduced while watching for the appearance of symptoms. The whole process may take months to complete. Elimination diets remain controversial and are often difficult to maintain. Headache diaries may be useful in identifying certain dietary triggers that can then be avoided or consumed in lower quantities [6]. Potentially offending foods are listed in Table 10.1. A balanced diet is generally recommended and given the relationship between hypoglycemia and headaches, skipping meals or consuming a low calorie diet should be avoided. Regular physical activity has also been found to reduce the frequency of migranes [9].

Nutrition-focused questions related to migraine headaches

1) Ask about the intake frequency of the dietary triggers listed in Table 10.1. A food frequency questionnaire may be useful for this purpose.

2) Assess overall diet quality and physical activity. Make appropriate recommendations.

3) Recommend the patient keep a headache diary to detect the possible association of certain foods or behaviors with the development of a migraine.

Source: Marion Vetter, MD, RD and Katherine Chauncey, PhD, RD, FADA. 2007. Used with permission.

Anemia (iron deficiency)

Iron deficiency anemia has an overall prevalence of 11% in the industrialized world. Populations most at risk include pregnant women and women of childbearing age, women with heavy menses or low socio-economic status, strict vegetarians and vegans, infants and toddlers, and adolescents. Low iron intake and decreased absorption are the most common etiologies.

Evaluation
Serum biomarkers are available for the assessment of iron status and are used to distinguish between the stages of iron deficiency: depleted iron stores, early functional iron deficiency, and iron-deficiency anemia [10].

Iron stores
Ferritin is the most sensitive marker of iron stores and levels less than 12 µg are suggestive of depleted stores. As ferritin is an acute phase reactant, infection, inflammation, and other disease states can produce falsely elevated levels. Chronic alcohol use and hyperglycemia also result in elevated ferritin levels.

Early functional iron deficiency
Serum transferrin saturation can be used to assess iron deficiency. Normal saturation falls between 30–35%, whereas levels less than 15% indicate decreased iron availability for erythropoiesis in the bone marrow. Erythrocyte protoporphyrin concentration can also be used to assess whether adequate iron is available for red blood cell synthesis. Protoporphyrin levels remain elevated when there is inadequate iron available to be integrated into hemoglobin

[10]. Normal protoporphyrin levels vary from 16–65 µg/dL in adults. Anemia produces levels of over 100 µg/dL.

Clinical signs and symptoms

Clinical signs of anemia include pallor, mouth changes such as glossitis, atrophy of the lingual papillae, angular stomatitis, and tachycardia. Symptoms are generally non-specific and may include fatigue, palpitations, or dyspnea [11].

Medical Nutrition Therapy for anemia

Oral iron supplements are usually first line therapy for iron-deficiency anemia, as it is an inexpensive, safe, and an effective means of repleting iron stores. Ferrous sulfate is the most common preparation and contains 60 mg of elemental iron per 300 mg tablet. It is water soluble and dissolves instantly when exposed to gastric juice. With a standard dose of 180 mg of elemental iron daily, reticulocytosis is expected within a week and hemoglobin should increase by 2 g/dL over the course of 3 weeks. Currently, there is no consensus on the duration of iron therapy [11]. A common side effect is constipation and adherence may be low.

If the anemia does not correct with iron supplementation, several causes must be considered including:
• Impaired absorption (may be seen with celiac disease, malabsorptive disease, or concomitant use of binders)
• Poor adherence due to side effects
• Excess iron loss or increased need
• Thalassemia

Parenteral iron therapy, which is administered via intramuscular or intravenous routes, may be required in patients with severe malabsorption, ongoing blood loss, those requiring chronic hemodialysis, and those who are unable to tolerate oral iron. Iron dextran is the most widely available parenteral form and contains 50 mg/mL of elemental iron. However, there are multiple serious side effects associated with parenteral iron including muscle necrosis, phlebitis, and in rare cases, anaphylaxis.

In addition to medication, high iron foods should also be prescribed. These include beef, liver, kidney, beans, nuts, green leafy vegetables, and fortified products. Breakfast cereals and infant formulas are the most frequently consumed fortified products, but usually contain only small amounts of added iron. Cornmeal, grits, and pasta products are also frequently fortified. In the United States, fortified iron accounts for 25% of total iron intake.

Factors influencing iron absorption

The bioavailability of dietary iron may be influenced by several factors. *Heme* iron, which is typically present in meat, fish, and poultry, is three times more readily absorbed than the *non-heme* iron present in fruits, vegetables, and grains. Non-heme and fortified iron absorption can be increased by the addition of ascorbic acid. Ascorbic acid can reduce ferric iron to its more soluble ferrous form, thus decreasing the formation of insoluble complexes with absorption inhibitors. Ascorbic acid can enhance iron absorption by forming soluble complexes with iron at low pH that remain soluble in the more alkaline environment of the duodenum. Drinking orange juice with supplements can therefore increase the iron absorption.

Conversely, several compounds in certain foods may decrease iron absorption. These include tannins (found in teas), phosphates (found in bran products), phytates, and oxalates. Many of these substances chelate iron, rendering it unavailable for absorption. Phytic acid is found in high amounts in many infant formulas and can substantially decrease the bioavailability of iron. However, ascorbic acid can overcome the inhibitory effect of phytic acid if present in sufficient amounts. Enzymatic degradation has also been used to decrease phytic acid and increase iron absorption [12].

Calcium has also been found to reduce iron absorption to such an extent that some researchers advise that cheese, milk, or milkshakes not be consumed with the meals providing most of the dietary iron [13]. The long-term impact of this interference is unclear [14].

Megaloblastic anemia

Megaloblastic anemia is characterized by an elevated mean corpuscular volume (MCV) greater than 100 fL (femtoliters). It is usually caused by a deficiency of vitamin B_{12}, folic acid, or both. As vitamin B_{12} has a long half-life, it takes several years for stores to become depleted. However, folate stores are depleted in 2–5 months if dietary deficiency is present.

Etiology
Folate deficiency may be caused by inadequate intake, increased requirements secondary to underlying conditions such as pregnancy, increased cell turnover, impaired metabolism seen with chronic alcohol ingestion, drug-induced disorders of DNA synthesis, and congenital disorders of DNA synthesis (ie. Lesch–Nyhan). Vitamin B_{12} deficiency may be caused by inadequate intake, decreased levels or lack of intrinsic factor (can be congenital or related to surgical resection) with subsequent pernicious anemia, achlorhydria, or *Diphyllobothrium latum*. Combined vitamin B_{12} and folate deficiency is seen in gluten-induced enteropathy and celiac disease.

Screening
Certain populations including the elderly, patients with malnutrition, and alcoholics, are at risk for B_{12} and/or folate deficiency. Screening should also be performed in patients with dementia or other neurologic symptoms.

Evaluation

Patients with an elevated MCV often warrant measurement of serum folate and cobalamin levels.

• *Folate levels.* Serum folate levels less than 4 ng/mL are suggestive of folate deficiency. However, serum folate levels are indicative of short-term folate balance and can be decreased by recent alcohol intake, pregnancy, medications, or several days of decreased dietary intake. Although red blood cell folate levels are more reliable indicators of tissue folate stores, it is an expensive test and is usually reserved for patients with borderline folate levels.

• *Cobalamin levels.* There are multiple assays for measuring vitamin B_{12} levels. In general, cobalamin levels less than 200 pg/mL (<148 pMol/L) suggests vitamin B_{12} deficiency and levels greater than 300 pg/mL make it very unlikely.

• *Metabolite levels.* Methylmalonate and homocysteine are useful measurements in patients with borderline cobalamin or vitamin B_{12} levels or in patients who are pregnant. Both metabolites are elevated in cobalamin deficiency due to decreased metabolism. Homocysteine is elevated in folate deficiency only.

• *Peripheral smear.* Hypersegmented neutrophils are seen with cobalamin and/or folate deficiency.

Medical Nutrition Therapy for folic acid deficiency

Even if malabsorption is present, daily oral supplementation of 1 mg folic acid is usually adequate. At this dose, stores are typically repleted in 1–2 months. Maintenance of folate stores can be achieved with daily intake of 50–100 μg. Excellent food sources of folate include dairy foods, green leafy vegetables and liver.

Pernicious anemia

Pernicious anemia is caused by a vitamin B_{12} deficiency. Most commonly this condition is secondary to a lack of intrinsic factor, which is produced in the antrum of the stomach and is necessary for the absorption of vitamin B_{12} in the ileum. Dietary deficiency is very rare, although strict vegans are at risk because they avoid all animal products.

Clinical and laboratory evaluation

Pernicious anemia can cause neurologic symptoms including paresthesias, decreased proprioception and dementia. Classically, the Schilling test was used in the past to confirm the presence of pernicious anemia. Given the difficulty in administering the test and the expense, it is now rarely used. Anti-intrinsic factor antibody tests are now available and are highly specific for pernicious anemia.

Medical Nutrition Therapy for pernicious anemia

Pernicious anemia is treated with intramuscular vitamin B_{12} injections given 1 mg daily for 1–2 weeks, followed by monthly doses. High doses of oral vitamin B_{12} are also effective (typically 1–2 mg daily.) Cobalamin can also be given sublingually or via a nasal spray. Food sources of vitamin B_{12} include liver, meat, eggs, dairy products and green leafy vegetables. Soy milk enriched with vitamin B_{12} can be recommended, especially for vegetarians.

Nephrolithiasis (kidney stones)

Kidney stones are often composed of calcium salts, uric acid, cystine, or struvite and are influenced by nutritional, environmental and genetic factors. Crystal formation often occurs under conditions of urinary supersaturation with crystallization promoters (e.g., calcium, oxalate, uric acid) or when the urinary level of inhibitors (e.g., citrate, glycosaminoglycans, nephrocalcin) is decreased. Calcium oxalate stones are the most common, followed by calcium citrate stones.

Medical Nutrition Therapy for kidney stones

Fluids

Regardless of the pathogenesis of kidney stones, increased fluid intake is the cornerstone of therapy. Higher fluid intake of 2–3 L/day increases urinary volume, resulting in decreased urinary supersaturation and lower levels of crystal-forming components [15]. Two large prospective studies found a significantly lower incidence of stone formation with increased fluid intake in subjects who had a prior calcium stone. However, the type of fluid may impact stone formation. Multiple studies have shown an increased risk of stones with apple and grapefruit juice consumption, although the mechanism is unclear [15]. Soda intake greater than 1 L per week was also associated with a higher risk of nephrolithiasis. This is thought to be secondary to phosphoric acid, which is used as an acidifying agent in soda. The increased acid load results in increased urinary excretion of uric acid and calcium and decreased excretion of citrate [16].

Oxalate

Although calcium and oxalate crystallize in a 1 : 1 ratio, recent evidence has shown that calcium stone formation is associated more with increased urinary oxalate levels as opposed to urinary calcium levels. Small increases in oxalate excretion dramatically raise the urinary saturation of calcium oxalate and can precipitate stone formation [15]. However, hyperoxaluria is rarely due to excessive consumption of oxalate-rich foods. Dietary oxalate accounts for only 20% of urinary oxalate, while the majority is endogenously produced as byproducts of glycine and ascorbic acid metabolism [17]. As considerable variation exists in oxalate absorption between individuals, patients susceptible to calcium oxalate stones may benefit from a low oxalate diet of 40–50 g/day. Additionally, adequate calcium intake is also essential to bind oxalate. (See Appendices G, H and N).

Calcium

As many patients with recurrent nephrolithiasis often have idiopathic hypercalciuria, excess calcium intake was initially implicated in the formation of calcium oxalate stones. In the past, restriction of dietary calcium was used to lower urinary calcium and prevent recurrent stones. However, multiple studies have shown that a low calcium intake has many detrimental effects and may actually increase stone risk by causing reciprocal hyperoxaluria [16, 17]. When lower levels of calcium are available, less calcium oxalate is formed in the intestinal lumen and overabsorption of dietary oxalate occurs. In turn, this causes increased urinary supersaturation of calcium oxalate, favoring stone precipitation. Additionally, calcium restriction in calcium stone formers with idiopathic hypercalciuria does not reduce urinary calcium levels to that of healthy controls [17]. Lastly, decreased calcium intake is also associated with negative calcium balance and bone loss. Given these findings, a calcium intake of 800–1200 mg/day should be adequate to prevent hyperoxaluria and maintain calcium balance.

Sodium

Given the relationship between the renal tubular handling of calcium and sodium, dietary sodium intake plays a role in the pathogenesis of stone formation. Calcium is passively reabsorbed in the proximal tubule and loop of Henle in conjunction with the gradient created by the reabsorption of sodium and water. Thus, higher levels of sodium intake are associated with increased urinary calcium. In addition, sodium intake has a direct and indirect effect on the distal tubule through its effects on parathyroid hormone. Sodium restricted diets, 80–100 mEq/day or 1840–2300 mg/day, have been found to increase proximal sodium and calcium re-absorption and decrease calcuria [16]. (See Appendix I for high sodium foods.)

Protein

Multiple studies have documented a strong correlation between excess animal protein intake and increased incidence of calcium and uric stones [17]. Protein metabolism generates a significant acid load, primary from the sulfuric acid generated by the catabolism of sulfur-containing amino acids. Subsequently, renal tubular calcium reabsorption is decreased, leading to increased urinary excretion of calcium, oxalate, and uric acid [17]. Urinary citrate (a potent inhibitor of stone formation) excretion is also decreased. Vegetarians were found to have a much lower prevalence of nephrolithiasis, presumably because vegetable proteins contain less sulfur-containing amino acids [15]. Modest protein restriction to 1 g/kg body weight has been recommended although clinical studies are lacking [16].

Citrate

Citrate functions as an inhibitor to stone formation by complexing with calcium ions to decrease urinary supersaturation, and by inhibiting the growth of calcium oxalate and calcium phosphate crystals. Lower urinary citrate concentrations have been associated with a high animal protein, high sodium, or combined high protein and high sodium intake [15]. Large quantities of orange juice consumption have also been associated with increased urinary citrate excretion [15].

Chronic kidney disease

Chronic kidney disease (CKD) is a permanent, progressive loss of kidney function characterized by a decline in glomerular filtration rate (GFR). The National Kidney Foundation (NKF) defines CKD as persistent kidney damage confirmed by a GFR <60 mL/min for >3 months [18]. CKD has replaced the former terminology of pre-ESRD (end-stage renal disease), predialysis, and chronic renal insufficiency, which were previously used to describe individuals with renal insufficiency not yet requiring dialysis or transplant.

Given the rising prevalence of diabetes and cardiovascular disease, corresponding increases in CKD have also occurred. Type 2 diabetes is the largest single contributor to CKD. Diabetic nephropathy due to type 2 diabetes constitutes the major reason for the rising incidence of ESRD in the United States. Hypertension is the second leading cause of CKD in the United States. The NFK recognizes that the rapid increase in CKD will require primary care physicians to provide medical care for patients with CKD, particularly in the early stages when intervention might slow the progression of the disease (control of blood sugar and blood pressure) [19].

Reduction of dietary protein intake can be a clinically cumbersome approach to halting progressive renal disease. Nevertheless, meta-analyses have consistently confirmed the value of dietary protein restriction as a maneuver for reducing progressive kidney injury across a relatively wide range of disease categories [20].

CKD has been formally classified into five stages under the 2002 Kidney Disease Outcome Quality Initiative (K/DOQI) of the NKF [18]. Prior to this initiative, there was no stratification upon which to diagnose and base care in a uniform manner. Stages 1–4 represent kidney disease categories where medical and nutrition management can impact and potentially delay progression to Stage 5 (chronic kidney failure). Staging of chronic kidney disease allows providers to talk more clearly with patients, and use of the word "kidney" rather than "renal" also facilitates communication (Tables 10.2 and 10.3) [19].

In addition to symptomatic relief and forestalling dialysis, the Modification of Diet in Renal Disease Study (MDRD) [21], demonstrated that moderate protein restriction (0.6 g/kg) also delayed the progression of renal disease. There has been some confusion about the benefit of protein restriction, but post hoc analyses of the MDRD study indicate that low protein diets definitely retard the progression of renal failure. Analysis of data showed that combined tight control of blood pressure and modification of protein (0.6 g/kg/day with a GFR <25) helped delay progression by as much as 41% [22].

Table 10.2 Classification stages of chronic kidney disease

Stages	GFR (mL/min/1.73 m^2)
Stage 1 Kidney damage with normal or high GFR	GFR $\geq$ 90
Stage 2 Kidney damage with mild decreased GFR	GFR 60–89
Stage 3 Moderate decreased GFR	GFR 30–59
Stage 4 Severe decreased GFR	GFR 15–29
Stage 5 Kidney failure	GFR < 15 or dialysis

Source: [18].

Given decreased intake (0.6–0.8 g/kg), protein quality is important and at least 50% should be of high biological value (HBV) [22]. HBV protein contains a larger percentage of essential amino acids. This allows a lower dietary protein content diet. HBV protein is found in meats, fish, poultry, dairy products, egg whites, and protein powder. Although guidelines for 0.6–0.8 gm/kg/day are recommended in CKD, maintaining appropriate body protein stores and translating the diet from theory into food reality often necessitates liberalization [22]. The distribution of remaining non-protein calories should embrace cardiovascular health principles controlling blood pressure and lipids [23].

Table 10.3 Selected nutritional parameters for normal kidney and for Stages 1–4 CKD.

Nutritional parameter	Normal kidney function	Stages 1–4 CKD
Calories (kcal/kg/day)	30–37	35 < 60 years 30–35 $\geq$ 60 years
Protein (gm/kg/day)	0.8	0.6–0.75 (50% HBV)
Fat (% total kcal)	25–35%	<7% saturated fat; <200 mg cholesterol
Sodium (mg/day)	Unrestricted	2400
Potassium (mg/day)	Unrestricted	Generally unrestricted unless serum potassium level is >5 mg/dL or potassium-sparing medications are used
Calcium (mg/day) and dietary intake	Unrestricted	<2000 including binders
Phosphorus (mg/day) phosphate level is >4.6mg/dL	Unrestricted	800–1000, if serum
Fluid (mL/day) urine output	Unrestricted	Unrestricted with normal

Source: [22,35].
CKD, chronic kidney disease.

Research indicates that CKD patients treated with a low-protein diet for prolonged periods before dialysis exhibit improved survival after they begin dialysis [24].

Moderate protein restriction is considered safe and reduces uremic symptoms in patients with chronic renal disease by decreasing nitrogenous waste products. Bernard confirmed that patients with mildly impaired renal function had decreased whole-body protein turnover and reduced amino acid oxidation on a moderately low-protein diet, which suggested a protein-sparing effect [25]. A low-protein diet also limits the intake of phosphates, acid, and salt, as well as precursors of uremic toxins, thus improving uremic symptoms and complications of CKD [24].

Medical Nutritional Therapy for chronic kidney disease
Given the impact of diet (specifically protein restriction) on the progression of renal disease, patients with impaired kidney function should undergo routine nutrition assessment and may benefit from early referral to a renal dietitian [22]. Medicare reimburses the services of a registered dietitian for renal disease [26]. Regular assessment of dietary compliance and protein stores is required. Compliance to the protein restriction by a CKD patient can be measured by the collection of a 24-hour urine specimen. A nitrogen balance calculation can determine if a patient is eating more (or less) than the prescribed amount of protein.

HIV and AIDS

HIV (human immunodeficiency virus) is a complex illness and has multiple nutritional implications, ranging from metabolic derangements to significant food–drug interactions. Nutritional status is one of the strongest predictors of functional status and survival in HIV-positive patients [27]. Multiple studies have shown that nutritional interventions may have positive effects on health outcomes [27, 28].

The use of highly active antiretroviral therapy (HAART) – antiretroviral drugs used in combination – has dramatically altered the lives of HIV and AIDS (acquired immunodeficiency syndrome) patients by preventing the progression of AIDS and increasing quality of life. Many AIDS patients live longer and thus need more help managing the complexities of the disease, including diet and nutrition education and counseling. Primary care physicians can provide most components of comprehensive HIV care [28].

Nutritional risk stratification
All patients with HIV should be periodically screened for nutritional risk, as multiple factors can lead to nutritional compromise at any stage of the disease. Screening should include information about weight history (specifically weight loss or gain), wasting, dietary intake, problems associated with intake (poor dentition, thrush, or esophagitis), gastrointestinal symptoms, and a

review of potential food–drug–nutrient interactions. Cardiovascular risk factors including dysplipidemia, diabetes, and hypertension should also be discussed. Although no standardized screening tools are available, the Revised Subjective Global Assessment is a validated form and has been the most extensively studied in the HIV population [29].

Ideally, all HIV patients should have access to a registered dietitian (RD) to perform the nutritional evaluation as part of the multidisciplinary team approach (See Table 10.5). However, continuing education and RDs trained in nutrition therapy for HIV and AIDS patients are available for consultation through the American Dietetic Association (www.eatright.org). In the absence of an RD, primary care providers can initiate early nutritional counseling and monitoring (see Box below.) Suggestions for managing symptoms of diarrhea, nausea/vomiting, fatigue, and taste changes are shown on pp. 214–215.

Early nutrition counseling and intervention in HIV patients

1) Nutrition counseling and intervention should begin as soon as someone is diagnosed as HIV positive. The goal is to encourage the patient to focus his/her attention on diet while still feeling well to maximize reserves and provide appropriate nutrition to the immune system.

2) Establish appropriate calorie intake and increase caloric intake with food and supplements as needed.

3) Recommend vitamin and mineral supplementation. Do not megadose, but start with a multiple vitamin and mineral containing 100–200% of the recommended dietary allowance (RDA) for most nutrients.

4) Antioxidant nutrients such as vitamins E, A, and C; selenium; and zinc may need to be supplemented in higher amounts. Do not exceed the tolerable upper limits (UL) established by the dietary reference intakes.

Source: [27].

Nutritional guidelines for HIV/AIDS symptoms

Diarrhea

Increase fluids especially water, broths, diluted fruit juices and sports drinks. Avoid caffeine and alcohol.

• Eat small servings every few hours.

• Initiate the BRAT (bananas, white rice, applesauce and white toast) diet if intolerant to other foods.

• Lactose-containing foods, high fiber foods, and high fat foods can make diarrhea worse.

Table 10.4 Food safety issues for persons with AIDS

- Avoid raw and undercooked proteins foods, especially rare meats, sushi, soft cheeses, unpasteurized milk or dairy products, or uncooked or cracked eggs.
- Use different cutting boards and utensils for raw and cooked meats.
- Maintain appropriate food temperatures:
  - Hot foods: cook at 165°F to 200°F and hold at 140°F to 165°F
  - Cold foods: refrigerator 40°F, freezer 0°F
  - Do not eat foods left at room temperature for more than 2 hours, especially mayonnaise, eggs, meat, or easily spoiled foods.
- Do not thaw foods at room temperature; thaw in refrigerator or cold water changed frequently.
- Wash fresh produce well before eating or peeling.
- Wash hands frequently with soap and warm water.
- Discard moldy or spoiled foods and foods that are past expiration date.
- Use paper towels in kitchen instead of dish towels.

Source: [37].

Nausea/vomiting
- Avoid strong smelling foods.
- Stay in upright position for at least 2 hours after eating.
- In addition to the recommendations for diarrhea, eat bland food like eggs, potatoes, rice, crackers, and pretzels.

Fatigue
- Have easy-to-prepare foods such as frozen dinners, crackers, peanut butter, cheese, pasta, and jarred sauces available.
- Refer to community home delivered meal programs, order delivery foods from restaurant, or ask family or friends to help with cooking duties.

Change in taste
- Marinate protein foods with fruit juices, Italian dressing, soy sauce, sweet and sour sauce.
- Try different spices.
- Suck on hard candies, especially sour balls.
- Add lemon or lime juice or vinegar to vegetables or meats.
- Use mouthwash and brush teeth and tongue before eating.

Nutrition assessment
As HIV has many specific risk factors for nutritional compromise and associated nutritional deficiencies, general screening protocols are often not adequate for persons with HIV. Nutrition assessment of these patients should

---

Table 10.5 Categories for registered dietitian consultation

Low risk – consult RD as needed
- Stable weight or appropriate weight gain and growth.
- Consuming adequate and well-balanced diet.
- Maintains regular exercise.
- Normal levels of cholesterol, triglycerides, albumin and glucose.
- Normal hepatic and renal function.
- Stable psychosocial issues.

Moderate risk – consult RD within one month
- Obesity or evidence for body fat redistribution.
- Elevated cholesterol (>200 mg/dL), triglycerides (>250 mg/dL), or low cholesterol (<100 mg/dL).
- Osteoporosis, diabetes mellitus – controlled or new onset, hypertension
- Oral thrush.
- Dental problems.
- Chronic nausea or vomiting, diarrhea, or eating disorder.
- Possible food–drug–nutrient interactions.
- Unstable psychosocial situation.

High risk – consult RD in one week or less
- 10% unintentional weight loss over 4–6 months.
- 5% unintentional weight loss within 4 weeks or in conjunction with thrush, dental problems, dysphagia, chronic nausea or vomiting, or diarrhea; central nervous system (CNS) disease, active opportunistic infection or concurrent illness.
- Poorly controlled diabetes mellitus.
- Pregnancy.
- Severe dysphagia.
- Enteral or parenteral feedings.
- Two or more medical comorbidities or dialysis.
- Complicated food–drug–nutrient interactions.
- Severely dysfunctional psychosocial situation.

RD = Registered Dietitian
Source: [29]. ADA & adapted from

---

include weight status, measurement of body composition (lean body mass and fat), biochemical assessment of serum micronutrients and proteins, dietary intake, and other conditions that may impact overall nutritional status [30]. Baseline nutrition assessment should be performed shortly after diagnosis with yearly follow-up sessions for patients without symptoms. Patients who are more symptomatic and are at nutritional risk should be seen more frequently [27].

Table 10.6 Components of a nutritional assessment.

History	Measurements	Laboratory tests
Weight history since developing HIV (expressed as a percentage of weight change).	Height and weight Body mass index (BMI) Waist circumference	Albumin and prealbumin Serum free testosterone Vitamin B_{12}/Folate (RBC)
Presence of opportunistic infections, fever, diarrhea or gastrointestinal distress or malabsorptioin.	Hip circumference Waist-to-hip ratio	Fasting lipid profile Fasting glucose
Factors affecting food availability (social, financial).		
Diet history and intake.		
Medication review.		
Use of nutritional or herbal supplements.		
Functional status.		

Source: American Dietetic Association. Adapted from [29].

Body composition measurements

A recognized complication of HAART therapy is a change in body shape referred to as "lipodystrophy" or "fat redistribution syndrome." This syndrome is characterized by loss of fat in the extremities, accumulation of visceral and abdominal fat, breast hypertrophy, and the emergence of an interscapular fat pad or "buffalo hump" [31,32].

In the past, nutritional status was monitored through body weight measurements. However, significant losses in lean body weight can be masked by relative increases in total body water [31]. Measurement of body composition (rather than body weight) is therefore critical in screening HIV patients who are at risk for malnutrition. Several methods are available to approximate body composition. Anthropometry is a noninvasive method of evaluating body composition and involves the measurement of multiple areas of subcutaneous fat. Lean body mass estimated by anthropometry has been shown to correlate well with lean body mass measurements performed by dual X-ray absorptiometry in patients with HIV [30]. Additional methods for characterizing body composition include bioelectric impedance analysis, hydrodensitometry, and dual X-ray absorptiometry. Minimal nutrition assessment components in HIV positive patients are given in Table 10.6.

Weight loss and wasting

Despite the advent of HAART, wasting remains a significant problem in the HIV population. Multiple studies have demonstrated a strong relationship between loss of lean body tissue and increased morbidity and mortality [31].

Classic wasting can be defined as the depletion of both lean body mass and fat stores. With the use of antiretrovirals, fat redistribution is more commonly seen in the truncal region with subsequent loss of subcutaneous fat from the face, buttocks and extremities. Factors thought to contribute to wasting include malabsorption (secondary to diarrhea or mucosal changes within the small intestine), decreased intake, hypogonadism, and cytokine derangement [33].

The Centers for Disease Control and Prevention defines significant weight loss as greater than 10% of body weight. Recently the Working Group on the Prevention and Treatment of Wasting and Weight Loss suggested an expanded definition to include patients with weight <90% of ideal body weight (or BMI < 18.5) and weight loss >10% from pre-illness maximum or >5% in the previous six months [33].

Evidence now suggests that nutrition counseling and support, appetite stimulants, progressive resistance training and anabolic hormones can increase lean body mass and reverse weight loss in patients with HIV [33].

Dyslipidemias

Although lipid abnormalities were noted in HIV patients prior to the era of antiretroviral therapy, the use of protease inhibitors (PI) has been associated with markedly elevated triglycerides and decreased HDL levels. Additionally, protease inhibitors have also been thought to cause the redistribution of fat to the truncal area with subsequent lipoatrophy in the face and extremities [32].

Evidence about cardiovascular risk in the HIV population is conflicting, but most experts argue that such patients are more predisposed to coronary heart disease given the combination of dyslipidemia, increased insulin resistance, visceral adiposity, and chronic inflammatory state secondary to HIV and should be treated aggressively to lower their risk [34].

Treatment guidelines for HIV-related dyslipidemia and truncal adiposity is similar to those recommended for the general population.

Intensive dietary and lifestyle modification is recommended initially, but if lipid levels remain elevated after a trial period of six months, then lipid-lowering medication should be initiated. However, medications should be selected carefully as there are many potential drug interactions.

References

1 Manges AR, Johnson JR, Foxman B, O'Bryan TT, Fullerton KE, Riley LW. Widespread distribution of urinary tract infections caused by a multidrug-resistant *Escherichia coli* cloonal group. *N Engl J Med* 2001;345(14):1007–13.

2 Howell AB, Foxman B. Cranberry juice and adhesion of antibiotic-resistant uropathogens. *JAMA* 2002;287(23):3082–3.

3 Reid G, Hsiehl J, Potter P, Mighton J, Lam D. Cranberry juice consumption may reduce biofilms on uroepithelial cells: a pilot study in spinal cord patients. *Spinal Cord* 2001;39 (1):26–30.

4 Kontiokari T, Laitinen J, Jarvi, L *et al.* Dietary factors protecting women from urinary tract infections. *Am J Clin Nutr* 2003;77(3):600–4.

5 Reid G, Beuerman D, Heinemann C, Bruce AW. Probiotic *Lactobaccillus* dose required to restore and maintain a normal vaginal flora. *FEMS Immunol Med Microb* 2001;32:37–41.

6 Millichap JG, Yee M. The diet factor in pediatric and adolescent migraine. *Pediatric Neuol* 2003;28(1):9–15.

7 D'Andrea G, Terrazzino S *et al.* Elevated levels of circulating trace amines in primary headaches. *Neurology* 2004;62(10):1701–5.

8 Jansen SC, van Dusseldorf M, Bottema KC, Dubois AE. Intolerance to dietary biogenic amines: a review. *Ann Allergy Asthma Immunol* 2003;91(3):233–40.

9 Wasiewski W. Preventive Therapy in Pediatric Migraine. *J Child Neurol* 2001;16(2):71–8.

10 Hambidge M. Biomarkers of trace mineral intake and status. *J Nutr* 2003;133(Supp 3):948S–55S.

11 Schrier S. Treatment of anemia due to iron deficiency. *UpToDate* Version 12.3; www.uptodate.com.

12 Davidsson L. Approaches to improve iron bioavailability from complementary foods. *J Nutr* 2003;133(5 Suppl 1):1560S–2S.

13 Hallberg L, Rossander-Hulten L, Brune M, Gleerup A. Inhibition of haem-iron absorption in man by calcium. *Br J Nutr* 1992;69:533-40.

14 Molgaard C, Kaestel P, Michaelson KF. Long-term calcium supplementation does not affect the iron status of 12-14-y-old girls. *Am J Clin Nutr* 2005 Jul;82(1):98-102.

15 Hess B. Nutritional aspects of stone disease. *Endocrinol Metab Clinic N Am* 2002;31(4):1017–30.

16 Rose B. Treatment of recurrent calcium stones. *UpToDate* Version 12.3 www.uptodate.com

17 Martini L, Wood R. Should dietary calcium and protein be restricted in patients with nephrolithiasis? *Nutr Rev* 2000;58(4):111–17.

18 National Kidney Foundation. K/DOQI clinical practice guidelines for chronic kidney disease: evaluation, classification, and stratification. *Am J Kidney Dis* 2002;39(2 suppl 1):S1–S266.

19 Johnson CA, Levey AS, Coresh J *et al.* Clinical practice guidelines for chronic kidney disease in adults: Part I. Definition, disease stages, evaluation, treatment, and risk factors. *Am Fam Physician* 2004;70(5):869–76.

20 Hostetter TH. Prevention of the development of progression of renal disease. *J Am Soc Nephrol* 2003;14:S144–S147.

21 Effects of dietary protein restriction on the progression of moderate renal disease in the Modification of Diet in Renal Disease Study. *J Am Soc Nephrol* 1996;7(12):2616–26.

22 Beto JA, Bansal VK. Medical nutrition therapy in chronic kidney failure: Integrating clinical practice guidelines. *J Am Diet Assoc* 2004;104(3):404–9.

23 Appel L. Lifestyle modification as a means to prevent and treat high blood pressure. *J Am Soc Nephro* 2003;14:S99–S102.

24 Mitch WE. Beneficial responses to modified diets in treating patients with chronic kidney disease. *Kidney International* 2005;67(s94): s133–s135.

25 Bernard J, Beaufrere B, Laville M, Fouque D. Adaptive response to a low-protein diet in predialysis chronic renal failure patients. *J Am Soc Nephrol* 2001;12:1249–54.

26 Hostetter TH, Lising M. National kidney disease education program. *J Am Soc Nephrol* 2003;14:S114–S116.

27 American Dietetic Association. Position of the American Dietetic Association and Dietitians of Canada: Nutrition Intervention in the Care of Persons with Human Immunodeficiency Virus Infection. *J Am Diet Assoc* 2004;104(9):1425–41.

28 Goldschmidt RH, Dong BJ. Treatment of AIDS and HIV-related conditions – 2002: Antiretroviral therapy. *J Am Board Fam Pract* 2002;15(4):319–31.

29 Nerad J, Romeyn M, Silverman E *et al.* General nutrition management in patients infected with the Human Immunodeficiency Virus. *Clin Infect Dis* 2003;36(Suppl 2):S52–S62.

30 Knox T, Zafonte-Sanders M, Fields-Gardner C *et al.* Assessment of nutritional status, body composition, and Human Immunodeficiency Virus-associated morphologic changes. *Clin Infect Dis* 2003;36(Suppl 2):S63–8.

31 Gerrior J, Kantaros J, Coakley E *et al.* The fat redistribution syndrome in patients infected with HIV; Measurements of body shape abnormalities. *Spinal Cord* 2001;101(10):1175–80.

32 Sattler F. Body habitus changes related to lipodystrophy. *Clin Infect Dis* 2003;36 (Suppl 2):S84–S90.

33 Grinspoon S, Mulligan K. Weight loss and wasting in patients infected with human immunodeficiency virus. *Clin Infect Dis* 2003;36(Suppl 2):S69–S78.

34 Dube M, Fenton M. Lipid abnormalities. *Clin Infect Dis* 2003;36(Suppl 2):S79–S83.

35 Kent PS. Integrating clinical nutrition practice guidelines in chronic kidney disease. *Nutr Clin Prac* 2005; 20(2):213–217.

36 Jepson RG, Mihaljevic L, Craig J. Cranberries for preventing urinary tract infections. *J Urol* 2005;173(1):111.

37 Food Safety and Inspection Service, US Department of Agriculture, Food safety for persons with AIDS. Available at: www.fsis.usda.gov/OA/pubs/aids.htm.

Vitamins, minerals, supplements and alternative nutrition

CHAPTER 11

Vitamins

Randee Silverman and Jeremy Brauer

Vitamins are required throughout all stages of life from infancy, to adulthood. They are classified as micronutrients: defined as chemical substances required for normal growth and metabolism.

Vitamins are organic compounds essential for a multitude of metabolic reactions *in vivo*. For the most part, humans rely on exogenous sources to supply their vitamin needs. Known exceptions are the production of vitamin K and biotin by certain intestinal microorganisms; the synthesis of vitamin D from its precursor, cholesterol; and the synthesis of niacin from its precursor, tryptophan (amino acid).

The importance of adequate vitamin and mineral balance for health and disease prevention has been increasingly discussed in recent literature. Clinicians must assume a stronger role in the education of their patients with respect to appropriate use of vitamin and mineral supplements. Dietary intake of vitamins and minerals should be the hallmark of these discussions.

In the US, the Food and Drug Administration (FDA) is the agency mandated to regulate dietary supplements. Under the Dietary Supplement and Education Act, supplements are regulated independent of foods and as such have a separate set of standards for labeling. In addition, the US government established the Office of Dietary Supplements at the National Institutes of Health to further evaluate scientific evidence for the use of dietary supplements as well as to monitor safety. Given the complexity of issues surrounding the use of dietary supplements, it is imperative that health care professionals identify and utilize reliable information resources in developing care plans for patients and clients.

Dietary reference intake

To address the changing nutritional needs of the American population, the Food and Nutrition Board of the Institute of Medicine established the first Dietary Reference Intakes (DRIs) in 1997 [1]. The new DRIs move beyond the traditional Recommended Daily Allowances (RDAs) to focus on the prevention of chronic disease. The DRIs provide a range of safe and appropriate intakes as well as tolerable upper limits based on the available research. DRI is a collective term that includes four nutrient-based dietary reference values for every life-stage and gender group. These include estimated average requirement, recommended dietary allowance, adequate intake, and tolerable upper intake level. At present, DRIs have been established for vitamin A, carotenoids the B vitamins, vitamin C, vitamin D, vitamin K, folate, calcium, choline, chromium, copper, fluoride, iodine, iron, magnesium, manganese, molybdenum, phosphorus, biotin, pantothenic acid, selenium, and zinc [1–5]. Recommendations regarding the intake of other nutrients will be available over the next decade as the scientific evidence is evaluated.

Estimated average requirement

The estimated average requirement (EAR) is the daily intake estimated to meet the requirement of 50% of the individuals in a particular life-stage and gender group. The EAR is the most useful DRI for assessing the nutrient intake of an individual.

Adequate intake

When the EAR is unavailable owing to lack of data, an adequate intake (AI) can be determined based on intakes of groups of individuals. It is an approximation of the average nutrient intake by a population or subgroup that appears to be healthy and not demonstrating the risks of the particular chronic disease.

Tolerable upper intake level

The upper intake level (UL) is the level of daily nutrient intake that is unlikely to pose risks of adverse health effects to almost all (97–98%) of the individuals in a specified life-stage and gender group.

Vitamin A

Vitamin A is a fat-soluble vitamin and refers to compounds or mixtures of compounds having vitamin A activity. In animals, vitamin A usually exists as a retinal, retinyl esters, retinol and retinoic acid. Retinoic acid is the most active form of vitamin A. Retinol is referred to as preformed vitamin A. In plants, vitamin A exists in its precursor form, provitamin A carotinoids (e.g. beta-carotene) and cryptoxanthin [6].

Forms and absorption

When we ingest provitamin A, such as beta-carotene from plants, the body converts these compounds to retinol, which is then reduced to retinal in the intestinal tract. Vitamin A is broken down by pancreatic and intestinal enzymes and absorbed in the ileum. This process requires bile salts. About 90% of the vitamin A absorbed from the intestine is stored in the liver. When a particular part of the body, such as the eyes, requires vitamin A, the liver releases a sufficient amount, which is carried through the blood bound to RBP (retinol binding protein) and delivered to cells and tissues that need it.

Functions of vitamin A

Vitamin A plays an essential regulatory role in the following bodily functions.
1) Vision where it is required for the formation of rhodopsin, a pigment located in the eye's retina. When stimulated by light, rhodopsin splits into two proteins, opsin and all-trans retinal. When it is dark, the reverse reaction occurs: the retinal and opsin combine to form rhodopsin, a reaction that requires a sufficient amount of vitamin A. In the absence of adequate amounts of vitamin A (retinal), regeneration of rhodopsin is incomplete and night blindness occurs.
2) Normal integrity and growth of skin and tissue cells, which moistens the linings of the eyes, mouth, stomach, and intestinal tract, respiratory tract, and genital and urinary tract, functioning as a barrier to bacteria and viruses [6,7].
3) Production of collagen, which is the primary component of teeth, bones, cartilage, tendons, and connective tissue.
4) Normal reproduction, by helping testicles and ovaries to function properly and aiding in the development of the embryo.
5) In the form of beta-carotene, it serves as an antioxidant, which may reduce the risk of certain cancers.

Causes and effects of vitamin A deficiency

Vitamin A deficiency is one of the most common forms of malnutrition in the world, with pregnant women, infants, and young children being most susceptible. Primary deficiency is due to inadequate intake of vitamin A and its precursors, whereas secondary deficiency occurs from poor absorption of fat-soluble vitamins, which may occur in people with cystic fibrosis, Crohn's disease, tropical sprue, liver disease or in those who abuse alcohol.

Clinical problems associated with vitamin A deficiency include xerophthalmia, (which causes, epithelial thickening of the conjunctiva, night blindness, corneal ulceration, and irreversible blindness), poor wound healing, and loss of epithelial integrity of the skin, gastrointestinal, urinary and respiratory tracts.

Causes and effects of vitamin A toxicity

Overdoses of vitamin A (>7500 retinal equivalents or 500,000 IU/day) are toxic and may cause flaking, itching and peeling rashes, blurred vision, hair loss, muscle and bone pain, headaches, nose bleeds, vomiting, irritability, and drowsiness. Taking large doses of vitamin A (>100,000 IU/day) may also lead to an enlarged spleen and liver, vision problems, hair loss, muscle, bone and joint pain, headaches, weakness and dry skin.

Consuming too much vitamin A during pregnancy can cause defects in the developing embryo. Women considering pregnancy should be told to discontinue vitamin A supplements, especially doses exceeding 5000 IU (800 retinal equivalents). The tolerable upper intake level for vitamin A has been established at 3000 µg/day.

Because only limited amounts of beta-carotene are converted to vitamin A, excessive intake has not been shown to produce these side effects. People who consume large doses of beta-carotene, either through dietary sources or supplements, may develop a yellow tinge to their skin.

Relationship to disease prevention

An association between beta-carotene and vitamin A and a lower risk of many types of cancer has been suggested. A controversial claim is that a higher intake of beta carotene and/or vitamin A food sources may decrease the risk of lung cancer [8]. A number of prevention studies that examined this using supplements did not find vitamin A to be protective [9].

Blood tests to measure deficiency or toxicity

Serum levels of vitamin A as retinol
Measurement of serum retinol binding protein levels, the carrier of retinol
Dark adaptation tests and Electroretinogram tests

Vitamin A requirements

Those taking birth control pills, which may increase the amount of retinal in the blood, are advised to limit vitamin A intake to no more than 5000 IU/day.

Table 11.1 DRI for vitamin A.

Vitamin A	DRI (μg/day)*
Males: ages 14–70+	900
Females: ages 14–70+	700

*μg/day = ug retinol equivalent.
Source: [4].

Retinol equivalents

Vitamin A or retinal is ingested either as vitamin A or a beta-carotene which can be split in the intestine to vitamin A. Beta-carotene is the most abundant carotenoid present in green, yellow or orange fruits and vegetables. The nutritional equivalent of 1 μg retinal or 1 μg retinal equivalent (RE) is 0.6 μg of beta-carotene. But this may vary by food source.

Vitamin A food sources including fortified sources

(See Appendix A).

Vitamin D

Vitamin D is a fat-soluble vitamin that occurs in two forms, vitamin D_2 and vitamin D_3. Vitamin D_2, or ergocalciferol, occurs in a small number of foods, while the body manufactures vitamin D or cholecalciferol, in the skin when exposed to sunlight.

Forms and absorption

Since vitamin D is a fat-soluble vitamin, bile salts are required for its absorption. Once absorbed via the ileum, vitamin D is converted in the liver to its hormonal form, where it acts upon the intestine, bone and kidney to regulate calcium and phosphorous absorption. Smaller reserves of the vitamin are located in the skin, brain, lungs, spleen, and kidneys. When calcium levels in the blood are low, the body releases parathyroid hormone (PTH), which stimulates the kidney to convert vitamin D to its active form. This is turn stimulates the gastrointestinal tract to increase calcium and phosphorous absorption.

Functions of vitamin D

Vitamin D plays an essential regulatory role in the following bodily functions.
1) Normal intestinal absorption of calcium and phosphorus.
2) Regulation of calcium and phosphorous in the bones, teeth, and cartilage in children and maintenance of healthy bones and teeth in adults.
3) Maintenance of blood calcium and phosphorus levels.

Causes and effects of vitamin D deficiency

Vitamin D deficiency is characterized by rickets in infants and children, and osteomalacia (softening of the bones) in adults. Rickets manifests as retarded growth, swelling and tenderness at the ends of the bones and malformation of the joints. Rickets in infants and children also leads to a delay in the closure of the skull bones, possibly leading to a larger skull, as well as bowed legs, pot belly, spinal curvature, and chest malformations (rickitic Rosary). Osteomalacia may lead to pain in the legs, ribs, hips and muscles, easily broken bones and difficulty getting up from a sitting position or climbing stairs. Older adults or seniors are at increased risk for vitamin D deficiency, especially those who are bed-ridden or who live in nursing homes and may not have adequate exposure to sunlight. Osteomalacia may occur when long-term anticonvulsant medications, such as phenobarbital or phenytoin are taken because they increase the breakdown of vitamin D by the liver. Individuals with chronic kidney disease often develop osteodystrophy, due to reduced renal conversion of vitamin D to its active form.

Causes and effects of vitamin D toxicity

High doses of vitamin D over a long period of time may lead to kidney stones, nausea, headaches, weakness, anorexia, frequent urination, weight loss, irregular heartbeat, and weak bones and muscles. Excess levels may also lead to calcification of soft tissues (kidney, lungs, joints, stomach and blood vessels) possibly resulting in irreversible damage. In infants and children, too much vitamin D can lead to retarded growth, rounding of the skull, mental retardation and death. However, these excess doses of vitamin D have been primarily reported from supplements rather than food or too much sun exposure. Explorers who consume polar bear liver have also been reported to have vitamin D toxicity. The tolerable upper limit for vitamin D has been established at 50 µg/day.

Relationship to disease prevention

Epidemiologic studies suggest that a higher dietary intake of calcium and vitamin D, and/or sunlight-induced vitamin D synthesis, correlates with lower incidence of cancer [10,11]. More specifically, recent studies have suggested that vitamin D has a role in the prevention of colon cancer [12]. Vitamin D researchers also point out relationships to cardiovascular disease, osteoporosis, and autoimmune disorders [13].

Blood test to measure deficiency or toxicity

The active form of vitamin D is 1,25-(OH) and can be measured in the blood as calcitriol.

Vitamin D requirements

Table 11.2 DRI for vitamin D.

Vitamin D	DRI (µg/day)
Males: ages 9–50	5
Females: ages 9–50	5

Source: [1].

Vitamin D food sources (including fortified sources)

(See Appendix B).

Vitamin E

Vitamin E is a fat-soluble vitamin made up of alcohol compounds called tocopherols and tocotrienols. Each series comes in alpha, beta, gamma and delta forms for a total of eight compounds with vitamin E activity. Of the various tocopherols, alpha-tocopherol is the most active form of vitamin E with the highest biological activity.

Forms and absorption

Vitamin E is absorbed passively in the ileum, requiring the presence of bile salts. Vitamin E absorption is enhanced in the presence of medium-chain triglycerides. Vitamin E binds with plasma lipoproteins, but it does not require a specific carrier protein, and red blood cells also participate in its transport. Vitamin E is stored primarily in the liver, fat, and muscle tissue.

Functions of vitamin E

Vitamin E plays an essential regulatory role in the following bodily functions.

1) Exerts a protective role in maintaining the integrity and function of fats and phospohlipids in cell membranes throughout the body by functioning as an antioxidant and protecting against free radicals.

2) Acts as an antioxidant by protecting vitamin A from being oxidized in the small intestine.

3) Protects red blood cells from being broken down and prevents blood clots.

Causes and effects of vitamin E deficiency

Vitamin E deficiency is rare, except in people who can not absorb fat. Clinical signs include neurologic dysfunction, loss of deep tendon reflexes, diminished vibratory and position sense, and hemolytic anemia, due to shortened survival of mature red blood cells. In infants diagnosed with protein-energy malnutrition, lack of vitamin E causes red blood cell lysis. Infants who are treated with oxygen are likely to develop retrolental fibroplasias, leading to vision impairment and possibly blindness. Treating these infants with vitamin E has had positive effects.

Causes and effects of vitamin E toxicity

Reports indicate that megadoses of vitamin E can interfere with the vitamin K clotting mechanism which may result in increased bleeding tendency, and impairment of white blood cell function and decreased immune function. Because of its involvement with blood clotting, large doses of vitamin E should be avoided 2 weeks before and after surgery and in those taking anticoagulant medications, such as coumadin or warfarin. The tolerable upper intake level for vitamin E has been established at 1000 mg/day.

Relationship to disease prevention

Apart from its other important biologic functions, vitamin E is also considered to be nature's most effective lipid-soluble, chain-breaking antioxidant, protecting cell membranes from oxidative damage. Recent studies have been performed to determine whether vitamin E could reduce the risk of heart attacks and thus deaths from heart disease. However, the data show little to no effect on reducing cardiovascular disease (CVD) risk [14].

Blood test to measure deficiency or toxicity

Serum alpha tocopherol levels 5–18 µg/dL

Vitamin E requirements

Table 11.3 DRI for vitamin E.

Vitamin E	DRI (mg/day)
Males: ages 14–70+	15
Female: ages 14–70+	15

Source: [3].

Vitamin E food sources (including fortified sources)

(See Appendix C).

Vitamin K

Vitamin K is a fat-soluble vitamin that is obtained from dietary sources and also produced by intestinal bacteria. Phylloquinone is the predominant form of vitamin K from dietary sources and menaquinone is produced by bacteria within the body.

Forms and absorption

Absorption of vitamin K occurs primarily in the proximal small bowel and requires bile salts. Following intestinal absorption, vitamin K is taken up and stored mostly in the liver.

Functions of vitamin K

Vitamin K is an essential component in the body's normal blood clotting process. Vitamin K is a required cofactor for enzymes involved in the synthesis of prothrombin in the liver. Osteocalcium in bone is also vitamin K dependent and is thought to play a role in bone mineralization.

Causes and effects of vitamin K deficiency

Deficiency of vitamin K is rare, since 90% of the required vitamin K is provided by the intestinal flora. However, deficiency may occur in people with intestinal malabsorption, tropical sprue, regional ileitis, cystic fibrosis, bile salt deficiency, and long-term antibiotic therapy, which destroys the intestinal microorganisms. Warfarin an anticoagulant is a specific vitamin K antagonist. Symptoms of vitamin K deficiency include prolonged clotting time resulting in bleeding problems which can occur in the mouth, genital urinary systems, gastrointestinal tract, and skin. Easy bruising of skin may occur (ecchymosis).

A recent observational study has suggested that there is a correlation between a low plasma level of vitamin K and a higher prevalence of osteoarthritis of the hands and knees [16].

Infants are given a vitamin K injection at birth as a precaution to prevent hemorrhagic disease of the newborn. Newborn infants are at risk for hemorrhagic disease because the placenta is unable to sufficiently transmit lipids, therefore vitamin K does not cross the placental membrane well. Infants do not begin to synthesize vitamin K in the intestinal tract until approximately one week after birth; breast milk is a very minimal source of vitamin K; and the liver of a newborn is unable to sufficiently produce prothrombin.

Causes and effect of vitamin K toxicity

Allergic reactions to megadoses of vitamin K have been reported, however toxicity is rare. Brain damage may occur in infants who are supplemented with unusually high levels of vitamin K. There is no tolerable upper level for vitamin K.

Vitamin K and blood thinning medications

High intake of vitamin K from the diet will alter the effectiveness of anti-coagulant medications because of vitamin K's ability to enhance or promote blood clotting. Therefore, patients taking anticoagulant medications, such as warfarin or coumadin, need to maintain their intake of vitamin K-containing foods fairly constant from day-to-day so that their blood does not clot faster than it should [16].

An understanding of the high, medium, and low dietary sources of vitamin K is necessary for people taking these medications. Higher amounts of vitamin K are found in dark green leafy vegetables such as spinach, kale and collard greens and in the outer peels of certain fruits, such as apples and grapes. Other significant dietary sources of vitamin K are found in certain oils including soybean, canola, cottonseed, and olive oil, although values fluctuate since these oils are highly susceptible to both daylight and fluorescent light. Animal foods, dairy products, breads, cereals and pasta products contain very little vitamin K. (See Appendix D)

Blood test to measure deficiency or toxicity

Testing clotting factors, such as prothrombin time

Vitamin K requirements

Table 11.4 DRI for vitamin K.

Vitamin K	DRI ($\mu g/day$)
Male: ages 19–70+	120
Female: ages 19–70+	90

Source: [4].

Vitamin K food sources

(See Appendix D).

Ascorbic acid (Vitamin C)

Ascorbic acid is a water-soluble vitamin commonly known as vitamin C. It is the least stable of all the vitamins, and is easily destroyed during cooking and food processing.

Form and absorption

The jejunum and ileum actively absorb vitamin C and its absorption increases as intake levels decline. The amount of vitamin C in tissues is modulated by renal excretion, therefore, when tissue concentrations are high, the kidneys excrete excess vitamin C.

Functions of vitamin C

Vitamin C plays an essential role in the following bodily functions:

1) Formation of collagen, responsible for strengthening bones and blood vessels, anchoring teeth into the gums, as well as forming the substances necessary for body growth, tissue repair and wound healing.

2) Protects cells by serving as an antioxidant for free radicals.

3) Enhanced immune function by enabling white blood cells to break down bacteria.

4) Plays a role in the production of hemoglobin and red blood cells.

5) Enhances the absorption of iron.

Causes and effects of vitamin C deficiency

Individuals who do not have access to or avoid citrus fruits and juices, may have insufficient vitamin C intake. In addition, individuals who are following a macrobiotic diet, which is lacking in night shade fruits and vegetables, typically will require a vitamin C supplement to prevent deficiency. Individuals with severe burns, fractures, pneumonia, rheumatic fever, and tuberculosis, as well as surgery, have increased requirements for vitamin C. Alcohol decreases absorption and cigarette smoking depletes tissue levels, thus alcoholics and smokers should increase their dietary intake or take supplemental vitamin C.

Vitamin C deficiency is characterized by the development of scurvy, a condition which leads to muscle weakness, joint pain, impaired wound healing, loose teeth, bleeding and swollen gums, bruised skin or perifollicular hemorrhages, fatigue and depression.

Causes and effects of vitamin C toxicity

Since vitamin C is a water-soluble vitamin, the body excretes the excess when intake exceeds the body's requirements. However, because vitamin C is metabolized to oxalic acid, consuming too much may cause increased excretion of oxalate, which may cause development of kidney stones. Megadoses of vitamin C can have other side effects including nausea, diarrhea, vomiting, insomnia, headaches, and abdominal cramps. Laboratory tests for glucose may also be false-positive in patients taking more than 1000 mg of vitamin C per day because the structure of ascorbic acid resembles glucose. The tolerable upper intake level for vitamin C has been established at 2000 mg/day. It is probably advisable to obtain vitamin C from dietary sources, and limit supplements, if desired, to less than 500 mg/day. Tissue saturation is reached at approximately 200 mg/day.

Relationship to disease prevention

Vitamin C is a powerful intracellular antioxidant. Vitamin C is also used commercially to prevent oxidation of foods, such as when lemon juice is used to prevent apples from turning brown [17].

Treating the common cold with vitamin C

The role of vitamin C in fighting viral infections has been controversial for decades. At the present time, it appears that vitamin C may have a mild antihistamine effect and if taken during a cold, may decrease the severity as well as duration of the symptoms.

Blood test to measure deficiency or toxicity
Serum levels and vitamin C in white blood cells ("buffy coat")

Vitamin C requirements

Table 11.5 DRI for vitamin C

Vitamin C	DRI (mg/day)
Male: ages 19–70+	90
Female: ages 19–70+	75

Source: [3].

Vitamin C food sources (including fortified sources)

(See Appendix E).

Thiamin (Vitamin B$_1$)

Form and absorption
Thiamin is readily soluble in water and not stored in the body to any great extent. It is primarily absorbed in the jejunum via active transport when intake levels are low and passive transport when intake levels are high. Absorption is significantly reduced in the presence of alcohol, as well as in individuals with a folate deficiency. Once absorbed, thiamin is stored in the muscle tissue.

Functions of thiamin
Thiamin plays an essential role in the following bodily functions.
1) Acts as a coenzyme in energy metabolism and is important for metabolic reactions which generate energy from carbohydrates and fat. Therefore, its requirements are based upon the caloric content of the diet and the amount of carbohydrate and fat that is metabolized.
2) Aids in normal growth and development.
3) Helps maintain proper functioning of the cardiovascular, nervous and gastrointestinal systems.

Causes and effects of thiamin deficiency
Primary thiamin deficiency, due to poor intake of thiamin-containing foods, is rare in the US because the majority of grain products are fortified with thiamin.

However, thiamin deficiency may occur in individuals who abuse alcohol, because excessive alcohol intake significantly decreases thiamin absorption and interferes with its metabolism.

Early thiamin deficiency is characterized by poor appetite, irritability, fatigue, and weight loss. As the deficiency progresses, individuals develop weakness, stocking and glove nerve damage, headaches, and a rapid heart rate. Beriberi, a form of thiamin deficiency, may affect 1) infants who are breast fed by mothers who have thiamin deficiency, 2) people who consume large amounts of carbohydrates, especially from polished rice, which removes the vitamin in processing, and 3) alcoholics [18]. Advanced stages of beriberi affect the nervous and cardiovascular system, causing abnormal heart rhythms and heart failure. Wet beriberi refers to the effects on the cardiovascular system, and dry beriberi refers to the effects on the central and peripheral nervous system.

Causes and effects of thiamin toxicity
Thiamin toxicity has not been described.

Relationship to disease prevention
Unlikely. None beyond treating deficiency.

Blood test to measure deficiency or toxicity
Serum thiamin levels

Thiamin requirements

Table 11.6 DRI for thiamin.

Thiamin	DRI (mg/day)
Men: ages 14–70+	1.2
Women: ages 19–70+	1.1

Source: [5].

Thiamin food sources (including fortified sources)

Beef	Rice (enriched)
Bread (enriched)	Pork
Cereals (enriched)	Sunflower seeds
Nuts	Whole grain cereals (enriched)
Liver	

Riboflavin (Vitamin B$_2$)

Riboflavin is a water-soluble vitamin that is an important component of many enzyme reactions related to carbohydrate metabolism.

Form and absorption
Riboflavin is readily absorbed in the jejunum. Due to chelation, absorption of dietary riboflavin is reduced in the presence of copper, zinc, tryptophan, vitamin C, dietary fiber and saccharine.

Functions of riboflavin
Riboflavin plays an essential role in the following bodily functions:
1) Aids in normal growth and development.
2) Helps glucose breakdown to yield energy.
3) Facilitates glycogen production and utilization of fats.
4) Helps change the amino acid tryptophan into niacin.
5) Serves to maintain normal mucous membranes and protects the nervous system, skin and eyes.

Causes and effects of riboflavin deficiency
Riboflavin deficiency can result from inadequate intake, poor absorption or lack of utilization, as well as increased excretion. Symptoms of riboflavin deficiency include cracked and red lips, inflammation of the mucosa of the mouth and tongue, chielosis, dry scaling skin, edema of the mucous membranes and anemia. The eyes may also become bloodshot, itchy, watery and sensitive to bright light. Riboflavin deficiency typically develops in conjunction with deficiencies of other water-soluble vitamins.

Causes and effects of toxicity
Riboflavin has demonstrated conflicting results in randomized trials for migraine prophylaxsis.

Relationship to disease prevention
None.

Blood tests to measure deficiency or toxicity
Measurement of the activity of erythrocyte glutathione reductase (EGR). Older techniques: fluorometric and microbiological assessment of riboflavin in blood cells and urine.

Riboflavin requirements

Table 11.7 DRI for riboflavin.

Riboflavin	DRI (mg/day)
Men: ages 14–70+	1.3
Women: ages 19–70+	1.1

Source: [5].

Riboflavin food sources (including fortified sources)

Asparagus	Milk
Broccoli	Milk products
Eggs	Oranges
Fish	Whole grains
Fortified cereals, breads, pastas, oatmeal, rice	Poultry
Meat	

Niacin (Vitamin B$_3$)

Niacin is a water-soluble vitamin, which exists in two forms; nicotinic acid and nicotinamide.

Form and absorption

Niacin and nicotinamide are absorbed in the stomach and duodenum, depending on intake levels. Niacin is also synthesized from the amino acid tryptophan, a reaction which requires a vitamin B$_6$-dependent coenzyme. Once absorbed, niacin is present in all cells.

Functions of niacin

Niacin plays an essential role in the following bodily functions:

1) Normal enzyme production in at least 200 reactions in the body involved in energy production. Most enzymes require niacin to accept electrons or donate hydrogen molecules.

2) Normal production and breakdown of glucose, fats, and amino acids, thereby helping the body to metabolize these substances.

3) Required for normal development, maintenance and function of the skin, gastrointestinal tract and nervous system.

4) Essential for DNA synthesis.

Causes and effects of niacin deficiency

Since niacin is found primarily in protein-rich foods, this deficiency is rare in the US. Historically, a deficiency was found in people whose diet consisted mainly of corn, which is lacking in the essential amino acid tryptophan. Vitamin B$_6$ deficiency can also contribute to niacin deficiency, as the synthesis of niacin from tryptophan requires a vitamin B$_6$-dependent enzyme. Individuals who abuse alcohol also are at increased risk of niacin deficiency because alcohol significantly reduces niacin absorption.

The initial signs of niacin deficiency, referred to as pellagra, include fatigue, loss of appetite, weakness, mild gastrointestinal disturbance, anxiety, irritability and depression. Mucous membranes in the mouth are affected which may result in inflammation, soreness, and burning of the tongue. Symptoms of advanced pellagra include severe diarrhea, symmetrical dermatitis (skin rashes), delirium, and death if left untreated.

Causes and effects of niacin toxicity

Consumption of niacin from a dietary supplement greater than 2000 mg per day over a long period has been associated with elevated liver enzymes and elevated blood sugar levels in some individuals. Supplements of niacin may cause flushing, itching and burning, particularly in the face and skin, and rashes. The tolerable upper limit for niacin has been established at 35 mg/day.

Relationship to disease prevention

Although excessive amounts of niacin may be toxic in some individuals, pharmacological doses of nicotinic acid (between 1–3 g/day) have been used to successfully treat individuals with hyperlipidemia [19]. Side effects of niacin at these dosages include flushing, itching and burning, particularly in the face and skin, which may be minimized by administering an aspirin prior to ingesting each dose of niacin or prescribing time-released niacin. Niacin has also been used to treat dizziness and ringing in the ears and prevent premenstrual headaches [20].

Blood tests to measure deficiency or toxicity

No satisfactory direct measurement of serum niacin is available.
Levels of urinary metabolites N'-methylnicotinamide (NMN) and N'-methyl-2pyridone-5carboxamine (2-pyridone) are decreased in niacin deficiency.

Niacin requirements

Table 11.8 DRI for niacin.

Niacin	DRI (mg/day)
Men: ages 14–70+	16
Women: ages 14–70+	14

Source: [5].

Niacin food sources (including fortified sources)

Bread (enriched)	Liver
Cereals (enriched)	Oatmeal (enriched)
Corn	Pasta
Fish	Red meat
Poultry	Rice (enriched)
Legumes	Wheat

Folate (folic acid)

Folate is a water-soluble B vitamin also known as folacin or folic acid. The term folic acid is the synthetic form of folate that is taken via supplements. Folate is found in food sources.

Functions of folate

Folate plays an essential role in the following bodily functions.
1) Synthesis of DNA and RNA, growth and development, and production of new cells.
2) Works in conjunction with vitamin B_{12} to form hemoglobin for the synthesis of red blood cells.
3) Functions as a methyl donor for the enzyme involved in the conversion of the amino acid homocysteine to methionine.
4) Regulation of nerve cell development in the growing embryo and developing fetus during pregnancy.

Causes and effects of folate deficiency

Folate deficiency in humans is attributed to sub optimal dietary intake of folate, behavioral and environmental factors, and genetic defects. Although folate deficiency is rare in the US it occurs in individuals who are unable to absorb folate from their intestinal tract, such as those with tropical sprue, Crohn's disease, ulcerative colitis, and short bowel syndrome.

Lack of folate results in abnormalities in red blood cell formation in the bone marrow, affecting cell division and protein synthesis [21]. As a result, the bone marrow releases megaloblasts into the bloodstream that cannot carry adequate amounts of oxygen to the tissues. Symptoms of folate deficiency include macrocytic anemia, sore mouth, diarrhea, weight loss, heartburn, constipation, and a burning, red tongue. Folate deficiency also results in elevated blood homocysteine levels. It is estimated that two-thirds of individuals with high homocysteine levels have poor folate intake.

Folate deficiency in the elderly may be the result of a poor diet or the use of drugs that impede the absorption of folate. Antacids hinder the absorption of folate by raising the pH levels of the upper intestine. Cimetidine, sulfasalazine, phenytoin, and alcohol also impede the absorption of folate. Methotrexate acts as an antagonist to folate. Supplements of folate can reverse the macrocytic anemia in pernicious anemia; however, they will not reverse the neurological damage caused by pernicious anemia (see vitamin B_{12}, below).

Causes and effects of folate toxicity

Excessive consumption of folic acid may mask a vitamin B_{12} deficiency, allowing the neurologic sequelae to progress even though the anemia associated with this deficiency resolves. Common symptoms seen with folate toxicity are diarrhea, insomnia and irritability. The tolerable upper intake level for folate has been established at 1000 µg/day.

Relationship to disease prevention
Researchers are continuing to investigate the relationship of folate to the prevention of heart disease and neural tube defects in pregnant women.

Prevention of heart disease
People with high blood levels of the amino acid homocysteine have been shown to have an increased risk of developing heart disease. Homocysteine levels are affected by the amount of folate in the blood, since folate is required for the conversion of homocysteine to methionine. Therefore, researchers have suggested that increasing folate, either through the diet or supplements, will reduce homocysteine levels in the blood and cut the risk of heart disease as well. However, recent findings suggest no beneficial vascular effects in high risk populations [22]. These secondary prevention studies do not rule out a potential role of folate in primary prevention.

Prevention of neural tube defects in pregnant women
Since folate is involved in the synthesis of DNA and proteins, adequate levels are particularly important at times of rapid cell growth, such as in fetal and placental development. It is thought that neural tube defects occur for a combination of reasons: dietary deficiency of folate and a genetic defect in the production of enzymes involved in folate metabolism [23].

The neural tube is formed early in pregnancy, between 18–30 days post-conception. This means that formation is initiated even before most women know they are pregnant. Defects in the formation of the neural tube can include anencephaly, spina bifida, meningoceles and myoceles. This early formation, and the detrimental effects of folate deficiency on neural tube formation, form the basis for the recommendation that folic acid supplementation should be begun prior to conception and continued at least through the first trimester of pregnancy. Recent comparison of US birth certificate data shows a 19% drop in the prevalence of reported neural tube defects from October 1998 to December 1999, after mandatory folic acid fortification of enriched grain products began, compared to the period between October 1995 and December 1996, before fortification. Greater decreases in neural tube defects (up to 75% lower) have been seen in studies using higher levels of daily folate supplementation than the average consumed by most Americans since fortification was instituted. In addition, studies of groups with a higher rate of neural tube defects also show a greater reduction in risk [24].

Blood test to measure deficiency or toxicity
Serum folate levels reflect very recent dietary ingestion rather than total body folate stores. Therefore, a normal serum folate test does not exclude folate deficiency. Red blood cell folate levels provide a better reflection of total body folate stores. Serum homocysteine levels also reflect folate status.

Folate requirements

Table 11.9 DRI for folate.

Folate	DRI (μg/day)
Men: ages 14–70+	400
Women: ages 14–70+	400

Source: [5].

Folate food sources (including fortified sources)

(See Appendix E).

Pyridoxine (Vitamin B$_6$)

Vitamin B$_6$ is a water-soluble vitamin that is one of a group of compounds known as the pyridines. These include pyridoxine, pyridoxal and pyridoxamine. All of these compounds are closely related and are easily converted to pyridoxal phosphate, a coenzyme involved in the metabolism of amino acids.

Forms and absorption

Vitamin B$_6$ and its related compounds are absorbed in the duodenum. Once absorbed, vitamin B$_6$ is widely distributed in the body, with muscle serving as an important storage site.

Functions of vitamin B$_6$

Vitamin B$_6$-dependent enzymes perform a number of bodily functions.
1) Production and degradation of amino acids.
2) Synthesis of insulin, antibodies, and neurotransmitters (including serotonin, dopamine, norepinephrine, and histamine).
3) Normal hemoglobin production and the binding of oxygen to the hemoglobin molecule.
4) Conversion of the amino acid tryptophan to niacin; breakdown of glycogen to glucose; and linoleic acid (a polyunsaturated fatty acid) to arachidonic acid.

Causes and effects of vitamin B$_6$ deficiency

Vitamin B$_6$ deficiency can occur in alcoholics and women who use oral contraceptive pills. Deficiency is characterized by oily, flaky skin, nausea, cracked lips, depression, confusion, diarrhea, and loss of appetite [25]. Because vitamin B$_6$ is required to convert tryptophan to niacin, symptoms of a niacin deficiency may also occur in people with a vitamin B$_6$ deficiency [25].

Certain medications can lower the level of vitamin B$_6$ in the body. For example, isoniazid (INH) and penicillamine bind vitamin B$_6$, rendering it inactive [26].

Medical conditions associated with a decrease in the blood levels of pyridoxal phosphate include asthma, renal disease, Hodgkin's disease, sickle cell anemia, diabetes, and cigarette smoking.

Causes and effects of vitamin B$_6$ toxicity

Megadoses of 2–6 g/day of vitamin B$_6$ for two months or more can cause a polyneuropathy characterized by failure of muscular coordination and severe sensory damage. The tolerable upper intake level for vitamin B$_6$ has been established at 100 mg/day.

Relationship to disease prevention

Vitamin B$_6$, in the form of pyridoxine hydrochloride, has been utilized to treat Down's syndrome, autism, high urinary oxalate levels, gestational diabetes, carpal tunnel syndrome, asthma, depression, and diabetic neuropathy. In addition, vitamin B$_6$ may play a role in the prevention of heart disease in people with high blood levels of homocysteine, since it is a required cofactor for enzymes involved homocysteine metabolism.

Blood tests to measure deficiency or toxicity

Serum vitamin B$_6$ levels
Urinary excretion of 4-pyridoxal acid
Activation of erythrocyte transaminases
Ability to metabolize test doses of tryptophan or methionine

Vitamin B$_6$ requirements

Table 11.10 DRI for vitamin B$_6$.

Vitamin B$_6$	DRI (mg/day)
Men: ages 14–50	1.3
Women: ages 19–50	1.3

Source: [5].

Vitamin B$_6$ food sources (including fortified sources)

Bananas	Pasta
Brussels sprouts	Peas
Cabbage	Potatoes
Carrots	Poultry
Cauliflower	Rice
Fish	Tomatoes
Meat	Whole grains

Vitamin B$_{12}$

Vitamin B$_{12}$ is a water-soluble vitamin and is also known as cobalamin or cyanocobalamin.

Form and absorption

Vitamin B_{12} first complexes with a binding protein, intrinsic factor (produced in the stomach), then it is absorbed in the terminal ileum.

Functions of vitamin B_{12}

Vitamin B_{12} plays an essential role in the following bodily functions:

1) Normal growth and development, especially in children.
2) In conjunction with folate, normal production of red blood cells.
3) Synthesis of nerves, cells and the myelin.
4) DNA synthesis.
5) Processing and burning of fat and carbohydrate.

Causes and effects of vitamin B_{12} deficiency

Those at greatest risk of a vitamin B_{12} deficiency include strict vegetarians, vegans, and patients who follow a macrobiotic diet, which avoid all animal products, including meat, chicken, fish, eggs, and dairy foods.

Pernicious anemia develops in people unable to produce intrinsic factor and in those who have had their terminal ileum surgically removed.

Many older people develop achlorhydria and lose their ability to secrete gastric acid and pepsin (an enzyme necessary to separate vitamin B_{12} from food protein), so they absorb less vitamin B_{12}. In addition, patients using acid-supressing medications, long-term, may have low vitamin B_{12} levels [27].

Symptoms of vitamin B_{12} deficiency include megaloblastic anemia, nerve damage (often felt as tingling in the hands and feet), and inflammation of the tongue and oral mucosa. Vitamin B_{12} deficiency, if not treated, can cause severe, irreversible nerve damage and dementia [27].

Causes and effects of vitamin B_{12} toxicity

No toxic or adverse effects have been associated with large intakes of vitamin B_{12}. When high doses of vitamin B_{12} are given orally only a small percentage is absorbed which may explain its low toxicity. There is no tolerable upper intake level.

Blood tests to measure deficiency or toxicity

Serum vitamin B_{12} levels
Urinary methylmalonic acid levels

Vitamin B_{12} requirements

Table 11.11 DRI for vitamin B_{12}.

Vitamin B_{12}	DRI (ug/day)
Men: ages 14–70+	2.4
Women: ages 14–70+	2.4

Source: [5].

Vitamin B$_{12}$ food sources (including fortified sources)

Vitamin B$_{12}$ is a product of bacterial fermentation. The only dietary sources are foods of animal origin such as meat, chicken, fish, eggs, and dairy products. Fortified foods, such as brewers yeast and soy milk, may also contain added vitamin B$_{12}$. Seaweed, algae, spirulina and fermented plant foods, such as tempeh and miso, do not provide adequate amounts of vitamin B$_{12}$ for vegans.

Dairy products	Meat (liver, heart, kidneys)
Eggs	Poultry
Fish	Shellfish
Fortified foods (brewers yeast, soy milk)	

Pantothenic acid

Pantothenic acid is a B-complex vitamin. It is a vitamin precursor of two components necessary for the metabolism of fats, carbohydrates and proteins called coenzyme A (CoA) and Acyl-carrier protein (ACP).

Functions of pantothenic acid
Pantothenic acid, as a component of CoA, is essential for the following bodily functions.
1) Synthesis of fatty acids, triglycerides, cholesterol, sphingosine porphyrin, and acetylcholine.
2) Metabolism of protein and amino acids, fat, and carbohydrates.
3) Synthesis of vitamin B$_{12}$ and hemoglobin.
4) Synthesis of cell membranes.

Causes and effects of pantothenic acid deficiency
Lack of pantothenic acid in the body is very unlikely and there is not enough evidence to conclude that a deficiency of this vitamin can occur naturally. However, by inducing a deficiency in test subjects, the following symptoms occur: indigestion, abdominal pain, burning sensation in the feet, arm and leg cramps, insomnia, and nerve inflammation (neuritis). Damage to the adrenal cortex (a gland located near the kidneys), nervous system, skin, and hair have also been observed. Alcoholics who exhibit neuritis may do so due to a lack of pantothenic acid; however, further evidence is needed for confirmation.

Toxicity of pantothenic acid
Unknown.

Blood tests to measure deficiency or toxicity
Serum and urinary levels.

Pantothenic acid requirements

Table 11.12 DRI for pantothenic acid.

Pantothenic acid	DRI (mg/day)
Men: ages 14–70+	5
Women: ages 14–70+	5

Source: [5].

Pantothenic acid food sources

Cereals	Liver
Eggs	Meat
Kidney	Whole grains
Legumes	Yeast

Biotin

Biotin is a member of the water-soluble B-complex of vitamins.

Forms and absorption
Biotin is absorbed in the proximal small intestine. Intestinal bacteria synthesize biotin which contributes to body stores.

Functions of biotin
Biotin is required for carbohydrate and fat metabolism. Biotin is also required for protein metabolism, although its role is less clear. Biotin deficiency will lead to decreased protein synthesis.

Causes and effects of biotin deficiency
Biotin deficiency in humans is rare. Experimentally, biotin deficiency has been induced in humans fed large quantities of raw egg whites containing the protein avidin. Avidin binds to biotin in the intestine preventing biotin absorption. Symptoms of biotin deficiency include inflammation of the skin, hair loss, muscle pain, abnormally increased sensitivity of the skin, lack or loss of appetite for food, nausea, mental problems, high cholesterol, and decreased hemoglobin levels.

Certain genetic conditions that respond to biotin have been identified, and children with those conditions display neurological abnormalities including seizures and developmental delays, as well as impaired immune systems.

Low levels of biotin have been found in pregnant women, alcoholics, and people who lack sufficient stomach acid.

Causes and effects of biotin toxicity

There is no evidence of biotin toxicity.

Blood tests to measure deficiency or toxicity

Serum biotin levels
Biotinidase activity
Organic acids in urine
Bacteriological assay tests

Biotin requirements

Table 11.13 DRI for biotin.

Biotin	DRI (μg/day)
Men: ages 19–70+	30
Women: ages 19–70+	30

Source: [5].

Biotin food sources

Cauliflower	Mackerel
Cowpeas	Nuts
Eggs	Sardines
Liver	Whole grain rice

Phytochemicals

Phytochemicals are naturally occurring compounds found predominantly in foods of plant origin. They are the molecules responsible for color and organoleptic properties of the food or spice. They also help plants to defend themselves against infection and damage caused by microorganisms insects and predators. It is estimated that there may be more than 100 different phytochemicals in just one serving of vegetables. Evidence has shown that those who consume a diet rich in fruits and vegetables, and thus phytochemicals, have a lower incidence of certain types of cancer, diabetes, heart disease and hypertension. Phytochemicals have an antioxidant effect protecting cells from cancer and/or coronary artery disease, as well as other illnesses such as urinary tract infections, rheumatoid arthritis, or immune suppressive states through a variety of mechanisms.

Foods containing phytochemicals include garlic, soybeans, dark-green leafy vegetables, broccoli, cauliflower, brussel sprouts, cabbage, onions, citrus fruits, berries, tomatoes, whole grains, black tea, green tea, wine, dark chocolate, soybeans and many herbs and spices including garlic, ginger, mint, rosemary, thyme, oregano, sage, basil, tumeric, caraway and fennel. Principle groups of phytochemicals found in fruits and vegetables include polyphenols, terpenes, sulfur and soponins. Phytochemicals in wine include anthocyanidins, proanthocyanidins, flavonols, phenolic acid and resveratrol.

Further research needs to be completed to better understand how and to what extent these protective chemicals may reduce the risk of certain diseases. The experimental and animal data for cancer and heart disease prevention are impressive. However, well-designed clinical trials to determine their effectiveness in people remain scarce. To ensure that your patients get a variety of phytochemicals, recommend a varied diet, with at least 7–9 servings of fruits and vegetables daily and including a wide range of food colors.

Recommended phytochemical intakes

The optimal levels for phytochemical and functional food intake have yet to be determined. However, since fruits and vegetables contain phytochemicals, at least 7–9 servings of fruits and vegetables is recommended daily.

References

1 Food and Nutrition Board. Institute of Medicine. *Dietary Reference Intakes for Calcium, Phosphorus, Magnesium, Vitamin D, and Fluoride*. National Academy of Medicine. National Academies Press: Washington, DC. 1997.

2 Food and Nutrition Board. Institute of Medicine. *Dietary Reference Intakes for Vitamin A, Vitamin K, Arsenic, Boron, Chromium, Copper, Iodine, Iron, Manganese, Molybdenum, Nickel, Silicon, Vanadium, and Zinc*. National Academy of Medicine. National Academies Press: Washington, DC. 2001.

3 Food and Nutrition Board. Institute of Medicine. *Dietary Reference Intakes for Vitamin C, Vitamin E, Selenium, and Carotenoids*. National Academy of Medicine. National Academies Press: Washington, DC. 2000.

4 Food and Nutrition Board. Institute of Medicine. *Dietary Reference Intakes for Vitamin A, Vitamin K, Arsenic, Boron, Chromium, Copper, Iodine, Iron, Manganese, Molybdenum, Nickel, Silicon, Vanadium, and Zinc*. National Academy of Medicine. National Academies Press: Washington, DC. 2001.

5 Food and Nutrition Board. Institute of Medicine. *Dietary Reference Intakes for Thiamin, Riboflavin, Niacin, Vitamin B6, Folate, Vitamin B12, Pantothenic Acid, Biotin, and Chlorine*. National Academy of Science. National Academies Press: Washington, DC. 2000.

6 Ross AC. Vitamins A and carotenoids. In: *Modern Nutrition in Health and Disease*. (10th Edition). Shils ME, Shike M, Ross AC, Caballero B, Cousins RJ. (Eds). Lippincott Williams and Wilkins: New York, 2006.

7 Harbige LS. Nutrition and Immunity with emphasis on infection and autommune disease. *Nutr Health* 1996:10:285–312.

8 Koo LC. Diet and lung cancer 20+ years later: more questions than answers? *Int J Cancer* 1997;Suppl10:22–9.

9 Albances D, Heinonen OP, Taylor *et al*. Alpha-tocopherol and beta-carotene supplement and lung cancer incidence in the alpha-tocopherol, beta-carotene cancer prevention study: Effects of base-line characteristics and study compliance. *J Natl Cancer Inst* 1996:88:1560–70.

10 Holick MF. Vitamin D: Its role in cancer prevention and treatment. *Prog Biophys Mol Biol* 2006 (Mar10).

11 Garland CF, Garland FC, Gorham ED *et al.* The role of vitamin D in cancer prevention. *Am J Public Health* 2006;96(2):252–61.

12 Lieberman DA, Prindiville S, Weiss DG, Willett W. Risk factors for advanced colonic neoplasia and hyperplastic polyps in asymptomatic individuals. *J Am Med Assoc* 2003;290: 2959–67.

13 Holick MF. Vitamin D: important for prevention of osteoporosis, cardiovascular heart disease, type 1 diabetes, autoimmune diseases and some cancers. *South Med J* 2005;98(10): 1024–7.

14 Lee IM, Cook NR, Gaziano JM *et al.* Vitamin E in the primary prevention of cardiovascular diseases and cancer: the Women's Health Study: randomized controlled trial. *JAMA* 2005;294(1):56–65.

15 Neogi T, Booth SL, Zhang YO *et al.* Low vitamin K status is associated with osteoarthritis in the hand and knee. *Arthritis Rheum* 2006;54(4):1255–61.

16 Nutescu EA, Shapiron L, Ibrahin S, West P. Warfarin and its interactions with foods, herbs and oher dietary supplements. *Expert Opin Drug Saf* 2006;5(3):433–51.

17 Finaud J, Lac G, Filaire E. Oxidative stress: relationship with exercise and training. *Sports Med* 2006;36(4):327–58.

18 Lonsdale D. A Review of the biochemistry, metabolism and clinical benefits of thiamin(e) and its derivatives. *J Evid Based Complement Alternat Med* 2006;3(1):49–59.

19 McCormack PL, Keating GM. Prolonged–release nicotinic acid: a review of its use in the treatment of dyslipidemia. *Drugs* 2005;65(18):2719–40.

20 Prousky J, Seely D. The treatment of migraines and tension-type headaches with intravenous and oral niacin (nicotinic acid): systematic review of the literature. *Nutr J* 2005;4(1):3.

21 Kamen B. Folate and antifolate pharmacology. *Semin Oncol* 1997;24:518–39.

22 Lonne Y, Arnold MJ. Homocysteine lowering with folic acid and B vitamins in vascular disease. *N Eng J med* 2006;354(15):1567–77.

23 Shaw GM, Schaffer D, Velie EM, Morland K, Harris JA. Periconceptional vitamin use, dietary folate, and the occurrence of neural tube defects. *Epidemiology* 1995;6:219–26.

24 Milunsky A, Jick H, Jick SS *et al.* Multivitamin/folic acid supplementation in early pregnancy reduces he prevalence of neural tube defects. *JAMA* 1989;262:2847–52.

25 Mackey AD, Davis SR, Gregory JF. Vitamin B6. In: *Modern Nutrition in Health and Disease* (10th edition). Shils ME, Shike M, Ross AC, Caballero B, Cousins RJ. (Eds). Williams and Wilkins: Baltimore, 2006.

26 Brent J, Vo N, Kulig K, Rumack BH. Reversal of prolonged Isoniazid-induced coma by pyridoxine. *Arch Intern Med* 1990;150:1751–3.

27 Carmel R. Megaloblastic anemias. *Curr Opin Hemaol* 1994;1:107–12.

CHAPTER 12

Minerals

Randee Silverman and Jeremy Brauer

Minerals are inorganic substances that occur in simple forms such as sodium chloride or in combination with organic compounds such as the iron in hemoglobin and the sulfur in almost all proteins. Minerals are classified as macrominerals or microminerals, based on their percentages of total body weight.

Macrominerals constitute more than 0.005% of the body's weight, or 50 parts per million (ppm). Macrominerals includes calcium, chloride, phosphorus, potassium, magnesium, sodium, and sulfur.

Microminerals fall into two categories:

• Minerals with identified roles in maintaining health include chromium, cobalt, copper, fluoride, iodide, iron, manganese, molybdenum, selenium, and zinc.

• Minerals with unestablished roles in health, such as arsenic, boron, cadmium, nickel, silicone, tin, and vanadium.

No single food is the best source for all minerals. Consuming a wide variety of foods usually ensures adequate and balanced mineral intake. Eating processed foods can decrease or increase mineral intake, depending on the food. Some minerals are deleted in processing. Iron and chromium, for example, are removed from whole grains during the refining process. As a result, select minerals may be replenished. Refined grains bearing the label "enriched" contain iron, which is added to compensate for the amounts lost during processing. However, other nutrients such as zinc are not routinely replenished. Sodium, mainly as sodium chloride, is added to numerous foods to enhance their taste and to serve as a preservative. Iodine is added routinely to table salt to prevent iodine deficiency. Orange juice, cereals, and other foods are commonly fortified with calcium.

Water contains varying amounts of numerous minerals. Fluoride is present naturally in many water sources, and many municipal water supplies are fluoridated. Hard water contains calcium and magnesium. These minerals can be ion-exchanged with sodium to produce soft water. Water is also a source of iron in some geographic regions.

General functions of minerals

Minerals function together for tissue synthesis and breakdown, and in the regulation of metabolism. Examples of their functions include:

1) Bone formation. Most of the body's calcium, phosphorus, and magnesium are deposited in the collagen matrix of bones. Bones provide a reservoir of minerals. Thus, although minerals are transported via the circulatory system, blood levels of minerals provide limited indication of the actual biochemical flux and body stores of minerals.

2) Tooth formation. Tooth enamel and dentine (hydroxyapatite) contain appreciable amounts of calcium and phosphorus. When fluoride is incorporated into the structure, the resulting fluoroappatite is less soluble in an acid medium and therefore more resistant to the development of dental caries.

3) Minerals are constituents of various regulatory compounds. Sulfur is part of the thiamin molecule. Cobalt is present in the vitamin B_{12} molecule. Some minerals serve as enzyme cofactors; for example, calcium activates pancreatic lipase, a digestive enzyme. Minerals may also catalyze reactions, e.g. copper is needed to incorporate iron into the hemoglobin molecule; zinc is necessary for the formation of insulin by the pancreas.

4) Exact amounts of sodium, potassium, calcium, and magnesium are necessary to regulate various cellular pumps and membrane ion channels. These elements control the passage in and out of cells of the materials that regulate the transmission of nerve impulses and muscle contractions.

Recommended mineral intake

The Food and Nutrition Board of the Institute of Medicine established the following intake parameters with regard to minerals.

• Dietary Reference Intakes (DRI) for calcium, magnesium, fluoride, phosphorus, chromium, copper, iodine, iron, manganese, molybdenum, selenium, and zinc [1,2,3].

• Estimated minimum requirements of healthy persons for sodium, chloride, and potassium [4].

Factors influencing mineral requirements and absorption

With proper selection from the abundant food and water supplies in the US, healthy individuals should be able to meet their mineral requirements. Because the bioavailability of minerals varies, recognition of factors favoring or hindering absorption is important. Factors that influence individual needs and the bioavailability of nutrients include:

Physiologic need

The amount of a mineral that the body absorbs depends on its needs. Women and growing children absorb a higher percentage of calcium and iron than adult males. Likewise, iron-deficient individuals absorb a higher percentage of ingested iron.

Bioavailability

Defined as the amount of an ingested nutrient that is digested and absorbed, bioavailability differs depending on the chemical form of the mineral. For example, calcium citrate is more bioavailable than calcium carbonate. Supplementation with lower doses of the more bioavailable form will achieve the desired physiologic outcome. Heme iron, found in animal flesh, is more available than the non-heme iron, found in eggs and plant foods.

Intestinal pH

Absorption of minerals occurs at various pH levels, depending on where it takes place in the intestine. The acid medium found in the stomach increases the solubility of calcium and iron salts in food, resulting in increased absorption. People suffering from achlorhydria, or individuals who take antacid medication may be at risk for poor absorption of calcium and iron.

Nutrient–nutrient interactions

1) Vitamin C enhances the absorption of calcium, iron, and zinc. Taking iron supplements with orange juice converts the iron from the ferric to the more absorbable ferrous form (this is true for all non-heme iron sources).
2) Long-term zinc supplementation has been shown to reduce serum copper levels; therefore, people who are taking zinc supplements should also increase their copper intake or consider copper supplementation as well.
3) Calcium supplements may be necessary to reduce undesirable increases in phosphorus levels for people who have kidney disease.

Causes of mineral deficiencies

The most prevalent mineral deficiencies in the US are iron (iron-deficiency anemia), calcium (osteoporosis), iodine (goiter), and fluoride (dental caries). Because the body stores and reuses minerals, deficiencies typically do not cause symptoms for years. Causes of primary deficiency include inadequate intake, poor absorption, or increased losses. Other examples include the following.

Chelating substances

Dietary oxalic acid (see Appendix N), phytic acid (whole grains), and tannins (tea, coffee) bind minerals and reduce absorption. Certain medications bind directly with minerals. For example, aluminum hydroxide antacids combine with food phosphates, and other antacids bind with bile salts, which indirectly may affect both vitamin and mineral absorption.

Intestinal motility

Mineral oil, laxatives, and diarrhea increase the motility of the intestinal tract, thereby causing the stool to move through the body quicker. As a result, the intestines have less time to absorb important minerals, such as iron and zinc.

Increased intestinal loss

People with Crohn's disease or those who have fatty stools or surgical resection of a portion of their small intestine can have significant reduction in the absorption of nutrients, vitamins and minerals. In developing countries, intestinal parasites harbored by many children are a major cause of mineral malnutrition.

Increased urinary loss

Excessive alcohol consumption can increase magnesium excretion. Certain medications, such as digoxin and steroids, increase urinary losses of calcium, magnesium, potassium, and zinc. While some medications increase sodium and water excretion, others increase the excretion of potassium, calcium, magnesium, and zinc.

Increased loss via perspiration

High body or environmental temperatures commonly cause loss of sodium, chloride, potassium, and magnesium, and secondarily, calcium and iron. People experiencing recurrent fevers, for example, as well as athletes, manual laborers, or those living in hot climates may lose significant minerals through sweating.

Causes of mineral toxicity

Toxic levels of minerals may result from excessive intake of copper, fluoride, iodine, iron, manganese, and selenium. Examples of toxicity include:
• Iron overload may occur in children as a result of taking excessive doses of children's multivitamins, or adult strength vitamins.
• People treated for ulcers may develop milk alkali syndrome caused by excessive intake of calcium and absorbable alkali from the antacids.
• Excessive intake of vitamin D can cause excessive calcium absorption and lead to possible soft tissue calcification.
• Dietary lead poisoning may result from storing orange juice or other acidic juices in unglazed ceramic ware or wine in lead crystal carafes. Currently, containers made from these materials carry warning labels to this effect.
• Allergic reactions: sulfite, used to prevent discoloration of salad bar vegetables and fruits and also as a reducing agent in some alcoholic beverages, can cause life-threatening pulmonary symptoms in people with asthma. A 1987 FDA mandate has restricted sulfite use in the US and requires food labeling.

MINERALS

Calcium

Calcium is the fifth most abundant mineral in the body, with 99% present in the bones and teeth. The remaining 1% is used for a variety of functions such as enzyme activation, blood clotting, and muscle contraction. Most calcium absorption occurs in the duodenum, but the jejunum and ileum contribute substantially to overall calcium absorption as well.

Vitamin D levels in the body regulate calcium absorption. The parathyroid gland responds to low serum calcium levels by releasing parathyroid hormone, which stimulates the kidney to convert vitamin D to its active form. Activated vitamin D in turn, increases absorption of calcium from the intestine and regulates calcium excretion. When calcium levels in the blood are elevated, the hormone calcitonin, released from the thyroid gland, prevents the bone from releasing calcium. Individuals who have problems absorbing vitamin D also have poor calcium absorption. Lactose, the sugar in dairy products, improves calcium absorption, whereas oxalate and phytate, which are present in certain foods, can reduce calcium absorption. Calcium excretion is related to dietary protein intake – high protein diets (>100 g/day) increase urinary excretion of calcium. People with a history of calcium oxalate kidney stones should be advised to limit their protein intake to the DRI level of 0.8 g/kg body weight/day.

Functions of calcium

Calcium plays an essential role in the following bodily functions:

1) Normal bone mineralization. Calcium maintains a dynamic equilibrium with the bone, characterized by the movement of 250–1000 mg of calcium in and out of bone tissue every day. Approximately 99% of the body's calcium is present in bones and teeth and is essential for bone strength.

2) Maintenance of cell membrane permeability.

3) Normal muscle contractions.

4) Normal blood clotting.

5) Nerve impulse conduction.

Causes and effects of calcium deficiency

Calcium deficiency usually remains undiagnosed for years because the bones continue to release normal amounts of calcium into the blood. Symptoms of calcium deficiency include bone pain, pins and needles in hands and feet, muscle cramps and twitching, convulsions, osteoporosis with accompanying bone fractures and loss of height. Calcium deficiency in children is characterized by stunted growth, muscle weakness, irritability, muscle cramps and twitching, and death. Problems related to poor calcium intake include:

1) Rickets is caused primarily by vitamin D deficiency, but lack of calcium and phosphorus influences the onset of this disease. Rickets is characterized by abnormal bone formation, bending and distortion of the bones, nodular enlargements of the boney epipheses and delayed closure of the fontanels and muscle pain.

2) Osteoporosis is defined as a reduction in bone density, rendering bones brittle and susceptible to fractures. Symptoms of osteoporosis include altered posture caused by deformity of the spine, or postural slumping due to acute pain; loss of height as a result of vertebral fractures; and kyphosis. The long bones are most commonly affected: hip, wrist and upper arm. A low calcium diet and lack of adequate physical activity are primary factors believed to contribute to the development of osteoporosis. Excessive alcohol intake, family history of osteoporosis, early menopause, short stature, and cigarette smoking are major contributors as well.

Causes and effects of calcium toxicity

Hypercalcemia, may be seen in people with a hyperactive parathyroid gland, excessive intake of vitamin D, or certain renal cancers which may lead to deposits of calcium in the kidneys. Hypercalcemia may result in dehydration, lethargy, nausea, vomiting, anorexia, and possibly death. The tolerable upper limit for calcium has been established at 2500 mg/day.

Bioavailability

Calcium absorption from different food sources and supplements varies considerably. For example, the percent absorption from beans is $1/2$ that of milk, while absorption from broccoli, kale, and bok choy is twice that of milk. Because these different foods all contain different amounts of calcium it takes 12 servings of beans or 15 servings of spinach to absorb the amount of calcium in one cup of milk.

Calcium requirements

Table 12.1 DRI for calcium.

Calcium	DRI (mg/day)
Men: ages 19–50	1000
Women: ages 19–50	1000

Source: [1].

Who is at risk of poor calcium intake: those who need it most

A study performed at the School of Public Health, University of Minnesota revealed that non-white women of low socioeconomic status tended to consume below the recommended dietary allowance (RDA) for calcium. Teenagers in particular were found to take in less than 68% of the RDA for calcium, making it likely that few teenage girls will reach their full potential bone mass, placing them at high risk for the development of osteoporosis later in life. In addition, approximately 30% of Asian-American females and 26% of African-American females reported consuming less than the RDA for calcium. Teenagers who diet or binge and purge to lose weight were also found to have low calcium intake, as were those who abused drugs and alcohol [5].

Relationship to disease prevention

More than 1.5 million fractures occur annually, costing the US health care system over 10 billion dollars each year. While osteoporosis is a multifactorial disorder, calcium intake during adolescence and throughout life is critical to achieving optimal peak bone mass and also may play a significant role in preventing degenerative bone diseases in later years. Adolescents need to be educated about the importance of calcium for health, as well as recommended intakes and good food sources of calcium, particularly lower-fat dairy products [6–8].

Calcium intake prevents hypertension

Evaluation of NHANES data published in 1980's first linked calcium intake to blood pressure [9]. While the impact of dietary calcium on blood pressure is clear from epidemiological studies, the role of calcium supplements is not clear [10].

Blood tests to measure deficiency or toxicity

Serum albumin (high levels bind calcium)
Serum levels of calcium for toxicity

Calcium food sources

(See Appendices G and H).

Iron

Iron is an essential element in all cells of the body. As a component of hemoglobin, myoglobin, and certain enzymes, iron plays a key role in oxygen transport and normal cellular respiration.

Forms and absorption

Iron is absorbed in the duodenum via iron-binding proteins which transfer it across the intestinal mucosa. Iron absorption requires an acidic gastric pH to convert it from ferric to ferrous forms. The absorption of iron from plants (non-heme iron) is also enhanced by vitamin C and increased in iron deficient individuals, such as pregnant women and adolescents, anemic individuals, or those who are bleeding. Amino acids and proteins can enhance absorption of iron.

Functions of iron

Iron plays an essential role in the following bodily functions:
1) Hemoglobin and myoglobin synthesis. About 70–75% of the body's iron is bound to hemoglobin and myoglobin, the other 25–30% is stored as ferritin and hemosiderin in the liver, bone marrow, and spleen. Iron is transported in

the serum bound to transferrin, which represents about 1% of the body's iron stores.

2) Necessary cofactor in many enzymatic reactions used to metabolize glucose and fatty acids.

Causes and effects of iron deficiency

Iron deficiency is one of the most prevalent nutritional problems in the world, with pregnant women, infants and children, menstruating females, and older adults at greatest risk. Iron deficiency is most frequently caused by inadequate dietary intake, or a diet with low bioavailable iron, such as vegetarians or infants who are not supplemented or given iron-fortified formula or cereal after the age of six months. In the US, iron intake of most boys and men exceeds the DRI, while intake of most girls and women (up to the age of 50) is less than the DRI.

Iron deficiency is characterized by weakness, fatigue, poor work performance, and changes in behavior. Symptoms of iron deficiency include pale skin, fatigue and feeling of faintness, cold or abnormal sensations of the extremities, shortness of breath, greater susceptibility to infections, concave shaped or brittle nails. Infants and young children with iron deficiency may have low IQ levels and learning and/or behavioral problems.

Causes and effects of iron toxicity

Excessive iron ingestion may cause deposition of iron in the tissues. Prolonged iron overload e.g. (hemochromatosis) may cause bronzed pigmentation to the skin, damage liver and pancreas tissue and possibly cause diabetes. The hemochromatosis gene is present in 1 in 200 non-Hispanic white Americans. The gene frequently is lower in homozygote individuals, Mexican-Americans and non-Hispanic blacks. Even among homozygote individuals, only 1% develop signs of iron overload. Tolerable upper limit for iron has been established at 45 mg/day.

Relationship to disease prevention

Iron deficiency anemia is an important cause of morbidity in special populations (i.e. infants, and menstruating women) and has been associated with learning difficulty in children.

In recent years there have been studies correlating serum ferritin levels and heart disease. Also, frequent blood donation (more than one unit per month), is associated with decreased incidence of heart disease. It was concluded that reducing iron levels may decrease the risk of cardiac events [11].

Iron requirements

Table 12.2 DRI for iron.

Iron	DRI (mg/day)
Men: ages 19–70+	8
Women: ages 19–50	18

Source: [2].

Blood tests to measure deficiency or toxicity

Hemoglobin and hematocrit blood levels
Mean corpuscular volume in the blood (MCV)
Mean corpuscular hemoglobin concentration (MCHC)
Transferrin
Ferritin
Total iron binding capacity (TIBC)

Iron food sources

(See Appendix L).

Zinc

Forms and absorption

Zinc absorption occurs throughout the small intestine, with the jejunum having a greater absorption rate compared to the ileum or duodenum. Zinc absorption is dependent on an individual's zinc status: the lower the body's stores, the greater the absorption. Zinc absorption is also reduced in the presence of copper, iron, oxalate, calcium, phytate, and fiber.

Once absorbed, zinc is widely distributed throughout the body, with highest levels found in the prostate, skin, brain, liver, pancreas, bone, and blood. Zinc levels are under homeostatic control, such that when intake levels are high, zinc is retained by the cells of the intestinal tract and excreted when those cells are sloughed off.

Functions of zinc

Zinc plays an essential role in the following bodily functions.
1) Acts as a coenzyme for over 100 enzymes, playing an important role in carbohydrate, fat, and protein metabolism.
2) Normal cell division, growth and repair at all stages of life, especially during fetal growth.
3) Synthesis of DNA and RNA and gene regulation.
4) Normal immune function including wound healing and skin integrity.
5) Sexual maturation, fertility, and reproduction.
6) Maintenance of normal sense of taste and smell.

Causes and effect of zinc deficiency

Zinc deficiency may be caused by inadequate dietary intake, increased requirements, decreased absorption, or increased loses of the mineral. Patients at high-risk include those who are HIV positive with chronic diarrhea, patients with Crohn's disease who have significantly increased loss of zinc, those with diabetes, uremia, inflammatory bowel disease, intestinal malabsorption, liver cirrhosis, and those who abuse alcohol.

Zinc deficiency will lead to impaired DNA, RNA and protein synthesis, thereby causing abnormal cell division, growth and repair [12]. Symptoms of a zinc deficiency include poor appetite, digestive problems, diarrhea, vomiting, night blindness, changes in perception of taste and smell, hair loss, skin problems, poor wound healing, impaired cell mediated immunity, growth retardation in infants, children and adolescents, decreased functioning of the sex organs resulting in delayed onset of puberty and sexual maturation in adolescents.

Causes and effect of zinc toxicity

Zinc is not considered to be a very toxic mineral, but large quantities in the body could cause decreased high-density lipoprotein levels and increased low-density lipoprotein levels. Zinc supplementation at 50 mg/day impedes copper absorption and lead to symptoms of copper deficiency. Toxic symptoms may include: gastrointestinal upset, specifically nausea and vomiting. Tolerable upper limit for zinc has been established at 40 mg/day.

Zinc requirements

Individuals with intestinal resection or surgical removal of all or part of their intestines may require zinc supplementation, as both transit time and surface area influence its absorption.

Table 12.3 DRI for zinc.

Zinc	DRI (mg/day)
Men: ages 14–70+	11
Women: ages 19–70+	8

Source: [2].

Relationship to disease prevention

Zinc is necessary to maintain normal blood testosterone levels and convert testosterone to estrogen. The testosterone to estrogen ratio in men declines with age, resulting in higher estradiol (estrogen) activity, which subsequently increases the risk of heart disease, weight gain, and obesity.

Blood tests to measure deficiency or toxicity

The laboratory criteria are not well established. Various laboratory procedures include: dark adaptation, taste acuity testing, activities of alkaline phosphatase and carbonic anhydrase. Zinc levels in the blood, red blood cells, white blood cells, hair, nails and urine can also be measured.

Zinc food sources (including enriched sources)

Chicken	Pork
Dried beans	Red meat
Eggs	Seafood
Legumes	Turkey
Liver	Wheat germ
Milk	Whole grains (whole wheat and rye
Nuts	bread, oatmeal)
Oysters	Yogurt

Magnesium

Forms and absorption

Magnesium is absorbed primarily in the jejunum and ileum and when intake is low, more magnesium is absorbed. Magnesium competes with calcium for absorption and its absorption is also enhanced by vitamin D. Once absorbed, magnesium is found in bone, muscle, cells, and extracellular fluid. Magnesium absorption is reduced when sections of the small intestine have been removed.

Functions of magnesium

Magnesium plays a role in the following bodily functions:
1) Formation of bones and teeth.
2) In conjunction with calcium, sodium, and potassium, magnesium is involved in transmitting nerve impulses and thereby eliciting muscle contractions.
3) Enzyme reactions used in fat and protein metabolism.
4) Protein synthesis.
5) Normal parathyroid hormone secretion when blood calcium levels are low.

Cause and effects of deficiency

While magnesium deficiency is rare, due to its presence in a wide variety of foods, deficiency can occur in individuals who have absorption or excretion problems. These conditions include intestinal malabsorption, surgical removal of the ileum, severe vomiting, and kidney disease. Individuals with protein–calorie malnutrition, chronic alcohol abuse, hyperparathyroidism, and liver cirrhosis may have low levels of magnesium in their blood. Patients taking diuretics may have increase magnesium excretion. Since magnesium is also required for normal parathyroid functioning, low magnesium levels may alter calcium and phosphorous homeostasis.

Symptoms of magnesium deficiency include low serum levels of calcium and potassium, as well as changes in the gastrointestinal, neuromuscular, cardiovascular and hematologic systems. Deficient individuals may also experience fatigue, lethargy, weakness, muscle cramps, poor appetite, impaired speech, anemia, irregular heartbeat, tremors, and failure to thrive. Advanced clinical signs of magnesium deficiency include rapid heart rate, fibrillations or muscle contraction of the heart, convulsions, and death.

Causes and effects of magnesium toxicity

Elevated blood magnesium levels may be seen in people with renal failure receiving high doses of magnesium. High blood levels may result in lethargy, decreased nerve transmission, nausea, vomiting, paralysis, cardiac arrest and death. The tolerable upper limit for magnesium has been established at 350 mg/day.

Relationship to disease prevention

Magnesium intake has been correlated with diabetes and heart disease risk in several studies of older Americans. A recent prospective study (CARDIA) demonstrated that low magnesium intake was associated with increased risk of developing metabolic syndrome [8]. Magnesium supplements have also been used successfully to treat patients with chronic headaches as well as muscle cramps.

Magnesium requirements

Table 12.4 DRI for magnesium.

Magnesium	DRI (mg/day)
Men	420
Women	320

Source: [1].

Blood tests to measure deficiency or toxicity

RBC magnesium levels accurately reflect the total body pool but do not reflect ionized magnesium which is most sensitive to deficiency states.

Magnesium food sources (including enriched sources)

(See Appendix K).

Iodine

Iodine is essential for humans as a component of thyroid hormones. Approximately 40% of the body's iodine is stored in the thyroid gland.

Forms and absorption
Iodine is absorbed in the gastrointestinal tract and travels through the bloodstream freely or bound to thyroxine-binding globulin (TBG). Excess iodine in the body is excreted via the urine.

Functions of iodine
1) Iodine is a constituent of all cells.
2) T_3 and T_4 control carbohydrate, protein, and fat metabolism.

Causes and effects of iodine deficiency
An iodine deficiency may result in a decrease in the production of the thyroid hormones (T_3 and T_4). To compensate for this lack of production of the thyroid hormones, the thyroid gland grows in size. Symptoms of iodine deficiency include, lethargy, dry skin, thick lips, enlarged tongue, reduced muscle and skeletal growth, and mental retardation (cretinism).

Causes and effects of iodine toxicity
Excessive dietary intake of iodine results in inhibition of thyroid hormone synthesis. Generally, the body will adapt to the higher intake but a few individuals will develop goiters due to reduced iodine absorption when iodine blood levels are too high. The tolerable upper limit for iodine has been established at 1100 µg/day.

Iodine requirements

Table 12.5 DRI for iodine.

Iodine	DRI (ug/day)
Men: ages 14–70+	150
Women: ages 14–70+	150

Source: [2].

Relationship to disease prevention
Iodine deficiency is a common worldwide cause of endemic goiter and cretinism in children who don't eat iodized salt and live in mountainous places where iodine is not found [13]. Deficiency of thyroid activity can also occur due to a congenital defect. One out of every 3000 children is born with this defect and early treatment with iodine is necessary to avoid mental retardation.

Blood tests to measure deficiency or toxicity
Serum and urine thyroids hormone levels
Thyroid function tests
Serum protein bound iodine levels

Iodine food sources (including enriched sources)

Seafood   Iodized salt
Seaweed

Copper

Form and absorption

Copper absorption occurs in the small intestine. Its absorption is enhanced in the presence of an acidic medium and decreased by calcium, cadmium, phytates, fiber, vitamin C, or zinc. About 30–40% of the copper in the diet is absorbed.

Functions of copper

Copper plays an essential role in the following.
1) Production of skin, hair and eye pigment (melanin).
2) Development of healthy bones, teeth, and vascular structures via its role in connective tissue synthesis.
3) Protection of cells from oxygen damage.
4) Maintenance of myelin sheath.
5) Metabolism of catecholamines.
6) Essential for iron metabolism.

Causes and effects of copper deficiency

Copper deficiency is rare though it can occur in malnourished infants. Copper deficiency results in anemia and connective tissue damage, which can result in lung damage or excessive bleeding. Low levels of copper in the blood are seen in nutritional diseases such as kwashiorkor, anemia, tropical sprue, celiac disease and the genetic disorder, Menke's syndrome.

Cause and effect of copper toxicity

Excessive copper intake or poisoning may occur with consumption of acidic beverages stored in containers made with copper. Symptoms of copper toxicity include: tachycardia, high blood pressure, jaundice, hemolytic anemia, uremia, and death.

The genetic syndrome, Wilson's disease, results in decreased amounts of blood copper levels, but increased copper deposits in certain organs such as the brain, kidney, cornea and liver. Untreated, it can result in nervous system and liver damage. The tolerable upper limit for copper has been established at 10,000 µg/day.

Copper requirements

Table 12.6 DRI for copper.

Copper	DRI (ug/day)
Men: ages 19–70+	900
Women: ages 19–70+	900

Source: [2].

Relationship to disease prevention
None.

Blood tests to measure deficiency or toxicity
Serum copper
Activity of the erythrocyte superoxide dismutase
Neutrophil count

Copper food sources (including enriched sources)

Barley	Organ meats
Cocoa products	Oysters
Dried legumes	Seafood, (crabmeat, lobster)
Kidney	Seeds (sesame, sunflower, pumpkin)
Liver	Whole grain cereals
Nuts (brazil, almond, cashews, peanuts, pistachio)	

Phosphorous

Phosphorus is an essential mineral present in bones and teeth. It is a constituent of lipids, proteins, carbohydrates, enzymes, DNA and ATP.

Form and absorption
Phosphorous is absorbed primarily in the small intestine. Absorption varies depending upon dietary phosphorous intake, as more is absorbed when intake is inadequate. During periods of growth phosphorous absorption is enhanced in the presence of calcium and vitamin D.

Function of phosphorous
Phosphorous plays an essential role in the following.
1) Normal construction of bones and teeth.
2) DNA and RNA synthesis.

(Functions of phosphorous continued)
3) Energy synthesis (ATP, ADP).
4) Aids in protein, fat, and carbohydrate metabolism.
5) In its ionic form, phosphate helps to maintain the body's normal pH levels.
6) Normal cell membrane structure.

Cause and effect of phosphorous deficiency

Phosphorous deficiency has been seen in individuals who consume excessive amounts of antacids for prolonged periods, which bind dietary phosphorous and prevent its absorption. Symptoms of phosphorous deficiency include weakness, anorexia, abnormal softness of an organ or tissue, and bone pain. Anemia, impaired red and white cells function, neurologic and psychiatric disorders, abnormal excretion of calcium in urine, and kidney stones may also result from phosphorous deficiency.

Cause and effect of phosphorous toxicity

Abnormal elevated blood phosphorus levels appear in individuals with renal failure or hypoparathyroidsm and is characterized by low blood concentrations of calcium and muscular spasms. Osteoporosis, arthritis, gout, dental problems, skin eruptions, lowered white blood cells, high risk of several cancers, and kidney stones have been associated with high blood levels of phosphorous. The tolerable upper limit for phosphorus has been established at 4000 mg/day. Unfortunately, there is inadequate evidence on the health effects of diets high in processed foods and carbonated beverages, both of which contain high amounts of phosphorous [14].

Phosphorous requirements

Table 12.7 DRI for phosphorous.

Phosphorous	DRI (mg/day)
Men: ages 19–70+	700
Women: ages 19–70+	700

Source: [1].

Relationship to disease prevention
None.

Blood tests to measure deficiency or toxicity
Serum phosphate levels (PO_4)

Phosphorous food sources (including enriched sources)

Brussels sprouts	Nuts
Cauliflower	Okra
Cheeses	Pork
Chocolate	Potatoes
Dairy products	Red meat
Fish (carp)	Salmon
Grains	Seafood
Ice cream	Shellfish
Legumes	Sprouts, Alfalfa
Lima beans	Swordfish
Liver	Whole milk
Mackerel	Yams
Milk chocolate	

Sulfur

Sulfur plays an essential role in the following.
1) Amino acid synthesis (cystine, cysteine and methionine).
2) Carbohydrates metabolism (sulfur is a component of insulin).
3) Synthesis of connective tissue, skin, hair, and nails.
4) Formation of thiamin, biotin, and coenzyme A.

Causes and effects of sulfur deficiency
Sulfur deficiency has never been diagnosed in humans.

Cause and effect of sulfur toxicity
Possible adverse effects of consuming sulfur containing foods or sulfur-containing supplements at higher amounts include bloating or flatulence.

Sulfur requirements
There are no established DRI for sulfur [4].

Relationship to disease prevention
Various studies have shown that 50–60% of test subjects with a variety of joint and muscular types of injuries or arthritis had a positive response from supplementing with sulfur. In addition, sulfur supplementation has been shown to improve hair growth, brilliance and thickness of hair fiber, as well as nail health (strength, thickness, and appearance).

Sulfur supplementation may promote faster wound healing, reduced parasitic infections, reduced severity of sun burns, reduced allergic reactions, and improved lung function including asthma. Along with vitamin C, sulfur helps to maintain elasticity of the skin. Food or supplement sources of sulfur should be avoided in Crohn's disease, Lou Gehrig's disease and Alzheimer's disease.

Blood tests to measure deficiency or toxicity
None.

Sulfur food sources (including enriched sources)

Cheese	Legumes
Chicken	Meat
Eggs	Milk
Fish	

Fluoride

Fluoride is found at varying concentrations in drinking water and soil. It is considered a beneficial nutrient and is present in trace amounts in the body. About 99% of the fluoride in the body is in bones and teeth.

Functions of fluoride
Fluoride promotes mineralization of body tissues. The use of topical and systemic fluoride for oral health has resulted in major reductions in dental caries. The role of high doses of fluoride for prevention of osteoporosis is undergoing active study.

When fluoride is consumed in optimal amounts from water and food, and used topically in toothpastes, mouth rinses, and professionally applied office treatments it performs the following functions:

1) Increase tooth mineralization and bone density.
2) Reduce the risk and prevalence of dental caries.
3) Promote enamel remineralization throughout life for individuals of all ages.

Causes and effects of fluoride deficiency
While controversial in some circles, fluoridation of public water supplies has been endorsed by over 90 professional health organizations as the most effective dental public health measure in existence. Still, about half of the US population fails to receive the maximum benefits possible from community water fluoridation and the use of fluoride products.

Water fluoridation
Fluoridation, by definition, is the adjustment of fluoride in a water supply to a concentration of between 0.7–1.2 ppm. The value of water fluoridation for the prevention of dental caries has been unquestionably demonstrated.

Causes and effects of toxicity
Fluoride can be toxic when consumed in excessive amounts, so concentrated fluoride products should be used with caution. To prevent the possibility of acute fluoride poisoning, fluoride products should be kept out of reach of small children. Fluorosis, a hypomineralization of tooth enamel results from

excessive fluoride ingestion during enamel development prior to tooth eruption. Fluorosis can range from very mild to severe. In cases of mild fluorosis, teeth are highly resistant to dental caries but may have chalky white spots or patches. Severe fluorosis can result in teeth with brown discoloration and is most often seen in areas of the country that have excessive concentrations of natural fluoride in water supplies such as wells.

Swallowing of fluoride toothpaste in early years, misuse of dietary fluoride supplements, or long-term use of infant formula (particularly powder concentrates reconstituted with fluoridated water) can lead to flourosis. To minimize the risk of excessive exposure The American Dental Association requires toothpaste manufacturers to include the phrase "use only a pea-sized amount (of toothpaste) for children under six."

Fluoride requirements

Table 12.8

Fluoride	mg/day
Men: ages 19–70+	4.0
Women: ages 19–70+	3.0

Source: [1].

Blood tests to measure deficiency or toxicity

There are new blood tests available to screen for early signs of fluorosis.

Fluoride food sources (including enriched sources)

The primary dietary source of fluoride is fluoridated water. The average child under age 6 consumes less than a half liter of water a day and would consume less than 0.5 mg/day of fluoride from drinking optimally fluoridated water. Additionally, beverages (such as bottled water, brewed tea, infant formulas) and commercially prepared foods (e.g. poultry products, seafood and powered cereals) can also supply varying amounts of fluoride to the diet. The fluoride content of food can range from 0.01–1.0 ppm. Brewed tea can contain from 1–6 ppm of fluoride depending on the amount of tea used, the fluoride in the water used, and the length of brewing. In bottled water, the fluoride content is highly variable and often low. Although the majority of bottled water in the market is low in fluoride there can be considerable consumption from drinking, meal preparation, and the reconstitution of soups and beverages. Because foods processed with fluoridated water can add significantly to total fluoride consumption (particularly in infants), potential sources of high fluoride intake in children's diets should be identified before any fluoride supplementation is recommended.

Selenium

Selenium is an essential trace mineral in the body that contributes to the antioxidant defence mechanisms.

Form and absorption

Selenium absorption is efficient and is not regulated. Selenium enters in the body from the diet bound to two amino acids: cysteine and methionine. It is absorbed in the gastrointestinal tract in the range of 50–100%. Extra selenium in the body is removed via urine, feces, skin, and through breathing.

Functions of selenium

1) Selenium is an essential component of the enzyme glutathione peroxidase which protects cells from the damaging effects of free radicals. For example, low density lipoprotein (LDL) oxidation is reduced by selenium.

2) Selenium is essential for normal functioning of the immune system and thyroid glands.

3) Epidemiological and animal studies have shown that selenium may have anti-cancer properties, possibly from its antioxidant function, as well as from its ability to inhibit many enzymes involved in cell division and growth.

Causes and effects of selenium deficiency

Selenium deficiency is not common in the US. However, selenium deficiency has been seen in people who rely on intravenous nutrition. People with gastrointestinal problems can have impairment of selenium absorption. Low selenium intake has been seen in children with kwashiorkor, since selenium is present in foods with protein. Selenium deficiency also has been noted in people with rheumatoid arthritis. Selenium deficiency is commonly associated with a high risk of death in people with HIV/AIDS.

Signs of selenium deficiency are seen in countries where the selenium content in the soil is very low and therefore selenium intake is poor. People living in areas of China, New Zealand, and Venezuela develop an enlarged heart and poor cardiac function as a result of selenium deficiency. Selenium deficiency also may affect thyroid function because selenium is essential for synthesis of thyroid hormone.

Causes and effects of selenium toxicity

Selenium toxicity is rare in the US and the few reported cases have been associated with industrial accidents and a manufacturing error that led to an excessively high dose of selenium in a supplement. High blood levels of selenium can result in selenosis. Symptoms of selenosis are gastrointestinal upset, hair loss, white spots on nails, mild nerve damage, fever, anemia and damage to the kidney, spleen and liver, hypotension, convulsions and death. The tolerable upper limit established for selenium is 400 µg/day.

Selenium requirements

Table 12.9

Selenium	DRI (μg/day)
Men: ages 14–70+	55
Women: ages 14–70+	55

Source: [3].

Relationship to disease prevention
None.

Blood tests to measure deficiency or toxicity
Urinary selenium levels
Serum selenium levels
RBC selenium levels
Glutathione peroxidase activity in red cells and in platelets

---

Selenium food sources

Beef	Oatmeal
Brazil nuts	Rice enriched
Bread enriched	Spaghetti enriched
Chicken	Tuna
Cod	Turkey
Egg (raw)	

Sodium

The predominant extracellular cation

Functions of sodium
Sodium functions together with chloride to regulate hydration and cell membrane potentials.

Causes and effects of sodium deficiency
Sodium deficiency is uncommon because most Americans take in about 8 g of sodium from the diet and 4 g from table salt a day. Fluid retention or sodium loss can cause a relative deficiency of sodium. Prolonged vomiting, diarrhea, excessive or persistent sweating (such as marathon or triathalon runners), and certain forms of kidney disease may cause sodium deficiency. Symptoms of hyponatremia include headache, nausea, vomiting, muscle cramps, fainting, fatigue and death.

Causes and effects of sodium toxicity

Sodium intake is high in most developed countries. Average sodium intake is about 20 times the requirement, which is about 4000–5000 mg/day. Symptoms of increased salt intake can cause nausea, vomiting, diarrhea, and abdominal cramps. High sodium concentrations result from excess water or fluid loss. Hypernatremia can result in edema, hypertension, difficulty breathing, congestive heart failure, and death.

Relationship to disease prevention

Hypertension

Hypertension affects about one in four adults, or about 50 million Americans. It is the leading cause of stroke and can contribute to heart attack, heart failure, and kidney failure. It is well known that diets high in sodium are associated with a higher risk of developing hypertension. Studies have shown that modest sodium restriction is effective in lowering blood pressure and can improve the action of diuretics in lowering blood pressure [15]. While many studies fail to support a blood pressure lowering effect of limiting sodium intake on a population basis, it is clear that limiting dietary sodium intake reduces blood pressure and stroke risk.

Osteoporosis

Along with decreasing the risk of hypertension, lowering an individuals' sodium intake may decrease their risk of osteoporosis because high salt intake has been shown to increase calcium excretion. Each gram of sodium excreted by the kidney takes substantial amounts of calcium along with it. By decreasing salt intake, more calcium remains in the body thereby decreasing the risk for bone density loss [16].

Minimum requirement for sodium

	Table 12.10

Sodium	mg/day
Male: ages 10–70+	500
Female: ages 10–70+	500

Source: [4].

The Food an Nutrition Board, American Heart Association and the US Dietary Guidelines all recommend adults should eat no more than 2400 mg of sodium a day [4]. This is the equivalent of about 1 teaspoon of sodium chloride (table salt).

Blood test to measure deficiency or toxicity

Since a balance between dietary intake and renal excretion regulates the total body sodium content. Hypo and hypernatremia are rare except in cases of impaired renal function, abnormal sodium losses from the skin, and or gastrointestinal problems.

Sodium food sources
Sodium is present in varying amounts in all foods and is a common additive in many prepared and processed foods. Approximately 75% of the sodium and chloride found in our diet comes from processed food (see Appendix I).

Potassium

The predominant intracellular cation

Functions of potassium
Potassium is an extremely important electrolyte that functions in the maintenance of the following:
1) Water balance and distribution.
2) Acid–base balance.
3) Muscle and nerve cell function.
4) Heart function.
5) Kidney and adrenal function.
6) Maintaining glycogen in its aqueous intracellular mellieu.

Causes and effects of potassium deficiency
Hypokalemia is most commonly a result of excess potassium losses, which can occur from vomiting, diarrhea, kidney disease, or metabolic disturbances. Patients who abuse laxatives and those with anorexia or bulimia may also exhibit hypokalemia. Since potassium is lost in sweat, prolonged exercise in a warm environment can result in low blood potassium levels. In potassium deficiency there may not be enough glycogen and fatigue and muscle weakness can occur. Since potassium is found mainly in fruits and vegetables, a diet lacking in fruits and vegetables can lead to potassium deficiency. Symptoms of potassium deficiency include fatigue, muscle weakness, cramps, constipation, and impaired renal function. Severe hypokalemia can lead to cardiac arrhythmias and death.

Causes and effects of potassium toxicity
Potassium toxicity is most often seen in patients with poor renal function or excessive supplementation. Hypokalemia can be seen in patients with trauma or severe burns that lead to tissue damage and release of potassium into the blood. Symptoms of hyperkalemia include tingling in the hands and feet, muscle weakness, and temporary paralysis. If left untreated, severe hypokalemia can cause an irregular heartbeat and eventually cardiac arrest.

Relationship to disease prevention
Potassium helps maintain proper function of both the heart and nervous systems. Potassium plays a vital role in people with high blood pressure. Regular consumption of high-potassium foods can help to lower and control blood pressure. A high potassium intake has also been linked to decreasing the risk of stroke, osteoporosis, and calcium-containing kidney stones.

Potassium requirements

Table 12.11 DRI for potassium

Potassium	DRI mg/day
Men: ages 19–70+	3500
Women: ages 19–70+	3500

Source: [4].

Blood tests to measure deficiency or toxicity
Serum potassium levels
Urinary potassium levels

Potassium food sources

(See Appendix J).

Chromium

Chromium potentiates the action of insulin and has been identified as a "glucose tolerance factor".

Form and absorption
Chromium exists in various inorganic forms with little biological activity. Most chromium found in food is in the trivalent chromium (III) form. The glucose tolerance factor (GTF) form of chromium is bound to nicotinic acid, glycine, cysteine, and glutamic acid. Chromium absorption depends upon the form and physiochemical reactions in the intestinal lumen. Fiber and phytates reduce absorption and a deficient diet results in higher fractional absorption rates.

Functions of chromium
Chromium potentiates the action of insulin via an oligopeptide that has been named "chromodulin" which binds to the insulin receptor stimulating its kinase activity. In diabetic subjects, chromium supplementation has been shown to lower blood sugar and improve serum lipids. Efforts to reproduce improvements in lean body mass, noted in a few small trials, have not been successful.

Causes and effects of chromium deficiency
A diet high in simple sugars promotes chromium excretion and may lead to long-term deficits. Since it is not possible to determine chromium status, it is difficult to determine the impact of low chromium intake.

Causes and effects of chromium toxicity
Chromium toxicity has been of concern due to the large number of patients who have been taking this popular dietary supplement. Chromium

picolinate demonstrated mutagenic potential in hamster ovarian cell line, while chromium chloride and chromium nicotinate did not. No tolerable upper limit (TUI) has been established. Chromium (III) has low toxicity as a supplement while industrial exposure to chromium (IV) has been demonstrated to increase the risk of lung cancer.

Relationship to disease prevention

Patients with glucose intolerance have been shown to benefit from supplements of 400 μg/day GTF chromium. These findings have not been universally reproduced.

Blood tests to measure deficiency or toxicity

No reliable indicator of chromium status exists. It has been suggested that pre-diabetic or diabetic patients with hypertriglyceridemia be prescribed chromium supplements to determine their glucose and lipid responses. More research in this area is needed.

Chromium requirements

Table 12.12 Adequate intake for chromium

Chromium	AI* (μg/day)
Men: ages 19–70+	35
Women: ages 19–70+	25

AI, adequate intake.
*No DRI.
Source: [2].

Chromium food sources

Chromium in small amounts is present in meats, unprocessed grains, fruits and vegetables, fats and oils. Good sources include brewer's yeast, oysters and liver.

References

1 Food and Nutrition Board. Institute of Medicine. *Dietary Reference Intakes for Calcium, Phosphorus, Magnesium, Vitamin D, and Fluoride.* National Academy of Sciences. National Academies Press. Washington, DC. 1997.

2 Food and Nutrition Board. Institute of Medicine. *Dietary Reference Intakes for Vitamin A, Vitamin K, Arsenic, Boron, Chromium, Copper, Iodine, Iron, Manganese, Molybdenum, Nickel, Silicon, Vanadium, and Zinc.* National Academy of Sciences. National Academies Press. Washington, DC. 2000.

3 Food and Nutrition Board. Institute of Medicine. *Dietary Reference Intakes for Vitamin C, Vitamin E, Selenium, and Carotenoids.* National Academy of Sciences. National Academies Press. Washington, DC. 2000.

4 Food and Nutrition Board. Institute of Medicine. *Dietary Reference Intakes for Water, Potassium, Sodium, Chloride, and Sulfate. National Academy of Sciences National Academies Press.* Washington, DC. 2004.

5 Larson NI, Story M, Wall M, Neumark-Sztainer D. Calcium and dairy intakes of adolescents are associated with their home environment, taste preferences, personal health beliefs, and meal patterns. *J Am Diet Assoc.* 2006;106(11):1816–24.

6 Gass M, Dawson-Hughes B. Preventing osteoporosis-related fractures: an overview. *Am J Med.* 2006;119(4 Suppl 1):S3–S11.

7 Department of Health and Human Services. *Bone Health and Osteoporosis. A Report of the Surgeon General.* US DHHS. Rockville, MD. Office of the Surgeon General. 2004.

8 Greer FR, Krebs NF. American Academy of Pediatrics Committee on Nutrition. Optimizing bone health and calcium intakes of infants, children, and adolescents. *Pediatrics.* 2006;117(2):578–85.

9 McCarron D, Reusser M. Finding consensus in the dietary calcium-blood pressure debate. *J Am Coll Nutr* 1999;18:398S–405S.

10 Allender PS, Cutler JA, Follmann D, Cappuccio FP, Pryer J, Elliott P. Dietary calcium and blood pressure: a meta-analysis of randomized clinical trials. *Ann Intern Med.* 1996;124(9):825–31.

11 Meyers DG, Jensen KC, Menitove JE. A historical cohort study of the effect of lowering body iron through blood donation on incident cardiac events. *Transfusion.* 2002;42:1135–9.

12 McClung JP, Scrimgeour AG. Zinc: An essential trace element with potential benefits to soldiers. *Mil Med.* 2005;170(12):1048–52.

13 Vanderpas J. Nutritional epidemiology and thyroid hormone metabolism. *Annu Rev Nutr.* 2006;26:293–322.

14 Sax L. DRI for Phosphorous: a critical perspective. *J Am Coll Nutr.* 2001;208:271–8.

15 O'Shaughnessy Km, Karet FE. Salt handling and hypertension. *Ann Rev Nutr.* 2006;26:343–65.

16 Heany RP. Role of dietary sodium in osteoporosis. *J Am Coll Nutr.* 2006;25(3 Suppl):271S–276S.

CHAPTER 13

Dietary and nutritional supplements

Joel S Edman and Elizabeth Horvitz

More than half of adults in the United States take nutritional supplements to increase their energy level, improve their health status, and treat or prevent disease. Sales of these supplements have grown to $23 billion annually [1]. The use of supplements may have a significant impact on the prevention and treatment of disease or, in some cases, cause unintended side effects. Therefore, it is important for primary care clinicians to know what supplements their patients are taking, and the potential influence these supplements may have on their patients' health, medical conditions or medication's [1,2].

The use of nutritional supplements in clinical practice is, to a certain degree, a question of philosophy and practice orientation. For practitioners of integrative or complementary medicine, supplements work well within the framework of natural approaches that include diet, exercise, stress management, and other modalities such as acupuncture or massage. For allopathic physicians, who may have inadequate training in nutrition, combined with time constraints in the office, the degree to which nutrition-related issues can be addressed is often limited. An important question for the clinician to ask is whether the patient is taking any supplements and if these or any additional supplements should be included in their treatment plan. This question is particularly valid because the supportive clinical research on nutritional supplements is often weak, especially compared to pharmaceutical research. This disparity is likely due to the lack of financial incentives to conduct research with dietary supplements and significant methodological problems based on mechanism of action.

The contrasting models of practice are magnified further because of the media attention focused on potential adverse effects of nutritional supplementation. Unlike pharmacological therapy, nutritional supplements typically seek to restore a degree of homeostatis. Thus, the effects may be mild and often take a significant time to manifest. While integrative medicine practitioners look at the controversial research to see if adjustments should be made to their supplement recommendations, others who may not be familiar with supplement recommendations and those who are already hesitant to recommend them use the negative press as a reason for discouraging their patients from using supplements. Regardless of the viewpoint, however, it is important to understand that nutrients and nutritional products are often used in therapeutic or pharmacological doses. While the result may be a significant benefit to the patient, the patient may also experience some unintended consequence or adverse side effects which would require changes in prescribing practices. Despite these periodic controversies, this chapter will focus on some nutritional supplements that clinicians can safely and effectively recommend to patients to improve their health.

Regulation and range of products

The Dietary Supplement Health and Education Act (DSHEA) passed by Congress in 1994 is the primary legislation that regulates all aspects of supplements, including manufacturing, quality control, labeling, and marketing. A central feature of the bill is that dietary supplements are not classified as drugs, and are therefore not regulated by the FDA in the same manner as food and drugs [3]. In addition, it is illegal for a supplement manufacturer to claim that its product can cure, mitigate, treat, or prevent a disease, although structure and function claims are permitted if they are supported by research [4]. This legislation has created an important controversy regarding the accuracy of product labeling and ingredient quantity, as well as product purity. While this issue needs to be monitored closely, there are many supplement companies that have provided good quality products for decades, are certified by reliable organizations, and are committed to the development and growth of effective nutritional medicines [5].

There are a vast range of supplements that practitioners may recommend or that patients may opt to try on their own. Categories of supplements include vitamins, minerals, fatty acids, amino acids, antioxidants, probiotics and prebiotics, herbs and botanicals, enzymes, hormones, glandulars, functional foods and food concentrates, homeopathic remedies, and others. This chapter will only address vitamin and mineral supplements, which are the products most commonly used by the general public [2].

Why prescribe supplements

There are many reasons why a supplement may benefit a patient, including replacing missing nutrients due to poor dietary choices; variations in soil nutritional content; micronutrient losses from food processing and cooking; and genetic polymorphisms leading to variations in individual nutrient requirements [6]. It is possible to use several models to understand how supplements can benefit the patient population, including (a) nutritional deficiency; (b) sub-clinical nutritional deficiency; (c) biological response modifiers; and (d) mass action effects [7]. It is only the overt nutritional deficiency that is well defined and most widely accepted in medical and nutritional practice. Classic examples are iron and vitamin B_{12} deficiencies that produce clinical symptoms, can be easily identified through laboratory analyses, and can be supplemented and monitored for symptom and assay changes. (See chapters 11 and 12)

More challenging is the evaluation of the other three models for which there are varying levels of supportive evidence from *in vitro*, animal, and clinical research. For example, a perceived sub-clinical magnesium deficiency is the reason why many integrative medicine practitioners recommend magnesium despite normal serum or red blood cell magnesium levels [8]. Epidemiological evidence supports increased risk of diabetes and metabolic syndrome in individuals with suboptimal magnesium intake [9]. The biologically active form of the nutrient is ionized magnesium, which is measured by a special probe that is not currently available for clinical use. Magnesium is a cofactor for over three hundred enzymes and is a calcium channel blocker. Research supports magnesium's influence in hypertension, diabetes, and glucose tolerance, allergies, migraines, muscle cramps, constipation, neurocognitive function, and possibly other disorders [9,10]. Magnesium has been used therapeutically to reduce cardiac arrhythmias and interuterine contractions. Because magnesium is often inadequate in the diet and can be depleted by chronic disease, it may be prescribed by primary healthcare providers to help address a range of symptoms.

Omega-3 fatty acids or fish oil supplements are a good example of biological response modifier effects. Supplements can enhance dietary effects, and effectively alter the synthesis of pro-inflammatory versus anti-inflammatory eicosansoids (see chapter 14). Similar research findings to those for magnesium show omega-3 fatty acids are potentially beneficial in a range of disorders due to their anti-inflammatory effects and impact on cellular membrane fluidity and function [11]. Like magnesium, there is no established nutritional status measure although some studies have quantified blood levels of specific omega-3 fatty acids or omega-3 to omega-6 fatty acid ratios [12].

These are two good examples (among many) in which there are not accurate nutritional status measures available. The lack of effective assessment measures and data makes it much more difficult to conduct research that can quantify supplement recommendation effects and lead to valid clinical protocols. With regard to "mass action" effects, Bruce Ames *et al.* have written an excellent review of the biochemical influences of high-dose vitamins on enzyme binding and activity [7]. As many as 50 genetic diseases and many genetic polymorphisms have shown improvement through nutritional supplementation, indicating that supplements may benefit other polymorphisms yet to be determined as their identification and clinical effects are more thoroughly understood.

Despite the challenges presented, supplements can be effectively utilized in patient care once a reliable source of products is identified. The following is an effective framework from which supplements can be recommended: (a) a healthy diet as a foundation; (b) an evidence base that includes a sound rationale and mechanism; (c) a positive benefit to risk ratio; (d) a defined dose and time frame to assess effects; (e) targeted populations to treat, such as patients with adverse or inadequate responses to medication, or patients or families who would like to try nutrition and/or natural therapies before taking pharmaceuticals; and (f) to alleviate drug-induced nutrient depletion.

Recommending supplements

A comprehensive discussion of the use of dietary and nutritional supplements is beyond the scope of this text, particularly as new information accrues daily. The following sections contain a table of vitamin and mineral benefits and cautions (Table 13.1), basic examples of supplements that could be safely considered for use in clinical practice (including a foundation supplement program), and nutrient–drug interaction information.

Supplements should be recommended with caution in specific patient populations. For example, extra caution and/or lower doses of nutrients should be suggested for pregnant women and children, as there is little or no research to evaluate optimal doses or possible risks. Additionally, for patients with significant stomach or intestinal problems, supplements should be limited and/or built up slowly to ensure that they are well tolerated.

The first three supplements listed could be considered a foundation approach and would include: (a) a multivitamin and mineral to insure adequate intake of nutrients; (b) a fish oil supplement and (c) a calcium, magnesium and vitamin D supplements – for bone and other health benefits.

Multivitamins and minerals. There are a number of patients who would benefit from taking a multivitamin and mineral supplement. These include pregnant and breast feeding women, those following a low-calorie diet or who have irregular eating habits, strict vegetarians (vegans), patients who are anemic or recovering from surgery, as well as those who smoke cigarettes and drink alcohol.

Also, despite some conflicting results, research has suggested that multivitamin and mineral supplements may reduce the risk for heart attacks and certain types of cancer, as well as reduce C-reactive protein, and infection rates in diabetics and the elderly [13–17]. Finally, taking a multivitamin and mineral every day can reinforce healthy behaviors that contribute to a healthy lifestyle. It is important to note that nutritional supplements should be viewed as an adjunct to a healthy diet.

Omega-3 fatty acids or fish oil. The health benefits of fish oil were described briefly in a previous section, see Table 13.1. It should also be noted that fish oil is now endorsed by the American Heart Association for the prevention of cardiovascular disease (CVD). There are at least six mechanisms by which omega-3 fatty acids reduce CVD risk including: (a) anti-inflammatory; (b) hypolipidemic; (c) anti-thrombotic; (d) cytokine inhibition; (e) anti-arrhythmic; and (f) endothelial-derived nitric oxide stimulation [18].

Calcium, magnesium and vitamin D supplement. The importance of these supplements are shown in Table 13.1. Also, new research suggesting that vitamin D may be involved in immune function and cancer, autoimmune disorders, insulin resistance and possibly other disorders, especially in the elderly [19]. The current DRI for vitamin D of 400 IU per day may be increased to 1000 IU per day.

Probiotics. The most common bacteria used as probiotic supplements are *Lactobacillus* species and *Bifidobacter* species, although there are many others. Probiotics have been shown to be helpful for symptoms such as constipation and diarrhea, and they are very safe [20]. They may also be helpful for irritable bowel syndrome (IBS), inflammatory bowel disease (IBD), atopic disease and clostridium dificile infections with a yeast supplement, saccharomyces boulardii [21]. At this point, however, an empirical trial is the most common approach since the methods for identifying imbalanced or potentially pathogenic gastrointestinal flora is not as well validated as it hopefully will be at some point in the future.

Glucosamine sulfate and chondroitin sulfate. Research suggests that glucosamine and chondroitin sulfate can help reduce stiffness and pain in osteoarthritis [22]. Multiple controlled studies have also documented benefits in patient with osteoarthritis of the knee.

Co-enzyme Q10. CoQ10, or ubiquinone, is an important part of the oxidative phosphorylation chain leading to mitochondrial ATP synthesis. HMG CoA reductase inhibitors (statins) lower circulating levels of CoQ10 but the consequences are not well understood. Perhaps the most common symptom is muscle soreness. Supplementation may be warranted especially in susceptible populations such as those over 65 years of age or those with congestive heart failure [23].

Digestive enzymes. Although little research has been done, digestive enzymes can be particularly helpful in patients with chronic gastrointestinal symptoms (e.g. IBS and IBD) or in the elderly.

Milk thistle or silymarin. This is a herb with specific therapeutic benefit for liver function. Although herbs are not discussed in this chapter, they do represent an important part of the dietary supplement field. Especially in Europe and Australia, herbal products are regulated by government agencies to assure product quality. Because many herbs are metabolized by liver enzymes that are also involved with pharmaceuticals, interactions need to be carefully monitored.

Table 13.1 Benefits and cautions of common vitamin and mineral supplements.

Supplement	Indications	Cautions
Vitamin A *Dietary Reference Intake:* Men: 900 μg Women: 700 μg/d *Tolerable Upper Intake:* 3000 μg/d *Note:* If given as retinol activity equivalents (RAE): 1 RAE = 1 μg/d retinol = 12 μg β-carotene/d	Patients with skin problems such as acne and psoriasis Patients with peritonitis Patients with osteoarthritis Patients with poor night vision	Avoid if patient is taking any vitamin A-derived medications for skin problems, oral contraceptives, or is pregnant Use Beta-carotene with caution in patients who smoke High doses (over 7.5 mg/day) can cause flaking, itching skin, blurred vision, and headache Long-term intake of high vitamin A diet is associated with osteoporotic hip fracture in women There are questions about the safety of retinal and many prefer carotene as a vitamin A source.
Vitamin B$_1$ (Thiamin) *Dietary Reference Intake:* Men: 1.2 mg/d Women: 1.1 mg/d *Tolerable Upper Intake:* Not established	Patients with a weakened immune system Regular alcohol drinkers or cigarette smokers	No known problems
Vitamin B$_2$ (Riboflavin) *Dietary Reference Intake:* Men: 1.3 mg/d Women: 1.1 mg/d *Tolerable Upper Intake:* Not established	Patients who are vegetarians Patients with migraine headaches Patients with skin problems such as acne, eczema, and ulcers Patients with carpal tunnel syndrome Athletes	No known problems
Vitamin B$_3$ (Niacin) *Dietary Reference Intake:* Men: 16 mg/d Women: 14 mg/d *Tolerable Upper Intake:* 35 mg/d	For patients with hypercholesterolemia, up to 3.0 g/d may be prescribed	Doses of 50 mg/day can cause skin flushing, itching, headaches, cramps, and nausea May be problematic for patients with gout and glaucoma Very high doses can cause liver damage, hyperglycemia, and aggravate irregular heart rhythm

Vitamin B6

Dietary Reference Intake: 1.3–1.7 mg/d for men and women

Tolerable Upper Intake: 100 mg/d

Patients who have a poor diet, such as heavy alcohol users, or older people, who may have difficulties absorbing vitamin B6 from food

Those sensitive to monosodium glutamate

Women taking a birth-control pill

Patients using the asthma medication Theophylline or the tuberculosis medication Isoniazide

Those with high blood levels of homocysteine

May be taken with vitamins B12 and folate

More than 100 mg/day can cause numbness and tingling in fingers and toes related to nerve damage and ataxia

Vitamin B12 (Cobalamin)

Dietary Reference Intake: 2.4 μg/d for men and women

Tolerable Upper Intake: Not established

Patients who are vegetarians (vegans)

Those who may have problems absorbing vitamin B12 from food, such as the elderly

Patients with macrocytic anemia

Patients recovering from intestinal surgery

Patients with high blood levels of homocysteine

Elderly with neuro-cognitive decline

May be taken with vitamins B6 and folate

It is possible that patients taking acid blockers for prolonged periods may be less able to absorb vitamin B12

Folate

Dietary Reference Intake: 400 μg/d both men and women

Tolerable Upper Intake: 1 mg/d

Pregnant women

Patients with problems absorbing folate from food

Patients with liver disease or on dialysis

Patients with high blood levels of homocysteine

Patients with depression

May be taken with vitamins B6 and B12

High doses can mask a vitamin B12 deficiency, especially as it relates to macrocytic anemia

High doses (>15 mg) may cause nausea, appetite loss, and interfere with the effectiveness of some medications for epilepsy

Vitamin C

Dietary Reference Intake:
Men: 90 mg/d
Women: 75 mg/d

Tolerable Upper Intake: 2000 mg/d

Regular drinkers or smokers should increase their intake by 35 mg/d

Patients with severe burns, fractures, pneumonia, rheumatic fever (in which there is inflammation of the joints and a high body temperature), or tuberculosis

Patients with immune-deficiency

Patients preparing for surgery

Do not prescribe for patients with kidney stones, gout, or iron-storage diseases

High doses (>10 gms) can cause nausea, vomiting, diarrhea, headaches, and abdominal cramps

(Continued)

Table 13.1 (Continued)

Supplement	Indications	Cautions
Vitamin D *Dietary Reference Intake:* 5–10 µg/d for men and women (200–400 IU) *Tolerable Upper Intake:* 50 mg/d (2000 IU) *Note:* 1 µg Vitamin D = 40 IU	Patients who avoid dairy foods Those who do not get enough sunlight or live north of the latitude connecting San Francisco to Philadelphia Patients with fat malabsorption, such as those with cystic fibrosis Patients with a family history of osteoporosis The elderly, especially homebound or in a nursing home with poor sun exposure Patients with autoimmune disease	High doses (exceeding 5000 IU/day) may lead to kidney stones, tissue calcification, nausea, headache, fatigue and frequent urination In infants and children, too much vitamin D can lead to retarded growth, rounding of the skull, and learning difficulties Assess blood work for hypercalcemia
Vitamin E *Dietary Reference Intake:* 15 mg/d for men and women (22.5 IU) *Tolerable Upper Intake:* 1000 mg/d (1500 IU) *Note:* 1.5 mg/d Vitamin E = 1 IU	Patients at risk of Alzheimer's disease Elderly patients, especially those with immune deficiency It is recommended to take a supplement of mixed tocopherols as opposed to alpha tocopherol	High doses may be problematic for patients taking blood-thinning medications Avoid for 2 weeks before surgery High doses may interfere with niacin's ability to lower high blood cholesterol levels and cause dizziness or fatigue. Supplements may reduce the efficacy of statin drugs
Vitamin K *Dietary Reference Intake:* Men: 120 µg/d Women: 90 µg/d *Tolerable Upper Intake:* Not established	Babies given vitamin K at birth to prevent bleeding Women during and after menopause, to improve bone mass Patients with liver disease, jaundice, fat malabsorption Patients prescribed long-term aspirin or antibiotic medications	Vitamin K interferes with the effects of anticoagulant drugs, such as Warfarin (see Appendix D) High doses may cause allergic reactions in babies

Calcium

Dietary Reference Intake:
Men: 1000 mg/d (19–50 yrs)
   1200 mg/d (51 + yrs)
Women: 1000 mg/d (19–50 yrs)
   1200 mg/d (51 + yrs)
Pregnant and lactating women: 1000 mg/d
Tolerable Upper Intake: 2500 mg/d

Pregnant and breastfeeding women
Patients at risk of osteoporosis
Should be recommended in a 2:1 ratio of calcium to magnesium
Patients who avoid dairy foods
Patients not ingesting 3-A-day dairy servings

Calcium can compete with or limit the absorption of iron, magnesium, zinc, and manganese
Most multivitamins do not contain 100% daily value of calcium
Test for hypercalcemia

Fluoride

Dietary Reference Intake:
Men: 4.0 mg/d
Women: 3.0 mg/d
Tolerable Upper Intake: Not established

Patients who do not have fluoride added to their public drinking water
Children susceptible to dental caries

Do not swallow fluoridated tooth products
Children under the age of 6 years should use only a pea-sized amount of fluoridated toothpaste and be supervised by an adult when brushing
20–40 mg/d can interfere with how the body uses calcium
40–70 mg/d can cause heartburn and extremity pain

Iron

Dietary Reference Intake:
Men: 8 mg/d
Women: 18 mg/d
Tolerable Upper Intake:
45 mg/d

Patients with a low dietary intake of iron, such as vegetarians
Patients with problems absorbing iron, or who have lost blood, from injury or women who have heavy menstrual periods
Take vitamin C with iron supplements to aid absorption of the iron

Patients with Hemochromatosis should avoid all supplements containing iron
Prolonged high doses can cause oxidative stress that may cause damage to the liver and pancreas, and lead to diabetes

Magnesium

Dietary Reference Intake:
Men: 400–420 mg/d
Women: 310–320 mg/d
Tolerable Upper Intake: 350 mg/d
Note: The tolerable upper intake for magnesium refers only to the amount obtained from dietary supplements, and not from food sources

Athletes
Patients complaining of muscle cramps
Pregnant women at risk of premature labor
Patients with high blood pressure or other circulatory diseases or irregular heart rhythm
Patients with asthma
Patients with diabetes and pre-diabetes
Patients with headaches or migraines
Patients with excessive urinary loss of magnesium, very low blood levels of magnesium, long-term problems absorbing nutrients, severe diarrhea, or long-term vomiting

For patients with renal disease, serious accumulation of magnesium can occur
High doses (1000–5000 mg) may cause diarrhea

(Continued)

Table 13.1 (Continued)

Supplement	Indications	Cautions
Zinc	Patients with poor taste and smell	Do not take with either calcium or iron supplements simultaneously as these interfere with zinc absorption
Dietary Reference Intake:	Those with a weakened immune system	Long-term high doses can lower high density lipoprotein (HDL) cholesterol, cause copper deficiency, produce brittle nails, and weaken immune function
Men: 11 mg/d	Patients with a cold, flu, or sore throat	
Women: 8 mg/d		Doses exceeding 40 mg per day may interfere with white blood cell function
Tolerable Upper Intake: 40 mg/d		
Multivitamin and mineral supplement	Pregnant or breastfeeding women	Carefully review total nutrient quantities when taking a multivitamin in addition to other supplements
	Patients recovering from surgery or severe injury	Many popular multivitamins on the market do not contain chromium, selenium, and zinc
	Patients with infections, such as HIV	
	Patients who are anemic or have a low red blood cell count (hemoglobin) levels	Many multivitamin products contain vitamin K and should not be taken by patients taking anticoagulant medications
	Regular drinkers and smokers	
	Patients who avoid entire food groups, such as dairy foods due to lactose intolerance	
	Patients following a low-calorie diet or those who have irregular eating habits and skip meals	
	Patients who are strict vegetarians (vegans) elderly patients with poor dietary intake	

Source: Refs [2,4] and Darwin Deen, MD, Albert Einstein College of Medicine and Lisa Hark, PhD. RD, University of Pennsylvania school of Medicine. 2007. Used with permission.

Drug–nutrient interactions

What are drug–nutrient interactions?
When food and medications are taken together, interactions may diminish the intended purpose of the drug, affect the nutritional status of an individual, or lead to acute drug toxicity. Drugs can affect individual nutritional status in various ways.

Intestinal absorption of nutrients
Nutrient absorption is affected by intestinal transit time which determines the bioavailability of the nutrient (if it is bound to a drug or free to be absorbed), as well as gastric pH, and the length of contact time available for absorption. When some drugs and certain nutrients are taken together, they may bind and form an insoluble complex in the gastrointestinal tract. This complex alters the absorption of both the drug and the nutrient. Binding resins used to reduce cholesterol absorption can affect the absorption of fat-soluble vitamins (A, D, E, and K). Because laxatives speed the movement of material through the digestive tract, they reduce the interaction time between nutrients and the intestinal wall, decreasing absorptive ability. As a result, excessive use of laxatives can deplete vitamins and minerals needed for normal body functions [24]. Other examples of nutrient–drug interactions include anti-neoplastic drugs that may cause damage to the intestinal wall, reducing nutrient absorption and therefore nutrient status [25].

Distribution, metabolism and excretion of the nutrient
Once absorbed into the bloodstream, the drugs and nutrients must be transported and distributed to their sites of action. Some herbal remedies can interact at this stage with anticoagulant medication by either enhancing or reducing their action. This fact is very important for drugs with a narrow therapeutic window.

After distribution, drugs are metabolized and excreted from the body by the kidney, liver, or both. Drugs have been shown to alter the metabolism of folic acid, vitamin D, vitamin B_6, or vitamin K, resulting in higher requirements or danger of deficiency for the patient. The interaction of some drugs and supplements will lead to a reduced metabolism of the drug, resulting in higher serum drug levels. Diuretic drugs affect nutrient excretion by the kidney, causing urinary loss of potassium and magnesium.

Specific drug–nutrient interactions
By its nature, information on drug-nutrient interaction is typically based on case reports or clinical experience [26,27]. While the information in Table 13.2 is based on the best available evidence, it is not based on randomized controlled trials and therefore should be used with caution [28–30]. The "Recommendation" column is based solely on our judgment. For example, while Metformin, fibrates, and cholestyramine have been shown to interfere with B vitamin metabolism and raise homocysteine levels, supplementation with

Table 13.2 Drug–nutrient effects and recommendations.

Drug	Nutrient/ Supplement	Effect	Recommendation
Tetracyclines	Dairy intake Calcium folate Antacids	Decreased absorption with long-term use	Do not take together
	Riboflavin Vitamin C Zinc	Vitamin levels may be depleted	Avoid long-term use, consider supplementation
Metformin	Vitamin B_6 Vitamin B_{12}	Decreased vitamin absorption	Do not take supplement and drug together
Bile acids sequestrants (Questran TM)	Fat-soluble vitamins Vitamin B_{12}	Decreased absorption	Allow 12 hours between taking the supplement and drug
Statins	Coenzyme Q-10	Decreased synthesis	Consider supplements, however little evidence
Aluminum-based antacids (Maalox, Mylanta TM)	Phosphate	Bound and excreted, causes calcium loss	Avoid when possible
Phenolphthlein laxatives (Exlax, Correctol TM)	Vitamin D and calcium	Interferes with vitamin D resulting in decreased calcium absorption	Avoid long-term use, consider vitamin D supplement
Mineral Oil (Haleys M-O TM)	Fat-soluble vitamins	Reduce absorption	Avoid long-term use
Aspirin	Vitamin C	Reduced intracellular levels	Significance unknown
	Folic acid	High dose aspirin reduces absorption	Consider supplementation
Indomethacin/ Aspirin	Iron	Increase intestinal losses	Monitor hemoglobin, hematocrit, MCV
Broad spectrum antibiotics (Bactrim, Neomycin)	Vitamin K	Reduce gut bacteria that produce vitamin K	Avoid long-term use
Alcohol	Folic Acid Thiamin	Interferes with metabolism	Drink only modestly, consider (MV) supplementations
	Vitamin B_6 Vitamin B_{12} Vitamin C	Reduced absorption	
	Iron	Increased absorption	
	Zinc	Decreased absorption	

(Continued)

Table 13.2 (*Continued*)

Drug	Nutrient/ Supplement	Effect	Recommendation
Accutane	Vitamin A	Increased toxicity	Avoid supplementation with vitamin A, no interaction with beta-carotene intake
Quinolones	Calcium Iron Zinc	Decreased antibiotic absorption	Do not take at same time
Penicillamine	Iron Magnesium Copper Zinc	Interferes with drug absorption	Do not take at same time
Thiazide diuretic	Potassium Magnesium, Zinc	Increased excretion	Consider supplementation
	Calcium	Decreased excretion	Reduced requirement
Loop diuretic	Potassium Magnesium Calcium	Increased excretion	Consider mineral supplementation
Triamterene diuretic	Folic acid	May produce deficiency	Supplement with folate
	Potassium	Conserves levels	Avoid supplementation
ACE Inhibitors	Potassium	Raises serum levels	Avoid supplementation
Hydralazine	Vitamin B_6	Depletes stores	Consider vitamin B_{12} supplementation
Blood thinners (Coumadin, Warfarin)	Vitamin E	May increase anticoagulant effect	Avoid supplementation
	Vitamin K	Reduces anticoagulant effect	Avoid supplementation (must read multivitamin labels) control dietary vitamin K
Colchicine	Vitamin B_{12} Beta-carotene Magnesium Potassium	Interferes with absorption	Consider supplementation
Antiepileptic Drugs/ Barbiturates (Phenobarbitol, phenytoin, phenobarbital, carbamazepine, and primidone)	Folic acid Vitamin B_6	Drugs induce vitamin deficiency Vitamin suplements reduce drug levels	Avoid supplementation
	Vitamin D Calcium	Interferes with absorption Reduces calcium stores	Impact of supplementation with vitamin D unknown

(*Continued*)

Table 13.2 Drug–nutrient effects and recommendations. (*Continued*)

Drug	Nutrient/ Supplement	Effect	Recommendation
Tranquilizers (chlorpromazine thorazine)	Riboflavin Vitamin B_{12} Vitamin C	Vitamin depletion	Consider multivitamin supplementation
Hormone replacement therapy	Vitamin B_6 Folic acid Vitamin E Vitamin C	Lowers serum levels	Consider multivitamin supplementation
Birth control pills	Vitamin B_6 Folic acid Vitamin E Vitamin C	Lowers serum levels

May increase drug levels | Significance unknown |
Iron	Calcium	Interferes with absorption	Do not take together
Etidronate	Calcium Iron Magnesium	Minerals interfere with drug absorption	Do not take together
	Vitamin D	Interferes with metabolism	Requires vitamin D supplement
Mysoline	Vitamin K	Reduces vitamin K levels	Consider supplementation
	Calcium Vitamin D	Alters vitamin D metabolism	Consider supplementation
LevoDopa	Vitamin B_6	Vitamin reduces drug effectiveness	Avoid supplementation
Potassium Chloride	Vitamin B_{12}	Interferes with absorption	Consider supplementation
Thyroid hormone	Iron	Interferes with absorption	Do not take together
Anti-tuberculous drugs (INH, Rifampin)	Niacin Vitamin B_6	Drug interferes with vitamin metabolism May reduce drug effectiveness	Unclear Provide vitamin B_6 supplementation
	Vitamin D Calcium Phosphate	Interferes with vitamin metabolism via cytochrome P3A4	Consider vitamin D supplementation
Para amino salicylic acid (PAS)	Vitamin B_{12}	Deficiency is possible	
H2-blockers	Vitamin B_{12}	May reduce B_{12} absorption	
	Iron	Reduced absorptions	Monitor hemoglobin
Nitrofurantoins	Folic acid	Drug interferes with vitamin metabolism	Usually not a problem with short-term use.
Methotrexate Sulfasalazine	Folate	Decreases folate absorption	Supplement with folate

Source: Darwin Deen, MD, Albert Einstein College of Medicine, 2007. Used with permission and adapted from [27–29].

these vitamins lowers homocysteine levels but has not been shown to lower cardiovascular disease deaths [31].

Conclusion

There are many important issues to be aware of in order to adequately advise patients about the use of dietary and nutritional supplements. With the switch from RDAs to DRIs, a paradigm shift took place that changed the focus from an adequate intake of nutrients to desired levels of intake that promotes optimal biochemical and physiological function. While more research is needed to clarify these issues, this change does illustrate the potential role of dietary and nutritional supplements as adjuvant therapy and for prevention of chronic illnesses such as osteoporosis.

With regards to product reliability, it is important that companies be certified by a reputable organization. For example, a USP stamp certifies the approval of the US Pharmacopeia testing organization for purity, strength, and dissolution [32]. Other certifying organizations include the National Science Foundation (NSF) and the National Nutritional Foods Association (NNFA). Practitioners and patients should not hesitate to contact companies to verify which organization certifies their supplements and/or what their quality control procedures entail. Nutritionists or registered dietitians have significant experience with dietary and nutritional supplements and can help patients make appropriate diet and lifestyle changes that may include nutritional supplements.

References

1 National Institutes of Health. State-of-the-Science Conference Statement, Multivitamin/ Mineral Supplements and Chronic Disease Prevention. Draft Statement. May 17, 2006. http://consensus.nih.gov.

2 Radimer K, Bindewald B, Hughes J, Ervin B, Swanson C, Picciano MF. Dietary supplement use by US adults: data from the National Health and Nutrition Examination Survey, 1999–2000. *Am J Epidemiol* 2004;160(4):339–49.

3 US Food and Drug Administration: Center for Food Safety and Applied Nutrition, (2002) Tips For The Savvy Supplement User: Making Informed Decisions And Evaluating Information. www.cfsan.fda.gov/~dms/ds-savvy.html basic.

4 Office of Dietary Supplements: National Institutes of Health, (2004). Dietary Supplements: Background Information. http://dietary-supplements.info.nih.gov/factsheets/ dietary-supplements.asp h1.

5 US Food and Drug Administration: Center for Food Safety and Applied Nutrition, (2006). Dietary supplements. www.cfsan.fda.gov/~dms/supplmnt.html

6 Oakley, GP Jr. (1998) Eat right and take a multivitamin. *N Engl J Med* 338:1060–1.

7 Ames B. Supplements and tuning up metabolism. *J Nutr* 2004;134(11):3164S–3168S.

8 Olerich MA, Rude RK. Should we supplement magnesium in critically ill patients? New Horiz. 1994 May;2(2):186–92.

9 Ueshima K. Magnesium and ischemic heart disease: a review of epidemiological, experimental, and clinical evidences. *Magnes Res* 2005;18(4):275–84.

10 Swain R, Kaplan-Machlis B. Magnesium for the next millennium. *South Med J.* 1999;92(11):1040–7.

11 Yehuda S Rabinovitz S *et al.* Essential fatty acids and the brain: from infancy to aging. *Neurobiol Aging.* 2005;26(1):98–102.

12 Tiemeir H, van Tuijl HR *et al.* Plasma fatty acid composition and depression are associated in the elderly: the Rotterdam Study. *Am J Clin Nutr* 2003;78(1):40–6.

13 Holmquist C, Larsson S, Wolk A, de Faire U. Multivitamin supplements are inversely associated with risk of myocardial infarction in men and women – Stockholm Heart Epidemiology Program (SHEEP). *J Nutr* 2003;133(8):2650–4.

14 Fuchs CS, Willett WC *et al.* The influence of folate and multivitamin use on the familial risk of colon cancer in women. *Cancer Epidemiol Biomarkers Prev* 2002;11(3):227–34.

15 Church TS, Earnest CP, Wood KA, Kampert JB. Reduction of C-reactive protein levels through use of a multivitamin. *Am J Med* 2003;115(9):702–7.

16 Barringer TA, Kirk JK *et al.* Effect of a multivitamin and mineral supplement on infection and quality of life. A randomized, double-blind, placebo-controlled trial. *Ann Intern Med* 2003;138(5):365–71.

17 El-Kadiki A, Sutton AJ. Role of multivitamins and mineral supplements in preventing infections in elderly people: systematic review and meta-analysis of randomized controlled trials. *BMJ.*2005;330(7496):871.

18 Holub DJ and Holub BJ. Omega-3 fatty acids from fish oils and cardiovascular disease. *Mol Cell Biochem* 2004;263(1–2):217–25.

19 Holick, M. Vitamin D. Its role in cancer prevention and treatment. *Prog Biophys Mol Biol* 2006 Mar 10.

20 Boyle RJ, Robins-Browne RM *et al.* Probiotic use in clinical practice: what are the risks? *Am J Clin Nutr* 2006;83(6):1256–64;quiz 1446–7.

21 Katz JA. Probiotics for the prevention of antibiotic-associated diarrhea and Clostridium difficile diarrhea. *J Clin Gastroenterol* 2006;40(3):249–55.

22 Richy F, Bruyere O *et al.* Structural and symptomatic efficacy of glucosamine and chrondroitin in knee osteoarthritis: a comprehensive meta-analysis. *Arch Intern Med* 2003;163(13):1514–22.

23 Witte KK, Nikitin NP *et al.* The effect of micronutrient supplementation on quality-of-life and left ventricular function in elderly patients with chronic heart failure. *Eur Heart J* 2005;26(21):2238–44.

24 Kinnunen O, Salokannel J. Comparison of the effects of magnesium hydroxide and a bulk laxative on lipids, carbohydrates, vitamins A and E, and minerals in geriatric hospital patients in the treatment of constipation. *J Int Med Res* 1989;17(5):442–54.

25 Brandi G, Dabard J, Raibaud P. *et al.* Intestinal microflora and digestive toxicity of irinotecan in mice. *Clin Cancer Res* 2006;15;12(4):1299–307.

26 Khatib MA, Rahim O, Kania R, Molloy P. CASE REPORT: Iron Deficiency Anemia: Induced by Long-Term Ingestion of Omeprazole *Digestive Diseases and Sciences* 2002;47:(11)2596–7.

27 Kirk JK. Significant drug-nutrient interactions. *Am Fam Physician* 1995;51(5):1175–82;1185.

28 Graedon J, Graedon T. Deadly Drug Interactions: *The People's Pharmacy Guide.* St. Martin's Press, New York, 1999.

29 White R, Ashworth A. How drug therapy can affect, threaten and compromise nutritional status. *J Hum Nutr Diet* 2000;13(2):119.

30 Farhat G, Yamout B, Mikati MA, Demirjian S, Sawaya R, El-Hajj Fuleihan G. Effect of antiepileptic drugs on bone density in ambulatory patients. *Neurology* 2002;58:1348–53.

31 Desouza C, Keebler M, McNamara DB, Fonseca V. Drugs affecting homocysteine metabolism: impact on cardiovascular risk. *Drugs* 2002;62(4):605–16.

32 Mayo Foundation for Medical Education and Research, (June 2004). Vitamin and mineral supplements: Use with care. from Mayoclinic.com: www.mayoclinic.com/health/supplements/NU00198.

Further reading

Dhesi JK, Jackson SH, Bearne LM, Moniz C, Hurley MV, Swift CG, Allain TJ. Vitamin D supplementation improves neuromuscular function in older people who fall. *Age Ageing* 2004;33(6):589–95.

Feskanich D, Singh V, Willett WC, Colditz GA. Vitamin A intake and hip fractures among postmenopausal women. *JAMA* 2002;287:47–54.

Giovannucci E, Stampfer MJ, Colditz GA *et al*. Multivitamin Use, Folate, and Colon Cancer in Women in the Nurses' Health Study. *Annals of Internal Medicine* 1998;129(7), 517–24.

Gruenwald J, Graubaum HJ, Busch R, Bentley C. Safety and tolerance of ester-C compared with regular ascorbic acid. *Adv Ther* 2006;23(1):171–8.

Holick MF. Vitamin D: importance in the prevention of cancers, type 1 diabetes, heart disease, and osteoporosis. *Am J Clin Nutr* 2004;79:362–71.

Heaney RP. Vitamin D: how much do we need, and how much is too much? *Osteoporos Int.* 2000;11(7):553–5.

Madiwale T, Liebelt E. Iron: not a benign therapeutic drug. *Curr Opin Pediatr* 2006;18(2):174–9.

Manoguerra AS, Erdman AR, Booze LL *et al*. Iron ingestion: an evidence-based consensus guideline for out-of-hospital management. *Clin Toxicol* 2005;43(6):553–70.

Miller ER, 3rd, Pastor-Barriuso R *et al*. Meta-analysis: high-dosage vitamin E supplementation may increase all-cause mortality. *Ann Intern Med* 2005;142(1):37–46.

Otoom S, Bakhiet M, Khan A, Sequeira R. Prolonged use of phenytoin, carbamazepine or valproate monotherapy on plasma levels of folate and B12: A comparison between epileptic patients with or without cardiovascular disorders. *Neuro Endocrinol Lett* 2006;27(1–2):85–8.

Robertson A, Tenenbein M. Hepatotoxicity in acute iron poisoning. *Hum Exp Toxicol.* 2005 Nov;24(11):559–62.

Ryder KM, Shorr RI, Bush AJ, Kritchevsky SB, Harris T, Stone K, Cauley J, Tylavsky FA. Magnesium intake from food and supplements is associated with bone mineral density in healthy older white subjects. *J Am Geriatr Soc.* 2005 Nov;53(11):1875–80.

Shils M (Ed). (2005). *Modern Nutrition in Health and Disease*. 10th edition New York, NY: Lippincott Williams & Wilkins.

CHAPTER 14

Considering the alternatives

Benjamin Kligler, Joel S Edman and Mary Beth Augustine

"Integrative medicine" is the new term for the effort to combine the use of complementary/alternative medicine (CAM) approaches with the best of conventional medical care. This is an emerging and evolving approach to the management of disease and to health and well-being in which nutrition has a central role. It is defined by the Consortium of Academic Health Centers for Integrative Medicine (CAHCIM) as "the practice of medicine that reaffirms the importance of the relationship between practitioner and patient, focuses on the whole person, is informed by evidence, and makes use of all appropriate therapeutic approaches, healthcare professionals and disciplines to achieve optimal health and healing." [1].

Most integrative medicine centers offer a combination of natural therapies such as massage, acupuncture/Traditional Chinese Medicine, stress management, homeopathy, Ayurveda, yoga, tai chi, meditation and/or others; and the opportunity to integrate these natural and supportive therapies with allopathic medical approaches and practitioners. Nutrition therapy, including the use of dietary supplements, is a core component of this approach which is addressed with all patients at some point in the course of the practitioner-patient interaction. Nutrition and other integrative therapies, when carefully applied, are safe and have the potential for bringing greater well-being to all patients.

An important challenge for broader acceptance of integrative medicine is to establish the safety and efficacy of its approaches in clinical practice. This can be a difficult task given the multi-factorial nature of chronic diseases, and the multiple-intervention strategies which are often recommended. While there is ongoing research to examine the influence of individual therapies on specific diseases, true integrative medical clinical practice (and research) must examine and quantify benefits derived from dietary changes, nutritional supplements, exercise interventions, mind-body strategies, and sometimes whole systems of care like Chinese or Ayurvedic medicine approaches, all utilized simultaneously. There are currently no simple research models that can do this, so new approaches are being developed and tested. As a result, while research results accumulate for individual interventions, outcomes of these integrative medicine models can not be considered "evidenced-based."

Dietary modification both for prevention and treatment of specific conditions has been used extensively as a core approach in the practice of complementary/alternative medicine and is a cornerstone of the integrative approach to health care. Every traditional system of medicine – from Ayurveda to Chinese medicine to indigenous systems of the Americas – uses dietary advice and nutritional manipulation for specific therapeutic purposes. This chapter will review three of the most useful and commonly-applied therapeutic diets, and their indications and applications to specific disease conditions. Elimination diets, specific carbohydrate diets and anti-inflammatory diets. There are, however, many other approaches that could be presented depending upon the practitioners' preferences such as macrobiotic or raw foods diets for cancer [2,3], the Ornish Diet for reversing cardiovascular disease [4], low carbohydrate diets for weight loss, diabetes or metabolic syndrome [5–7], and fasting followed by vegan diets for rheumatoid arthritis and other auto-immune diseases [8,9] (see chapter 13).

Regardless of the specific diet, an important tenet of integrative medicine is that the nutritional quality should be maintained. Therefore, most practitioners recommend that food be as unprocessed as possible and free from additives, chemicals and environmental contaminants when feasible (e.g. organic or locally grown).

As is discussed in Chapter 15 (It's All About Changing Behaviors), and as every clinician knows, making a significant and durable dietary change can be difficult for many patients – and seemingly impossible for some. Our choices and decisions regarding what we eat are emotionally complex. Helping patients change involves encouraging them to develop an awareness of the connection between their emotions, psychological well-being, and their eating behavior. A supportive relationship with the health care practitioner is critical. Family structure and relationships must not be ignored, especially when applying therapeutic dietary change in children. Without a doubt the most important factors for adherence are patient motivation and support.

Elimination diet

The elimination diet is based on a principle still not totally well-defined or completely accepted within conventional medicine: the concept of food sensitivity. Conventional teaching describes how to diagnose and treat food allergy – a response to certain food antigens via skin testing or RAST (radioallergosorbent) blood testing. A certain number of patients manifest symptoms as a result of this type of allergy mechanism, and once the offending food is identified, symptoms are usually greatly improved by avoidance of this food. Food sensitivity, however, which can impact health conditions from asthma to irritable bowel syndrome to eczema, is not typically identified using conventional allergy testing and can be difficult to diagnose other than through a process of food elimination with concomitant symptom monitoring. Rather than being mediated by specific antibodies or by a well-defined T-cell response which will be detected by skin testing, food "sensitivity" is thought to be triggered by exposure of the gut-associated lymphoid tissue (GALT) to particular food antigens and then mediated by inflammatory cytokines, interleukin, and tumor necrosis factor (TNF). This type of sensitivity is not reliably measured by any current laboratory test – although there are certainly many unvalidated tests available which claim to accurately detect food sensitivities. This leaves only the clinical/empiric approach for diagnosis.

Elimination exclusion phase

The elimination diet consists of two phases: the elimination/exclusion phase, and the reintroduction/provocation (or food testing) phase. During the elimination period, the patient is advised to absolutely avoid the categories of foods that are the most common causes of food sensitivity: dairy, soy, eggs, corn, wheat, citrus, nuts, shellfish, pork, and chocolate. Foods not on this list which the patient eats frequently – more than three times per week, in general – are also eliminated. (See Table 14.1).

The exclusion/elimination phase generally lasts from 14–30 days. If food sensitivity is contributing to the patient's symptoms, by the end of this time period they will notice a significant improvement in those symptoms. In some disease conditions, such as rheumatoid arthritis, a much longer exclusion phase (up to 2–3 months) may be needed to see an effect. In conditions with a periodic or intermittent presentation of symptoms – such as migraine or asthma – the same may be true. In patients with significant pre-existing structural damage from a chronic illness – like rheumatoid arthritis, for example – such dramatic improvement may not take place. In these cases, though, the patient will sometimes nevertheless experience a partial but still significant improvement. Such a change, even if it does not represent a complete symptom remission, is an acceptable sign that food is contributing to the illness.

A "food/mood/symptom diary" kept by the patient is a critical component of the elimination diet protocol. This diary is used to record significant symptoms so they can be linked to the correct food(s). The diary should be started at the beginning of the elimination phase and continued through to the end of the testing phase. It is worth noting here that if at the end of the elimination phase the diary and/or the patient's report do not show any sign of significant improvement in symptoms, the protocol can be discontinued. At this point the assumption is made that the symptoms in this case are not triggered by food sensitivity. If there has been no improvement during the elimination phase, proceeding to the testing phase is not likely to be helpful.

Provocation/reintroduction phase

The provocation/reintroduction phase follows the elimination phase. During this period, each of the excluded food groups are reintroduced one at a time and eaten 2–3 times daily for a 3–7 day period, while the patient actively monitors for the recurrence of symptoms. It is critical to reintroduce only one suspected food at a time so that if symptoms recur, it is clear what food is responsible.

If there is no reaction after 7 days, another food may be reintroduced. If a "positive" reaction occurs as evidenced by worsening of symptoms, then that food should be removed again and at least a four-day period be allowed to pass before the next food is reintroduced.

Patients often ask in what order they should test the foods that they put back into their diet. Common sense dictates that the foods eaten most frequently are the foods most likely to be the culprit. A food which the patient eats only occasionally is not likely to be the trigger of an ongoing or chronic problem. Thus it makes sense to start the testing with the food groups the patient has been consuming most often.

Table 14.1 Sample allergy elimination diet

Foods to avoid

Dairy products Milk, cheese, butter, yogurt, sour cream, cottage cheese, whey, casein, sodium caseinate, calcium caseinate, and any food containing these.

Wheat Most breads, spaghetti, noodles, pasta, most flour, baked goods, durum semolina, farina, and many gravies, etc.

Corn Including any product with corn oil, vegetable oil from an unspecified source, corn syrup, corn sweetener, dextrose, glucose, corn chips, tortillas, popcorn.

Soy products Including tofu, soybean oil, soy sauce, soy milk.

Eggs Avoid whites and yolks, and any product containing eggs.

Citrus fruits Oranges, grapefruits, lemons, limes, tangerines and foods or drinks containing citrus.

Nuts Avoid all nuts including peanuts. This includes nut oils, milks and butters.

Pork Avoid any product made with pork or pork fat; some elimination diets also exclude beef.

Food additives Including artificial colors, flavors, preservatives, texturing agents, artificial sweeteners, etc. Most diet sodas and other dietetic foods contain artificial ingredients and must be avoided. Grapes, prunes, and raisins that are not organically grown contain sulfites and must be avoided.

Any other food you eat more than 3 times a week Any food you are now eating 3 times a week or more should be avoided and tested later.

Known allergens Avoid food you know you are allergic to, even if it is allowed on this diet.

Read labels! Hidden allergens are frequently found in packaged foods. "Flour" usually means wheat; "vegetable oil" may mean corn oil; and casein and whey are dairy products.

Source: Benjamin Kligler, MD, Continuum Center for Health and Healing, Beth Israel Medical Center. 2007. Used with permission.

(Continued)

Table 14.1 Sample allergy elimination diet (Continued)

Foods allowed

Cereals: Hot-Oatmeal, oat bran, cream of rye.
  Dry-Puffed rice, puffed millet, Oatio's (wheat-free), Good Shepherd (wheat-free), Crispy brown rice cereal. Diluted apple juice with apple slices and nuts go well on cereal.
Grains and flour products 100% rice cakes, rice crackers, rye crackers; any 100% rye or spelt bread with no wheat; oriental noodles, such as 100% buckwheat Soba noodles; rice, potato, buckwheat, and bean flours; rice or millet bread (as long as they do not contain dairy, eggs, sugar, or wheat); cooked whole grains including oats, millet, barley, buckwheat groats (kasha), rice macaroni, spelt (flour and pasta) brown rice, amaranth, quinoa.
Legumes (beans) Includes lentils, peas, chickpeas, navy beans, kidney beans, black beans, string beans, and others. Dried beans should be soaked overnight. Pour off the water and rinse before cooking. Canned beans often contain added sugar or other potential allergens. Some cooked beans packaged in glass jars, sold at the health food store, contain no sugar. Read labels. May also use bean dips without sugar, lemon, or additives. Canned soups include split pea and lentil soup (without additives).
Vegetables Use a wide variety. All vegetables except corn are permitted.
Proteins Poultry and fowl, fresh fish, (such as tuna and salmon, packed in spring water). Shrimp and most canned or packaged shellfish (such as lobster, crab, oysters) may contain sulfites and should be avoided. Canned tuna, salmon and other canned fish are OK. Lamb rarely causes allergic reactions, and may be used even when other meats are restricted. Also recommended are grain/bean casseroles (recipes in vegetarian cookbooks).
Oils and fats Sunflower, safflower, olive, sesame, flaxseed (edible linseed), canola oils. Do not use corn oil or "vegetable oil" from an unspecified source, as this is usually corn oil.

Source: Benjamin Kligler, MD, Continuum Center for Health and Healing, Beth Israel Medical Center. 2007. Used with permission.

Elimination diets in children

In children, especially those younger than 8 years old – who tend to be somewhat more limited in their willingness to change food choices than older children or adults – the classical elimination diet approach described above may not be practical. In particular, it can be very difficult for parents to find foods that young children will eat that fit the requirements of the elimination phase. In this situation, we often use a modified "sequential" elimination approach, where each of the major categories of foods removed during the elimination phase are removed one at a time, each for a period of two weeks. In this approach, for example, dairy foods would be eliminated for a two week period, and symptoms during that time documented. If symptoms improve significantly, then the assumption is that dairy is a cause of sensitivity, and it is kept out of the diet. If there is no change during that two week period, then dairy is resumed and a second food group – wheat, or soy perhaps – is removed, and the cycle is repeated. If the parents are in doubt at the end of a two week period, then they should reintroduce the food with close attention to symptoms, and do a 1–2 week "provocation" phase with that particular food. Although still challenging for families, and generally more time-consuming than the classical approach, this type of food elimination protocol can be helpful in young children.

Almost any unresolved complaint unresponsive to conventional medical approaches can be potentially responsive to an elimination diet approach, including migraine, bowel disturbances, nausea and indigestion, joint pain, or fatigue. Although the quality is highly variable, there are studies in the medical literature of elimination diet approaches to asthma, autism, arthritis, gastroesophageal reflux, recurrent abdominal pain, diarrhea, eczema, psoriasis, headache, recurrent otitis media, recurrent mouth ulcers, stomach or duodenal ulcers, urticaria, rhinitis, menstrual complaints, inflammatory bowel disease, weight loss resistance, and mood disorders.

As one case in point, the literature on asthma provides a number of studies on the use of elimination diets in both children and adults with asthma [10–14]. Results are generally mixed, with the biggest impact found in children with asthma, particularly when food elimination is combined with the use of nutritional supplements [15]. Some authors feel that the role of food sensitivities has been overstated, and that most reported sensitivities do not stand up to the "gold-standard" test of randomized double-blind food challenge [16]. However, in clinical practice the elimination diet remains a useful tool in the treatment of asthma. Common causes of food sensitivity in children with asthma include dairy foods, eggs, citrus, peanuts, soy, wheat, and chocolate [17].

Specific carbohydrate diet

Conventional medicine has typically had little to offer in terms of dietary advice for patients with inflammatory bowel disorders including diverticulitis, Crohn's disease (CD), and ulcerative colitis. There is, however, a therapeutic diet which can be extremely helpful to certain patients with this type of condition: The Specific Carbohydrate Diet (SCD). The SCD, described in detail in Elaine Gottschall's book "Breaking the Vicious Cycle," [18] is a low disaccharide diet, in which almost all foods containing disaccharides and polysaccharides are eliminated – including lactose-containing dairy, all grains, and all legumes.

The theory behind the use of the SCD diet in these disorders centers on the concept that part of the cause of diseases characterized by inflammation of the gastrointestinal tract may be a hypersensitive cellular immune response to certain components of the intestinal flora. Several studies have shown that specific foods can trigger symptoms in patients with both ulcerative colitis and

CD – and it may be that this is linked to the way in which these foods influence the intestinal flora. Carbohydrates have the greatest influence on the intestinal microbial population – much more than do proteins and fats. Certain types of carbohydrates – monosaccharides in particular – are easily digested and absorbed, leaving behind minimal residue for potentially pathogenic intestinal bacteria to feed on. Disaccharides and other more complex sugars tend to be more difficult to digest and absorb, leaving behind more breakdown products in the gut.

In the "vicious cycle" of carbohydrate malabsorption promoted by the disaccharides in susceptible individuals, pathogenic microbes proliferate due to their preference for the breakdown products of the complex sugars. This results in changes in intestinal pH, accompanied by disruption of digestion. The pathogenic bacteria also promote a "leaky gut" through their impact on intestinal mucosa, leading to the inappropriate absorption of certain food particles and their presentation to the gut-associated lymphoid tissue. This in turn leads to systemic inflammation and immune dysfunction. The pathogenic bacteria also promote fermentative degradation of certain hard-to-digest foods, leading to excessive gas, mucous in the stool, and bloating.

According to SCD proponents, the main dietary culprits in this "vicious cycle" are disaccharides, polysaccharides, and other enzymatically-resistant carbohydrates found in grains, certain starchy vegetables, fruits, table sugar, and lactose-rich dairy products. These foods are therefore the main targets for elimination in the SCD diet (see Table 14.2). In fact some studies do confirm that carbohydrate consumption is significantly higher in inflammatory bowel disease (IBD) patients than in healthy controls [19–21], although the significance of these findings in the pathogenesis of the disease remains unclear. Many patients with CD do have a higher dietary intake of sucrose, refined carbohydrates and omega-6 fatty acids, and reduced intake of fruit and vegetables.

Specific carbohydrate diet research

Research on the SCD diet to date is limited. In one study of 204 patients with CD, 69 were randomized to a low carbohydrate diet (84 g/day). Fifty-four percent of these benefited significantly for as long as they maintained the diet [22]. Elemental and exclusion diets have also been shown to be effective in some patients with CD [23], lending credence to the exclusion of disaccharides and polysaccharides. In a study of 33 patients with CD, 29 patients reported specific food intolerances, and 21 of these remained in remission on diet alone (elimination diet or elemental diet), with the mean length of remission being 15.2 months [24]. The most important foods provoking symptoms were wheat and dairy products. In another study a group of 20 patients with CD were followed for several years using variations on the SCD approach; all of these patients demonstrated a decrease in symptoms and reduction in medication use [25], and six patients experienced complete clinical remission, discontinued all medication, and maintained remission for five to 80 months.

Table 14.2 Specific carbohydrate diet guidelines

Foods to avoid

Grains, not even rice, sucrose, sugar including molasses, liquid milk, some beans including soy, white potatoes, corn, margarine, malt, fructose crystals (made from corn). The lists here are incomplete. There are extensive lists of allowed and not-allowed foods in Gottschall's *Breaking The Vicious Cycle: Intestinal Health Through Diet*. The book includes recipes, as well as suitable infant foods and formulas.

Foods allowed

The only carbs allowed are the simple sugars – fructose, glucose and galactose. Disaccharide sugars, made up of two molecules are not allowed, because they do not break down easily. Sucrose (or table sugar) is a disaccharide, so is lactose in milk.

Also, certain starch molecules, called amylose starch, are easily broken down and are completely digested. Amylose is found in most vegetables. Another type of starch, amylopectin, is found in grains. It is much more difficult to digest, and any food containing it is not allowed.

The diet is kept natural and unrefined as much as possible, since sugars and starches are added to just about everything that has been processed.

All natural meats, fish, fowl, eggs, cheese, nuts, fats, butter and oils are allowed, and fish canned in water or oil. As well, home-made yogurt is encouraged for its benefit to bowel health. Non-starchy vegetables, and whole fruits (no juices). Honey may be used, if obesity is not a concern. Zero-carb sweeteners may be used, without filler (maltodextrin is made from corn or barley), or stevia.

Typical menu:

Breakfast Baked apple sweetened with honey if allowed, scrambled eggs, muffin made from almond flour, coffee (no cream)
Lunch Tuna salad with home-made mayonnaise, dill pickle, radishes, chives on a bed of lettuce, pumpkin custard, beverage
Dinner Home-made spaghetti sauce with mushrooms and meat on a bed of steamed spaghetti squash, green salad with oil and vinegar dressing, fresh fruit, tea

Sources: [18 and 26].

In addition to its uses in patients with inflammatory bowel disease, the SCD is also often used for treating irritable bowel syndrome, celiac disease, diarrhea, and other digestive disorders. It has also recently become popular as one of the dietary approaches to autistic spectrum disorders. While a significant body of research evidence for the SCD in the management of IBD is lacking, anecdotal evidence is overwhelmingly positive. Generally a six week trial of the diet is adequate to determine if it is going to be helpful in a given patient.

Anti-inflammatory diet

As concerns about the safety of anti-inflammatory pharmaceuticals has grown, awareness of the potential of nutritional manipulation to influence inflammation in the body has grown as well. Because inflammation is caused by and mediated through a variety of mechanisms and systems in the body, the most effective approach to treating inflammation with diet consists of a combination of strategies aimed at multiple mechanisms. While any single one of these approaches may be only mildly effective, the combination has the potential to be much more so.

An anti-inflammatory diet is characterized by modifying intake in five crucial dietary categories: fat, sugar, antioxidants, allergenic foods, and anti-inflammatory herbs (used as culinary spices). Although some of the individual components of this diet – particularly the use of omega-3 fatty acids (FA) – have been studied and shown to be effective in reducing inflammation in some circumstances, the diet as a whole has not been evaluated to date. The diet is based, however, on a sound theoretical rationale which holds that if we combine a variety of dietary interventions, each of which has at least some anti-inflammatory potential, the additive effect will be helpful to many patients with inflammatory disorders. In fact, although studies of the anti-inflammatory diet as a whole are badly needed, the application of this approach in clinical practice to date does seem to bear out its effectiveness. The anti-inflammatory diet is commonly recommended for a wide range of disorders characterized by increased systemic inflammatory activity, including chronic pain syndromes; metabolic syndrome; type 2 diabetes mellitus; auto-immune diseases particularly rheumatoid arthritis and systemic lupus erythematous; and allergic disorders.

Anti-inflammatory fats

Probably the most important dimension of the anti-inflammatory diet approach is the area of dietary fat modifications. These modifications aim to increase omega-3 fatty acids (FAs), and decrease omega-6 FAs, saturated fat, and trans fatty acids. Because of their impact on the cascade of chemical reactions leading to the synthesis of prostaglandins and leukotrienes, omega-3 FAs form a central part of the anti-inflammatory diet approach. As illustrated in Figure 14.1, the omega-3 FAs move the prostaglandin cascade away from the pro-inflammatory group of prostaglandins and leukotrienes and toward the group considered anti-inflammatory.

Extensive research supports the role of the omega-3 FAs in the prevention and management of heart disease, stroke, hypertension, type 2 diabetes, ulcerative colitis, CD, depression, and various pain syndromes. Where omega-6 FAs increase inflammation, platelet aggregation, vasospasm, and vasoconstriction, and decrease bleeding time, omega-3 FAs are anti-thrombotic, anti-arrhythmic, hypolipidemic, and anti-inflammatory.

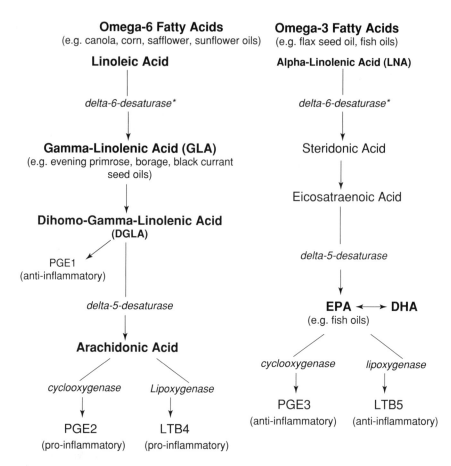

*Factors thought to impair delta-6-desaturase activity include Magnesium (Mg), Zinc (Zn) and vitamin B_6 deficiency: aging; alcohol; trans fatty acids; and high cholesterol levels.

Figure 14.1 Metabolic pathways of essential fatty acids.

Both omega-3 and omega-6 FAs are essential to life, and so the relevant question is not how to replace all omega-6 FAs with omega-3 FAs, but rather what balance between the two is most health-promoting. In many cultures felt to have healthy diets in general, the omega-6 to omega-3 FA ratios are in the 1 : 1 to 4 : 1 range – the traditional Greek diet of Crete (1 : 1); the Mediterranean diet (4 : 1); and the Okinawan diet (1 : 1) are examples. The standard American diet, emphasizing as it does fried and processed foods with minimal consumption of fish and high consumption of polyunsaturated vegetable oils, has an omega-6 to omega-3 ratio of 20–30 : 1. A further contributor to this imbalanced picture is the fact that domesticated animals fed omega-6-rich grains (as opposed to omega-3-rich grass) have been found to have altered lipid composition in their meat, resulting in lower omega-3 FAs than in grass-fed animals. Farm-raised fish and chicken eggs also have also been shown to be lower in omega-3 FA than wild fish and eggs from free-range hens respectively, probably due to the same difference in feed content.

An imbalanced omega-6: omega-3 ratio such as the one which exists in the typical American diet negatively influences prostaglandin synthesis, leading to increased pro-inflammatory prostaglandin E2 series (PGE2). This imbalance in prostaglandin synthesis may contribute to an increased risk of chronic degenerative and inflammatory diseases. Altered prostaglandin function, such as deficiency of PGE1 and excess of PGE2, may also play a major role in autoimmunity [27]; preliminary animal and human research suggests that supplementing with omega-3 FA rich-fish oil may delay the onset and progression of certain autoimmune diseases [28–33].

A final important aspect of modifying fats for the anti-inflammatory diet is the notion that when polyunsaturated fatty acid-rich vegetable oils are used, they should be used only in cold dishes. These oils are not heat stable, and heating them causes chemical and molecular changes which can promote inflammation and possibly even carcinogenesis. Trans-fats and partially hydrogenated fats typically found in highly-processed foods should also be limited in this diet.

Anti-inflammatory carbohydrates

The second major category for modification in the anti-inflammatory diet is sugar intake. This consists mainly of eliminating foods with high glycemic index (GI), and moving to more foods low and moderate glycemic index. The theory is that the low GI diet allows us to minimize the contribution of high insulin levels to systemic inflammation. High GI foods lead to a blood glucose response which is rapid and significant, and therefore to an insulin response which is also dramatic. Carbohydrates that break down slowly release glucose more gradually into the blood stream, leading to a more moderate insulin response.

High carbohydrate, highly refined diets, lacking in fiber, increase post prandial insulin levels and promote inflammation by their effect on essential fatty acid metabolism and prostaglandin synthesis. One of the many effects of elevated insulin levels is the upregulation of the enzyme delta-5-desaturase, which converts di-homo-gamma linolenic acid (DGLA) into arachidonic acid (AA). DGLA is a potent anti-inflammatory FA, (converted to PG1 series prostaglandins) while arachidonic acid is a pro-inflammatory FA (converted to PG2 series prostaglandins). A low GI diet can increase insulin sensitivity – thus reducing levels of circulating insulin and thereby reducing the potential pro-inflammatory impact of high insulin levels.

In low GI diets, refined grains are eliminated and whole grains are emphasized in limited amounts. Low-fat dairy is restricted due to its high carbohydrate content. Starchy vegetables are restricted but other vegetables are unrestricted. Fruits with a high glycemic index are eliminated and low and moderate glycemic index fruits are allowed in restricted amounts to minimize glycemic load. Legumes are emphasized due to their low GI. Lean proteins, fatty fish, low GI vegetables and fruits, and nuts are emphasized.

Anti-inflammatory antioxidants

The theory behind the antioxidant aspect of the anti-inflammatory diet is that many, if not all, inflammatory conditions do some of their damage to the affected body systems through the production of excessive amounts of free radicals by overly active inflammatory cells and mediators. There is some evidence that asthma, rhinitis, and atopic dermatitis are at least partially mediated by oxidative stress, and that augmenting endogenous antioxidant defenses might be beneficial [34]. In exercise-induced asthma, for example, supplementing daily with vitamin C may reduce the likelihood of asthma exacerbations [35]. It has been demonstrated that low serum levels of antioxidants result in enhanced cytokine production and effects [36].

The anti-inflammatory diet aims to mitigate this effect by increasing the amount of foods in the diet with potential antioxidant activity. Dietary antioxidants can be increased through emphasis on highly pigmented fruits and vegetables (yellow-orange-red, red-purple-blue vegetables and fruits), dark leafy greens and cruciferous vegetables, allium vegetables (onions and garlic), and citrus fruits. Green and black teas are also an excellent source of antioxidant substances. Although many practitioners will add the use of antioxidant supplements to this aspect of the diet, recent literature has raised some questions about the safety and effectiveness of indiscriminate use of antioxidant vitamin preparations (i.e. vitamin E and beta-carotene).

Anti-inflammatory herbs and spices

Research suggests that many common culinary spices exhibit anti-inflammatory, analgesic, and thrombolytic activity. Including such spices in one's diet on a regular basis may help reduce systemic inflammation. Important anti-inflammatory food herbs include ginger, rosemary, turmeric, oregano, cayenne, garlic, onion, clove, and nutmeg [37–41]. These culinary spices should be used liberally in the anti-inflammatory diet.

Food sensitivities/elimination trial

The "allergy-elimination" diet is described in Table 14.1. We mention it here again because of its important role as one of the elements in the anti-inflammatory diet approach. First, if a person has allergies as defined by conventional allergy testing, clearly these foods should be eliminated. Second, a trial elimination diet, may be considered as a way to discover other types of food which may be contributing to the patient's symptoms through the mechanism of food sensitivity as these foods may trigger inflammatory responses. The elimination diet should be strongly considered especially in patients who manifest with gastrointestinal and/or skin complaints in addition to their inflammatory condition.

The anti-inflammatory diet described above is a relatively new therapeutic approach and thus has not been well-researched to date. However, many of the individual components of the approach – such as the use of omega-3 FA in rheumatoid arthritis and other conditions, the impact of low GI diets on insulin metabolism, and the impact of vitamin C and other antioxidant substances on exercise-induced asthma – have been validated in clinical research. We look forward to clinical research examining what we feel is the even greater potential of the combined approach described here for patients with inflammatory disorders.

Conclusion

The importance of nutrition in the prevention and treatment of diseases such as cardiovascular disease and cancer is undeniable. What is not yet clear is the extent to which dietary guidelines and nutritional or dietary supplements can and should be recommended for a wide range of diseases, and what level of evidence is necessary before broad recommendations can be made. Integrative medicine practitioners make extensive use of nutritional therapies based on good clinical responses or experience, and an understanding that when appropriately applied they may be helpful. The integration of diet advice into the treatment plan also helps patients take responsibility and initiative in improving their well-being or healing.

Integrative medicine practice that includes nutrition and possibly a number of other natural therapies creates a focus on wellness, and attention to individual requirements and preferences. While significant research is required to establish safety and efficacy, there is growing interest in, and demand for, these approaches by the public.

References

1 Consortium of Academic Health Centers for Integrative Medicine website, http://www. imconsortium.org/cahcim/about/home.html.
2 Kushi LH, Cunningham JE, Hebert JR, Lerman RH, Bandera EV, Teas J. The macrobiotic diet in cancer. *J Nutr* 2001;131:3056S–64S.
3 Adzersen KH, Jess P, Freivogel KW, Gerhard I, Bastert G. Raw and cooked vegetables, fruits, selected micronutrients, and breast cancer risk: a case-control study in Germany. *Nutr Cancer* 2003;46:131–7.
4 Ornish D, Scherwitz LW, Billings JH, *et al*. Intensive lifestyle changes for reversal of coronary heart disease. *JAMA* 1998;280:2001–7.
5 Foster GD, Wyatt HR, Hill JO, *et al*. A randomized trial of a low-carbohydrate diet for obesity. *N Engl J Med* 2003;348:2082–90.
6 Yancy WS, Jr., Foy M, Chalecki AM, Vernon MC, Westman EC. A low-carbohydrate, ketogenic diet to treat type 2 diabetes. *Nutr Metab* 2005;2:34.
7 Aude YW, Agatston AS, Lopez-Jimenez F, *et al*. The national cholesterol education program diet vs. a diet lower in carbohydrates and higher in protein and monounsaturated fat: a randomized trial. *Arch Intern Med* 2004;164:2141–6.

8 Muller H, de Toledo FW, Resch KL. Fasting followed by vegetarian diet in patients with rheumatoid arthritis: a systematic review. *Scand J Rheumatol* 2001; 30:1–10.

9 Fuhrman J, Sarter B, Calabro DJ. Brief case reports of medically supervised, water-only fasting associated with remission of autoimmune disease. *Altern Ther Health Med* 2002; 8:112, 110–1.

10 Bock SA. Prospective appraisal of complaints of adverse reactions to foods in children during the first 3 years of life. *Pediatrics* 1987;79:683–8.

11 Oehling A, Garcia B, Santos F, *et al.* Food allergy as a cause of rhinitis and/or asthma. *J Investig Allergol Clin Immunol* 1992;2:78–83.

12 Onorato J, Merland N, Terral C, Michel FB, Bousquet J. Placebo-controlled double-blind food challenge in asthma. *J Allergy Clin Immunol* 1986;78:1139–46.

13 James JM, Bernhisel-Broadbent J, Sampson HA. Respiratory reactions provoked by double-blind food challenges in children. *Am J Respir Crit Care Med* 1994;149:59–64.

14 Pelikan Z, Pelikan-Filipek M. Bronchial response to the food ingestion challenge. *Ann Allergy* 1987;58:164–72.

15 Woods RK. Thien FC. Abramson MJ. Dietary marine fatty acids (fish oil) for asthma in adults and children. *Cochrane Database of Systematic Reviews.* (3):CD001283;2002.

16 Manteleone CA, Sherman AR. Nutrition and asthma. *Arch Int Med* 1997;157(1):23–34.

17 Baker JC, Ayres JG. Diet and asthma. *Resp Med* 2000;94:925–34.

18 Gottschall EG. *Breaking the Vicious Cycle: Intestinal Health Through Diet.* Kirkson Press 1994.

19 Persson PG. Ahlbom A. Hellers G. Diet and inflammatory bowel disease: a case-control study. *Epidemiology.* 1992;3(1):47–52.

20 Mayberry JF. Rhodes J. Newcombe RG. Increased sugar consumption in Crohn's disease. *Digestion,* 1980;20(5):323–6.

21 Tragnone A. Valpiani D. Miglio F. *et al.* Dietary habits as risk factors for inflammatory bowel disease. *Europ J Gastro Hepat* 1995; 7(1):47–51.

22 Lorenz-Meyer H. Bauer P. Nicolay C, *et al.* Omega-3 fatty acids and low carbohydrate diet for maintenance of remission in Crohn's disease. A randomized controlled multicenter trial. *Scand J Gastro* 1996;31(8):778–85.

23 Sanderson IR. Boulton P. Menzies I. Walker-Smith JA. Improvement of abnormal lactulose/rhamnose permeability in active Crohn's disease of the small bowel by an elemental diet. *Gut* 1987;28(9):1073–6.

24 Workman EM. Alun Jones V. Wilson AJ. Hunter JO. Diet in the management of Crohn's disease. *Human Nutrition - Applied Nutrition* 1984;38(6):469–73.

25 Galland L. "Dietary Approach to Inflammatory Bowel Disease" Poster presentation at the Fourth Annual Sympoium on Alternative Therapies at the New York Marriott World Trade Center March 28, 1999 by Leo Galland, M.D.

26 www.lowcarb.ca/atkins-diet-and-low-carb-plans/specific-carbohydrate-diet.html

27 Das UN. Prostaglandins and immune response. *J Assoc Phys India* 1981;29(10):831–3.

28 McCarty MF. Upregulation of lymphocyte apoptosis as a strategy for preventing and treating autoimmune disorders: a role for whole-food vegan diets, fish oil and dopamine agonists. *Medical Hypotheses.* 2001;57(2):258–75.

29 Venkatraman JT. Chu WC. Effects of dietary omega-3 and omega-6 lipids and vitamin E on serum cytokines, lipid mediators and anti-DNA antibodies in a mouse model for rheumatoid arthritis. *J Am Col Nutr* 1999;18(6):602–13.

30 Aug Ergas D. Eilat E. Mendlovic S. Sthoeger ZM n-3 fatty acids and the immune system in autoimmunity. *Isr Med Assoc J* 2002;4(1):34–8.

31 Jolly CA. Muthukumar A. Reddy Avula CP. Fernandes G. Maintenance of NF-kappaB activation in T-lymphocytes and a naive T-cell population in autoimmune-prone

(NZB/NZW)F(1) mice by feeding a food-restricted diet enriched with n-3 fatty acids. *Cell Immun* 2001;213(2):122–33.

32 Fernandes G. Troyer DA. Jolly CA. The effects of dietary lipids on gene expression and apoptosis. *Proc Nutr Soc* 1998;57(4):543–50.

33 Fernandes G. Dietary lipids and risk of autoimmune disease. *Clin Immun Immun* 1994;72(2):193–7.

34 Bowler RP. Crapo JD. Oxidative stress in allergic respiratory diseases. *J Aller Clin Immun* 2002;110(3):349–56.

35 Ram FS. Rowe BH. Kaur B. Vitamin C supplementation for asthma. *Cochrane Database of Systematic Reviews.* (3):CD000993,2004.

36 Grimble RF. Nutritional modulation of cytokine biology. *Nutrition* 1998;14(7-8):634–40.

37 Petersen M. Simmonds MS. Rosmarinic Acid. *Phytochemistry* 2003;62(2):121–5.

38 Katiyar SK, Agarwal R, Mukhtar H. Inhibition of tumor promotion in SENCAR mouse skin by ethanol extract of Zingiber officinale rhizome. *Cancer Research* 1996;56(5):1023–30.

39 Rao UJ. Lokesh BR. Presence of an acidic glycoprotein in the serum of arthritic rats: modulation by capsaicin and curcumin. *Molec Cell Biochem* 1997;169(1–2):125–34.

40 Olajide OA. Ajayi FF. Ekhelar AI. Awe SO. Makinde JM. Alada AR. Biological effects of Myristica fragrans (nutmeg) extract. *Phytother Res* 1999;13(4):344–5.

41 Sharma JN. Srivastava KC. Gan EK. Suppressive effects of eugenol and ginger oil on arthritic rats. *Pharmacology* 1994;49(5):314–8.

Successful changes to the environment

CHAPTER 15

It's all about changing behaviors

Darwin Deen and Alice Fornari

Counseling to change a patient's diet and physical activity has the potential to play an important role in the nation's health promotion and disease prevention efforts in the twenty-first century. Both *Healthy People 2010* [1] and the US Preventive Services Task Force [2] reports enumerate specific recommendations regarding nutrition and lifestyle counseling. Recent clinical guidelines for hypertension, hyperlipidemia, obesity, and diabetes include specific nutrition and exercise related recommendations to be implemented by primary care clinicians [3]. Of the ten most commonly diagnosed chronic diseases in primary care, seven are nutrition-sensitive conditions [4,5]. *Healthy People 2010* nutrition objectives for primary care clinicians focus on including nutrition counseling in 75% of physician office visits for hyperlipidemia, cardiovascular disease, or diabetes mellitus [1]. Studies support the premise that brief nutrition counseling in the primary care setting can be effective in improving risk factors [6]. While many consultations should include a nutritional aspect, physicians do not discuss nutrition with their patients as often as they could. Major barriers include short visit length, competing demands, the paucity of nutrition education in medical schools, and perceived poor compliance of patients with physicians' dietary prescriptions [7]. It has been demonstrated that "obese patients who receive counseling and weight management from physicians are significantly more likely to undertake weight management programs than those who do not" [8].

Practical considerations for nutrition counseling

One of the many challenges in providing nutritional care to patients is that simply providing the patient with accurate information regarding the relationship between their diagnosis and their diet is only the beginning of the process of helping them to change their behavior. In this chapter we review the process of behavior change as it applies to nutritional advice for patients with chronic disease treated in the ambulatory care setting. We will consider agenda setting, interview strategies that promote lifestyle behavior change, tools to assess the patient's dietary intake, and methods that can make primary care clinicians more successful at helping patients change behaviors.

The first visit

A brief diet and lifestyle assessment is a key component of the patient's medical and social history and should be ascertained during the first non-acute visit. Given the large number of diseases encountered in primary care for which nutrition interventions are relevant, diet and lifestyle advice is an important part of routine care [9]. Evidence supports medical nutrition therapy provided by dietitians is more effective when reinforced by other members of the health care team as part of their evaluation and management. Ongoing clinician involvement in the patient's efforts to initiate and maintain a healthy weight and lifestyle cannot be over emphasized. Thus, a brief assessment of dietary intake and lifestyle should be considered a key component of the medical and social history for physicians, physician assistants, and nurses as well as dietitians. Through assessments of body mass index (BMI), waist circumference, co-morbidities of overweight and obesity, as well as ongoing counseling, encouragement and monitoring, primary care physicians have an effective opportunity to educate patients about the importance of maintaining a healthy weight [8].

The appropriate place to begin a discussion of a recommended lifestyle behavior change is with the patient's understanding of the health implications of their current behavior. Just because a patient is aware of their diagnosis does not mean that they understand what implications that diagnosis has for their health. A discussion of potential outcomes based on potential behavior changes is essential to help motivate patients to make changes. This process differs from patient education as it involves eliciting information from the patient about their expectations rather than providing information to the patient. It is helpful at the earliest stages of an intervention to determine the patient's understanding of their illness and what he or she wishes to get out of the session. This will provide the practitioner and the patient with a common language to use in determining what changes to make and how to go about the process of making changes. Next, an assessment of the patient's readiness to change will guide the clinician in determining how best to proceed and to provide an atmosphere of patient-centeredness. Since nutrition intervention requires active involvement of the patient, formulating a joint agenda will make it possible to include effective advice and guidance for patients [9].

Dialogue for dietary assessment: primary care in action

Just as a medical assessment is initiated by querying a patient about their "chief complaint" or the reason for the medical visit, a nutrition assessment needs to begin by asking the patient about how their dietary intake and lifestyle are related to their current health status and treatment goals. Such a query can provide valuable insights for addressing readiness to make dietary changes. Promoting overall health by promotion of healthy eating should be a part of health maintenance visits. It is important to institute advice and counseling over consecutive consultations. This reflects the 5As model of change which supports the patient putting advice into effect, and not just telling them what you think they should do (discussed on p. 315 and Chapter 2). [10]. When patients are being seen for a chronic disease follow-up visit, dietary advice can be less general and more specific to their individual disease state or risks.

Helping patients make changes

Stages of change: the transtheoretical model

The transtheoretical model [11] was developed by Prochaska and DiClemente [12] in an effort to identify a unifying theory of how people with addictions change behavior. Prochaska initially reviewed existing psychological treatment modalities to find common themes. These themes were then tested with patients trying to quit smoking and six distinct stages were identified that described the path through which patients moved to successfully change behavior [12].

Prochaska and DiClemente [13] developed a treatment model based on identifying the stage that the patient was in and using a stage-appropriate intervention. They tested this model in patients with alcohol dependency and found it to be effective. It has since been applied to tobacco cessation and for other drug addictions with very good results. The use of the model for diet and exercise behavior change is still in its infancy, but many studies have shown positive results. It is important to recognize that behavior change is not always a linear process where patients move smoothly from one stage to the next. Sometimes a patient will relapse back to old habits and be unable to move forward again until they are able to successfully address whatever barriers interfered with their continued progress.

The transtheoretical model [13] of behavioral change has been used to assess patient's motivation and readiness to make lifestyle changes to address obesity, diabetes and cardiovascular related risks [14–16]. The stages that individuals go through in the transtheoretical model begin with precontemplation (not considering making a change in the target behavior), and advance through contemplation (considering the pros and cons of making a behavioral change), preparation (planning steps to make changes), action (actually changing the targeted behavior), maintenance (making the changed behavioral habitual), and relapse (when a formerly altered behavior pattern returns) though not always in a typical pattern or order. See Table 15.1.

Discussing past experiences with weight loss efforts or attempts to make other dietary changes can be helpful in opening the dialogue. As eating is a social and cultural activity, effective dietary change is promoted when the entire family makes changes together. It may therefore be necessary to address concerns about the health effects of a given dietary intervention on other members

Table 15.1 Using the Transtheoretical Model in Dietary Assessment.

Behavioral stage	Key assessment focus	Clinician's goal
Precontemplation	Patient is not yet considering dietary or lifestyle changes to reduce health risks or prevent disease.	Determine patient's knowledge and understanding of relationship of behaviors to risk.
Contemplation	Patient is considering making some lifestyle changes.	Identify short and long-term goals and select one change to try first.
Preparation	Patient is planning to make a specific lifestyle change.	Support patient's decision and review potential obstacles to success.
Action	Patient initiates new behavior change.	Ensure follow-up for problem solving and reinforce commitment.
Maintenance	Patient becomes comfortable with new behavior pattern.	Congratulate and support patient's commitment and recognize potential for relapse. Begin to identify new behaviors to modify.
Relapse	Patient has abandoned new behavior or returned to previous behaviors.	Discuss patient's emotional state and frame relapse as a learning opportunity.

Source: Adapted from [12,13].

Determining stages of change

An assessment of readiness to change can be obtained with a self-administered questionnaire or by interview [13].

1) Have you *ever* (tried to) changed the way you eat to lose weight or improve your health?
   No: skip to question 4
   Yes: question 2
2) Are you currently following a dietary plan for any reason?
   No: skip to question 4
   Yes: question 3
3) How long have you been following this plan and why?
   Less than a month (*action stage*)
   Longer than six months (*maintenance stage*)
4) During the past month, have you thought about dietary changes you could make to lose weight or improve your health?
   Yes: (*contemplation stage* or if plan is specific and to be implemented within a month *preparation stage*)
   No: (*precontemplation stage*)

The 5 A's model

The 5 A's model, was developed by the National Cancer Institute [10] (as the 4 A's) to help physicians provide smoking cessation counseling to their patients. The model has since been refined to be applied to any health behavior change (see below for an example of nutrition counseling). The A's stand for Assess, Advise, Agree, Assist, and Arrange. The following is a brief description of the recommended content for each step.

Assess: Identify specifics of the patient's current behavior: their specific health risk factors, their level of knowledge, level of interest/commitment to change, and their social supports that will influence the change process.

Advice: Review specific primary and secondary goals for behavior change, such as reducing fat intake or reducing the use of trans-fatty acid containing foods and the expected long- and short-term health outcomes that might result.

Agree: Seek a collaboration between the practitioner and the patient such that together you negotiate a plan that makes sense to both parties. This facilitates behavior change.

Assist: Use whatever methods are available and appropriate to accomplish change, consider available resources, and shepherd the patient through the process of change. This includes monitoring the plan and modifying specific aspects as needed.

Arrange: Follow-up, Ensure adequate follow-up with patients, whether by repeat visits or telephone reminders from staff members. This is an important part of most successful behavior change strategies. Behavior change does not occur immediately and requires time to translate into new habits.

The 5 A's program provides an easily understood skeleton of the process of behavior change and can be integrated easily with motivational interviewing and the transtheoretical model. It may be useful for practitioners to think of an individual visit in terms of which of the A's is being focused on.

Source: Adapted from [10].

of the family. Patients need to be assured that potential benefits may impact all family members who for example may chose to reduce their intake of sugar or saturated fats. This information provides a foundation for assessing a patient's current stage of behavioral change. The stage of behavioral readiness is fluid, e.g., life stressors can easily move a person from maintenance to precontemplation. The risk of relapse is greater for the "veteran" dieter, who may be quite knowledgeable about food composition, than for the novice who may be ready for change and seeking food composition information. Making dietary changes is often fraught with ambivalence and conflict over the commitment to behave differently in eating situations and to change food choices.

Motivational interviewing

Motivation is a state that varies from one moment to the next. Motivational interviewing [17] is an approach that has been shown to be effective at helping patients modify addictive behaviors and is increasingly being applied to lifestyle problems. To some degree, habitual behavior patterns such as unhealthy eating and sedentary lifestyle are addictive behaviors. The goal of motivational interviewing is to understand what the motivational state of the client is at the time and to act appropriately. For example, in the precontemplation stage a person needs information and feedback to better understand the problem and to begin to imagine that change is possible. Giving advice at this point is not helpful.

Motivational interviewing is characterized by eliciting motivation from the client, not trying to impose it from the outside. It has been defined as a directive, client-centered counseling style for eliciting behavior change by helping clients to explore and resolve ambivalence [18]. Resolving ambivalence is a key to motivational interviewing. When people move into the contemplation stage, when they are thinking about changing vs. not changing – balancing out the pros and cons – they are more susceptible to real change. However, a helping professional who starts pushing behavior change at the client at this stage will meet resistance.

It is the client's task, not the counselor's, to identify and resolve his or her ambivalence. What the client needs is help listing pros and cons and a professional who really listens. The client determines whether their current behavior is consistent with their goals and then makes choices to move him or herself. Direct persuasion is not an effective method to resolve ambivalence. Presenting arguments for the pro change side will leave the client the role of defending arguments for the con side of change: the counselor must leave room for the client to provide both the pros and cons. The counseling style is generally a quiet and eliciting one. In this setting, effective patient education requires more listening than talking. Readiness to change is not a client trait but a fluctuating product of interpersonal interaction. The therapeutic relationship is more like a partnership than one of expert and recipient. Patient motivation requires establishing a therapeutic relationship from which motivation can grow.

Motivation as a behavioral probability

The counselor can never really know what the client is thinking and feeling. We infer these things from what clients say, the emotions they show, and what they do. If clients adhere well to a prescribed plan, we expect they are more likely to do well than if they don't. We can turn this around and say, " 'motivation' can be defined as *the probability that a person will enter into, continue, and adhere to a specific change strategy*" [19]. This shifts the emphasis from "motivated" as a passive adjective to the active verb "motivate," which it is the counselor's job to perform. The counselor does not just give advice, but motivates, and increases the likelihood that the client will understand and perform all the little parts of action towards change. The client cannot be blamed for being unmotivated:

it is the counselor's job to provide the appropriate pieces at each stage of the process. Motivation is a part of the helping professional's job.

The goals of a motivational interviewing session will be achieved when the patient's self esteem has been maintained or enhanced, when the practitioner has used active listening, when the interview focuses on specific behaviors that are steps to an overall goal, and when incidental goals are set that will create progress toward an overall outcome. For example, if the client usually drinks several cups of coffee with half-and-half each day and one of their goals is to cut down on the saturated fat content of their diet, then they must first recognize that half-and-half is an important source of saturated fat. They must then refine that overall statement to recognize how much of an impact changing to whole or low-fat milk could have on their saturated fat intake. Considering how best to institute that change, they might decide to use whole milk when they are getting coffee at a restaurant but buy 1% low-fat milk to use at home. This would be a good step toward changing their taste preference for half-and-half.

Using motivational interviewing to identify ambivalence

Developing and maintaining motivation is crucial to making lifestyle changes. The assessment should be focused on addressing the internal ambivalence about giving up "unhealthy" habits associated with increased risk e.g., smoking or poor eating habits. The questions listed below can be used to identify sources of ambivalence and can help enhance the motivation to make desired dietary changes.

Understanding of current "unhealthy" lifestyle and poor eating patterns (*topics for probing questions*)
• What do you like about the way you eat now? (*Convenience, flavor, feelings.*)
• What changes do you feel are necessary in the way you currently eat? (*Which behavior is the patient most ready to change at the present time?*)
• What benefits do you gain from the way you eat? (*Visualize eating situations and feelings after eating.*)
• How does your eating relate to bad feelings? (*Anger, frustration, anxiety, stress.*)
• How does your eating relate to your method of coping? (*Examine coping style for various stressors and how that relates to eating.*)
• What would your life be like if you changed the way you eat? (*Visualize lifestyle changes and explore potential feeling of loss, concern about being hungry.*)
• What foods that you *like* do you think you would have to give up or be "told" to eat less of? (*Favorite foods, foods at social events, snacking pattern.*)
• What foods do you *dislike* that you think you "should" or will be "told to" eat? (*"Diet food" perceptions, food groups not currently eaten e.g., vegetables, etc.*)

Benefits of changing lifestyle and eating patterns
• What benefits to you think you might gain from changing the way you eat? (*Brainstorm the range of potential benefits e.g., fit into clothes, feel better, keep family from nagging.*)

- How does your eating (and lifestyle) pattern relate to "chronic" health problems (e.g., diabetes, hypertension)? (*Explore how medical nutrition therapy may affect control of cardiovascular disease (CVD) risk factors, and medication dosage/side effects e.g. sexual function, etc.*)
- How could changing your lifestyle improve your long-term health and ability to function? (*Explore important personal events.*)
- How could lifestyle changes improve your every day functioning, now? (*Explore fatigue, energy, ability to concentrate, stamina, etc.*)
- What food or lifestyle changes do you think you may like? (*Explore potential misperceptions of restrictions, or how some of the dislikes may be addressed e.g., feeling hungry.*)
- How do you think you could change your lifestyle to get the potential benefits without feeling deprived? (*List some of the reasons given for not changing intake.*)

While readiness to lose weight may be fairly global, the stage of readiness for specific food items or behaviors may vary widely. For two individuals who want to lose weight, one may be ready to substitute lower fat or skim milk for whole milk, while the other may be reluctant to make the milk substitution. However, these individuals may switch roles on another food behavior such as reducing portion sizes. Thus, assessing why a change may be difficult can facilitate the development of the solution. At a precontemplation or contemplation stage, open-ended questions provide valuable information about how the patient views dietary changes. Thus, the interviewer asks "why" questions about eating rather than "what" questions that can be used to quantify food intake. Much of the dialogue will focus on the ambivalence elicited regarding the perceived pros and cons of making dietary changes. At the preparation or action stage, "what" questions can identify food items that can be targeted for behavioral change. At the maintenance stage, "when" questions can be used to identify situations producing risk of relapse.

Practitioner factors that facilitate change

Relationship-centered care and behavior change

Considerable research supports the idea that the therapeutic relationship is the most important factor in the counseling process [20,21]. In a client-centered helping relationship, the client/patient feels safe enough to explore change. The counselor/practitioner is not directive, problem solving, or analytical. The counselor/practitioner must provide empathy, warmth, and genuineness.

Active listening

Active listening is a technique that increases the bond between practitioner and patient [22]. It is an important part of creating an environment where behavior change is more likely. The techniques of active listening include: observing the patient, remaining quiet to let the patient talk, listening to the words the patient uses particularly relating to their understanding of what the problem is, listening to how that patient describes their problem and noting discrepancies between what the patient says and how the patient says it, and listening for the patient's interpretation of what is going on.

Empathy

Empathy is not the same as sympathy. It involves active listening: restating what the patient has said in a way that makes clear that the listener understands what the client has said. It can be most easily demonstrated in the following formula. "You *feel*...[name the correct emotion expressed by the client] ... *because* [or *when*] ... [indicate the correct experiences and behaviors that give rise to the feelings]...." [22]. This is a beginner's tool that helps the clinician to learn how to understand and perform the expression of empathy.

Warmth

Warmth is the second factor that enables a therapeutic relationship to exist. The client must feel that the practitioner accepts him or her and has a positive regard and respect for him or her. Practitioners are professionals, and are obligated to maintain a professional attitude, but this does not mean a chilly demeanor. The patient will feel the provider's cold attitude if it exists.

Genuineness

Genuineness is the third essential element of the therapeutic alliance. The provider must tell the patient what he or she thinks and feels about what the patient says and does. It means telling the patient as much as you think he or she is ready to hear at that moment in words he or she will understand. This statement seems ambivalent; a mixed message. But being "genuine" is both difficult and essential. To be too honest and say too much may bruise emotions. To hold back may not convey enough of the truth to help the client move along. This is a continuum, and how close one can get to it is a measure of a practitioner's skill.

Barriers to change

Being judgmental, talking too much and not listening enough are severe barriers to change that many helping professionals exhibit. Five basic principles suggested by Miller [23] can help the professional work with barriers the patient exhibits.

Express empathy

By using the empathy formula, and later expressing empathy without the formula, the provider makes clear that the patient is being understood and accepted. Acceptance does not mean that the practitioner agrees with the patient or approves of the patient's behavior. It means that the provider accepts and understands the patient's perspective without judging it. Paradoxically, accepting people as they are creates opportunities for them to become something else.

The ambivalence patients' feel about change is normal, not pathological. If it were easy for them to change they would have done so already. Listening to their ambivalence and reflecting it back to them helps get them "unstuck."

Develop discrepancy

The goal of motivational interviewing is to have the patient present the reasons for change, rather than the provider. People persuade themselves better than any other person can. In discussion, point out discrepancies between what the patient says he or she wants and the consequences of their current behavior. Discrepancies between their current behavior and their own goals are motivational. It is also important to avoid direct confrontational messages.

Avoid argument

The practitioner should avoid direct confrontations. If the provider argues that the client has a problem and needs to change, it makes the patient feel defensive which may cause them to take the other side of the argument. The purpose of motivational interviewing is to get the client to become aware of problems and the need to change. Gentle persuasion or "soft confrontation" is often necessary. Resistance is a signal to the practitioner to consider strategies for change.

Roll with resistance

Confronting resistance directly only increases the likelihood that it will continue. It is important that the provider does not impose new viewpoints or goals, but rather encourages the patient to consider new information and offers new perspectives. "Take what you want and leave the rest" is the permissive kind of advice that is embodied in the motivational interviewing approach. The counselor exaggerates the patient's point of view, or turns a question or problem back to the patient, directing resistance back to the patient, and allowing the patient to find solutions.

Support self-efficacy

Self-efficacy is a person's belief that they can carry out a change or a task [24]. The practitioner must take any opportunity to convey messages that he/she has confidence in the patient's ability to carry out tasks leading to change. If the patient has made some changes, build on these early successes. If the patient has experienced setbacks, emphasize that there are many paths to the goal and the best approach still needs to be uncovered.

The importance of self-efficacy

Self-efficacy predicts when knowledge will influence behavior [25]. Self-efficacy is the patient's perception of their ability to exert control. Once knowledge gaps have been identified, addressing self-efficacy may be the most effective method of promoting behavior change. Self-efficacy is assessed by inquiring about who the patient feels is most in control of their diet, who was responsible for any past failures, and how the patient has responded to obstacles in the past. If the patient does not feel in control of his/her behavior, helping them to identify those areas where they can gain control will make behavior change more likely. If the patient blames themselves for past failures (low self-efficacy), they need a plan to address how to make this time different. If the patient feels that external factors were responsible for past failures, ask them to describe what has changed in the environment that will prevent this from happening again. To address self-efficacy, patients must be asked to make a realistic appraisal of their abilities.

There are four main sources of self-efficacy:
1) verbal persuasion (including self-talk);
2) performance accomplishment;
3) vicarious performance; and
4) physiologic arousal.

Activities that have been shown to influence self-efficacy include:
1) modeling behavior (such as cooking classes);
2) reflection on past accomplishments (positive reinforcement);
3) role plays (practicing potential difficult situations); and
4) placing emphasis on effective benefit (short-term benefits).

For example, rather than concentrating on the health benefits of a new dietary regimen, which are long term, advise the patient to think instead about how good they will feel about accomplishing a short term goal that they set for themselves. For example, fitting into an old suit that used to fit, or buying a new item in a smaller size.

The Health Beliefs Model to understand why people change

The Health Beliefs Model (HBM) [26] seeks to explain what motivates patients to change health behaviors. Patients vary greatly in their interest in health and in their willingness to change personal habits in the pursuit of improved health. The HBM considers perceived susceptibility, perceived severity, outcome efficacy, and cost vs. benefit in explaining why people choose to change.

Perceived susceptibility
Perceived susceptibility means that the patient considers himself or herself to be at-risk from their current behavior. For example, many patients discount the health risks associated with saturated fat consumption. They are not willing to change their diets because they do not acknowledge that dietary saturated fat leads to increases in serum cholesterol and low density lipoprotein (LDL) levels.

Perceived severity
Perceived severity describes that the patient believes that their outcome is bad enough that it needs to be prevented. For example, if an overweight patient feels that being overweight does not increase their risk for complications from

a chronic disease, they will not be interested in making dietary and lifestyle changes in an effort to control their weight and decrease risk.

Outcome efficacy

Outcome efficacy reflects the relationship between the behavior to be changed and the expected outcome. Very often we hear from clients: "I've been eating this way for my whole life, how much difference will it make if I change now?" Unfortunately, no one can say for sure what the outcome of any specific dietary change will be. The best we can do is to offer the patients the benefit of our experience and the assurances of the scientific literature.

Cost vs. benefit

Cost vs. benefit reflects the internalization of the belief that the outcome is worth the effort expended. This may be the hardest challenge to address for any given individual. Any change is difficult and some changes are more difficult than others. The things that we routinely expect of people may seem small to us but may represent a real challenge to the patient due to the fact that food is more than just a vehicle for sustenance. Dealing with the impact of dietary modifications on holiday meals, parties and other special occasions, eating with friends, etc. all impact the perceived costs of change for the individual.

Other methods for promoting behavior change

Choices and changes

A model for practitioners seeking to influence health behaviors, Choices and Changes, has been described by Keller & White [27]. It was designed as an adjunct to the transtheorectical model and proposes that patients change when they have conviction and confidence (and fail to change when they lack either). Conviction reflects the client's belief that making a certain change will influence their health. Confidence reflects their belief that they have the ability to make a given change (Fig. 15.1). The practitioner uses the therapeutic relationship to help identify the patient's levels of both conviction and confidence and provides counseling to move them toward being more convinced and more confident regarding a specific behavior change. The therapeutic relationship is established by eliciting the patient's experiences with open-ended questions, using reflective listening and empathy (providing acceptance for the patient's perspectives).

Practitioners can determine levels of conviction using questions such as: "How important do you think this change is to your health?" or "How committed are you to making this change?" When the practitioner identifies a patient who has conviction ("I know this is important") but lacks confidence, counseling proceeds in an effort to identify the source of this helplessness and addresses ways to improve their confidence. For example, by reviewing past accomplishments in other areas, by presenting change as a choice rather than a mandate, and by breaking larger changes into small steps that can be

SUCCESS

		High conviction/Low confidence **STUCK** Patient is frustrated	High conviction/High confidence **CHANGING** Patient is committed
C O N V I C T I O N	Convinced		
	Ambivalent	Low conviction/Low confidence **STUCK** Patient is unaware or cynical	Low conviction/High confidence **STUCK** Patient is skeptical
		Helpless	**Powerful**

CONFIDENCE

Figure 15.1 Choices and Changes Model, adapted from [27].

accomplished and reinforced along the way to the greater change, confidence may improve. A major shift is for a patient to begin the day with a high fiber breakfast that is low in fat. This could consist of high fiber cereals with non-fat milk, or whole grain bread with low-fat cheese. For many people this requires no longer eating bagels or rolls or sugar-rich cereals. The process to achieve this goal can be broken down into small steps and achieved over a few weeks. The patient can first begin with a once weekly change in breakfast and then increase to two to three times weekly before reaching the desired daily change. Exploring their ambivalence is important at this point ("What are the benefits of/problems with changing? What are the benefits of/problems with not changing"?). For example remembering to buy apples at the supermarket may be considered as a goal in itself although it is really only one step on the path to eating more fruit and vegetables. Practitioners can determine patients' level of confidence by asking: "How confident are you that you can make this change? How important is it for you to make this change?" Patients who feel confident of their ability to make change ("I know that I can do this"), but lack the conviction about a specific change will benefit from discussions focused on the ambivalence this represents and any discrepancies between the outcome that the patient desires and their current behavior (e.g. it will be very difficult to lower your cholesterol level if you continue to eat hot dogs or cheeseburgers for lunch every day). Help the patient to clarify what is most important to them and whether their current behavior is consistent with their goals.

Patients who lack both conviction and confidence may benefit from new information. They may not be ready for change at this time and they need their clinician to accept them without judgment while offering support for the potential for change at some later date. Patients are ready to change when both confidence and conviction are high. Discussions with these patients can focus on barriers and situations that may cause setbacks. Using the example above: as a person becomes more knowledgeable about the benefits of a fiber-rich diet, they can experiment with small purchases of appropriate items, either cereals or breads, and use different low fat accompaniments for each item to add flavor and increase satisfaction; an example is low-fat milk or yogurt with cereal or a tasty low-fat cheese with whole grain bread. Either of these requires that a patient either purchases these foods to have at home or finds an accessible breakfast establishment that has them. Either of these can easily represent a barrier requiring some brainstorming or alternative planning to surmount.

Conclusion

Brief nutrition counseling provided by primary care clinicians can produce beneficial changes in diet, risk factors (BMI, blood pressure), waist circumference and lab values Hgb (glucose, A1C, lipids). Research demonstrates that the combination of primary care-based programs training in patient-centered counseling intervention for nutrition change, and a low-cost office support system, has beneficial effects on patient's dietary fat intake, weight and blood lipid levels despite an environment where physicians practice under time pressure [28].

Models for multidisciplinary care vary depending on whether they are designed for an individual medical practice or as part of the health care services of a larger facility. For example, lifestyle changes for healthy weight management must be permanently incorporated into a patient's daily lifestyle to reduce obesity and its associated risks [8]. Continued use of registered dietitians to complement multidisciplinary approaches to patient education and chronic disease prevention and management is needed [5]. In practices that are teaching sites for medical students and residents, faculty expect students to discuss lifestyle change, i.e. smoking cessation and nutrition with patients, but few faculty preceptors provide feedback to the learners about how they carried out this patient advice/counseling session. Ongoing feedback from faculty should be given to learners regarding their patient advice and counseling activities, in addition to a greater mentorship role from faculty interested in nutrition. Widespread limited familiarity with current nutrition, health and disease guidelines indicates opportunity for preceptor education. This is also important for the medical education curriculum for students and residents.

Within the current organization of primary care, it could be argued that there is limited time to give detailed dietary advice. To be effective, acceptable and useful, dietary interventions need to fit into this primary care model as described by van Weel [4] to achieve as much effect as possible by an individualized intervention. Patients who are seen frequently and on a continuous basis benefit from the effectiveness of individual lifestyle interventions [29].

A well-motivated, informed and educated Primary Health Care Team can play a major role in facilitating dietary change in patients, translating nutritional guidelines into meaningful and practical terms, and offering advice that reflects the social and cultural mix of the local community. Group practices could connect with local community agencies/advocates to help address specific local issues and increase the relevance to community members who may or may not be patients [29].

"In these times of changing health care priorities there are great opportunities to maximize the health gain possible with diet. The potential contribution that diet could make to the nation's health is significant and it therefore needs to be put firmly on the health care agenda" [29].

Brief nutrition counseling tools are needed to help clinicians optimize nutrition counseling within the context of time constraints found in real-world primary care practice. Future research is warranted to determine how to optimize the use of registered dietitians in partnership with other health professionals to result in improved outcomes from dietary and lifestyle intervention, given the short time spent on nutrition counseling by physicians. The need is pressing in light of the epidemic of chronic diseases, hypertension, diabetes, hyperlipidemia and obesity [30] [see Chapter 2].

References

1 Healthy People 2010. US Department of Health and Human Services. www. HealthyPeople.gov

2 US Preventive Services Task Force Guide to Clinical Preventive Services. *Report of the US Preventive Services Task Force*. 2nd Ed. Baltimore: Williams and Wilkins, 1996.

3 Wylie-Rosett J, Mossavar-Rahmani Y, Gans K. Recent Dietary Guidelines to prevent and treat cardiovascular disease, diabetes, and obesity. *Heart Dis* 2002;4:220–230.

4 Van Weel C. Morbidity in family medicine: the potential for individual nutritional counseling, an analysis from the Nijmegen Continuous Morbidity Registration. *Am J Clin Nutr*. 1997;65(6 Suppl):1928S–1932S.

5 Wong V, Millen BE, Geller AC, Rogers AE, Maury J, Prout M. What's in store for medical students? Awareness and utilization of expert nutrition guidelines among medical school preceptors. *Prev Med*. 2004;39: 753–759.

6 Eaton CB, Goodwin MA, Stange KC. Direct observation of nutrition counseling in community family practice. *Am J Prev Med*. 2002 Oct;23(3):174–9.

7 Truswell AS. Family physicians and patients: is effective nutrition interaction possible? *Am J Clin Nutr*. 2000 Jan;71(1):6–12.

8 Rippe JM, McInnis KJ, Melanson KJ. Physician involvement in the management of obesity as a primary medical condition. *Obesity Res*. 2001;(Suppl 4):302S–311S.

9 van Weel C. Dietary advice in family medicine. *Am J Clin Nutr.* 2003;77(4 Suppl):1008S–1010S.

10 Whitlock EP, Orleans CT, Pender N, Allan J. Evaluating primary care behavioral counseling interventions: an evidence based approach. *Am J Prev Med.* 2002;22:267–284.

11 Prochaska JO, DiClemente CC, Norcross JC. In search of how people change: Applications to addictive behaviors. *Amer Psychol* 199247:1102.

12 Prochaska JO, Norcross JC, DiClemente CC. *Changing for Good.* New York, NY: William Morrow; 1994.

13 Prochaska, JO, and DiClemente, CC. Transtheoretical therapy toward a more integrative model of change. *Psychotherapy: Theory, Research and Practice.* 1982;19(3): 276–287.

14 Sutton K , Logue E, Jarhoura D, Baughman K, Smucker W, Capers C. Assessing dietary and exercise stage of change to optimize weight loss interventions. *Obesity Res* 2003;22:641–652.

15 Vallis M, Ruggiero L, Greene G, Jones H, Zinman B, Rossi S, Edwards L, Rossi JS, Prochaska JO. Stages of change for healthy eating in diabetes: relation to demographic, eating-related, health care utilization, and psychosocial factors. *Diabetes Care* 2003;26:1468–74.

16 Molaison EF. Stages of change in clinical nutrition. *Nutr Clin Care* 2002;5:251–257.

17 Miller WR and Rollnick S, *Motivational Interviewing: Preparing People for Change,* 2nd *ed.* New York, NY: Guilford Publishing; 2002.

18 Miller WR and Rollnick S, *What is MI?* http://www.motivationalinterview.org/clinical/whatismi.html (accessed 07/07/2006).

19 Miller WR. Motivation for treatment: A review with special emphasis on alcoholism. *Psych Bull.* 1985;98:84–107.

20 Rogers CR. A theory of therapy, personality, and interpersonal relationships, as developed in the client-centered framework. *Psychology: The Study of a Science* 1959;3:184–256.

21 Egan G. *The Skilled Helper: A Problem-Management Approach to Helping.* 7th ed. Pacific Grove, CA: Brooks-Cole Publishing Co; 2001.

22 Coulehan JL Block MR. *The Medical Interview: Mastering Skills for Clinical Practice.* 4th Ed. F.A.Davis, Phila; 2001.

23 Miller LE, Seltzer J.A test of the relationship between self-efficacy and burnout. *J Health Hum Resour Adm* 1991;13(4):483–8.

24 Zimmerman GL, Olsen CG, Bosworth MF. A 'Stages of Change' approach to helping patients change behavior. *Am Fam Physician* 2000;61:1409–16.

25 Rimal RN. Closing the Knowledge-Behavior Gap in Health Promotion: The Mediating Role of Self-Efficacy. *Health Communication* 2000;12(3):219–37.

26 Becker MH. *The Health Beliefs Model and Personal Health Behavior* Thorofare, NJ: CB Slack, Inc., 1974.

27 Keller VF, White MK. Choices & Changes: A New Model for Influencing Patient Health Behavior. *J Clin Outcomes Manage* 1997;4(6):33–36.

28 Ockene IS, Hebert JR, Ockene JK, Saperia GM, Stanek E, Nicolosi R, Merriam PA, Hurley TG. Effect of physician-delivered nutrition counseling training and an office-support program on saturated fat intake, weight, and serum lipid measurements in a hyperlipidemic population: Worcester Area Trial for Counseling in Hyperlipidemia (WATCH). *Arch Intern Med.* 1999 Apr 12;159(7):725–31.

29 Moore, H, Adamson AJ, Gill T, Waine C. Nutrition and the health care agenda: A primary care perspective. *Family Practice.* 2000;17:197–202.

30 Eaton CB, Goodwin MA, Stange KC. Direct observation of nutrition counseling in community family practice. *Am J Prev Med.* 2002 Oct;23(3):174–9.

CHAPTER 16

Community counts

Kathryn M Kolasa

Physicians have a tradition of social advocacy and primary care physicians have a record of achievement in advocating for policies that impact the quality and quantity of life of their patients. Primary care clinicians often advocate for patients in conflicts with managed care companies and many are involved in the political process advocating for health care reform. They have helped achieve significant reductions in tobacco, motor vehicle, and bicycle morbidity and mortality by testifying before policy makers, advocating to the public and advising patients [1]. Family medicine specialty has long recognized its responsibility in the realm of nutrition for the prevention and treatment of disease, and recognition of that responsibility has required nutrition training in residency [2]. Research confirms that family physicians recognize that nutrition counseling is their responsibility, even when they are not entirely comfortable and confident with the advice they give for lifestyle change.

The chronic diseases that represent the majority of the office visits to primary care doctors are not going to be cured simply by what happens in the clinician's office. Communities, families and individuals have to be involved in creating an environment that promotes healthy lifestyles. Physicians can play an important role in helping to shape community policies.

In order to address the lifestyle-related health problems of today, physicians must act in more than just the office setting. The socio-ecological model (Fig. 16.1) describes the areas (e.g. public policy, community, organizations, family and individual) where change is needed. Primary care providers have a role within the office practice but this usually falls at the "individual level". For example, reports that highlight the childhood obesity epidemic have heightened the visibility and credibility of healthy eating and physical activity as public health issues, and the need for policies and environments that support these behaviors at the organization, community and public policy levels.

Effective lifestyle counseling by the primary care physician

This chapter focuses on the role of the healthcare provider in promoting and supporting the environmental and policy changes needed to ensure that individuals can make desired lifestyle changes for health. However, it is important to reflect on the traditional role of the primary care physician in the office setting

Ecological Model

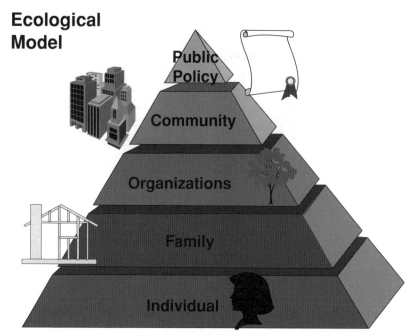

Figure 16.1 Socio-ecological model representing the positive and negative influences on the eating and physical activity behaviors of an individual.

where nutrition and lifestyle assessment, and prescriptions, are provided. Most office-based nutrition and physical activity interventions are delivered to the individual or family. Physicians, nurses, and nutritionists assess dietary and physical activity habits of patients, and then counsel them on potential modifications (such as increasing fruits and vegetables or decreasing saturated fat intake, etc.). Usually this occurs in one-on-one counseling, but can also occur in group visits or classes. Those health care providers who report the most success are those who first routinely assess diet, physical activity, and weight and then endeavor to tailor the lifestyle prescription to the ability and willingness of the patient to follow recommendations.

To effectively counsel patients on healthy eating and physical activity, physicians and their staff need current, evidence-based information to provide to their patients. They need to follow practice guidelines that include annual monitoring of patients' weight, plotting the body mass index (BMI) of children on growth charts, measuring waist circumference, and encouraging the DASH (Dietary Approaches to Stopping Hypertension) diet for patients with prehypertension. Culturally sensitive and language appropriate patient education materials need to be available and utilized. When appropriate, physicians can refer patients to a nutrition specialist, the registered dietitian. As health care advisors, clinicians have the access and authority to influence families' awareness of obesity as a health concern and to offer guidance on pursuing healthful dietary habits and regular physical activity [3].

Unfortunately, physicians rarely engage in continuing medical education programs covering nutrition topics [4]. Physicians need to become committed to obtaining and providing evidence-based nutrition and physical activity advice with the steady stream of newly published dietary studies. Careful study of dietary fads or trends is required so that physicians do not inadvertently add to patients' confusion about healthy eating. Additionally, primary care physicians need to adopt effective counseling techniques, such as motivational interviewing, that aim to help patients change behavior [5]. Styles of questioning that are non confrontational and focused on problem solving and goal setting help patients think of ways to overcome difficulties in changing targeted behaviors. (See Chapter 15.)

The healthcare environment

It requires more than a skilled clinician and a motivated patient to achieve diet and physical activity changes. The environment, including the health care environment, must support healthy behaviors. Primary care physicians can audit their office and health care environment to see if change is warranted. Environmental change describes changes to physical and social environments that provide new or enhanced supports for healthy behaviors. An environmental change is one that makes it easier for people to be aware of their health and to make health promoting choices. Are weight scales, measuring tapes, BMI charts or tools readily available? Do electronic medical records have templates for nutrition and physical activity data entry and teaching? Are behavioral goals charted so they can be followed up on? Is there a commitment to weigh, measure, and chart the height, weight, BMI and waist circumference of patients as vital signs? Do available patient education materials support changes being recommended? Do waiting room magazines, videos or television programming support evidence-based healthy eating and physical activity messages? Is water available in the waiting room? Is there a room for women to breastfeed or pump?

The American Academy of Family Physicians (AAFP) initiated a three year plan to make the family doctor's office the healthiest office in America. During year one, the focus was on the physician as a role model. In year two, the office staff was challenged to walk more and eat less. And in the years leading up to 2010, the plan is to extend to these efforts to the patients [6] (www.aafp.org). AAFP has set important goals for its membership to achieve by 2010, including to (1) improve their own personal level of fitness as a role model for their patient and practice population; (2) gain the necessary knowledge to help patients make positive changes in their health status, and, (3) know how to access tools and resources to combat the obesity epidemic. The AAFP program is connected to the nationwide Americans in Motion [7] (www.AIM.com) effort which encourages people to walk an extra 2000 steps per day and eat 100 fewer calories. Even though the AAFP program is limited to its membership, anyone can join AIM.

An assessment of all aspects of the practice environment is important. What foods and beverages are available during the workday or in vending machines? Are non-food or non-candy rewards given to pediatric patients? Are water and other healthy food options available for conferences and staff meetings? If sales representatives and vendors provide lunches or snacks, is there a policy that they provide health-promoting meals or, as a minimum, provide a piece of fruit along with the pizza? Are there incentives for staff to participate in health promoting activities (e.g. complimentary pedometers, reduced health insurance premiums, vacation days)? Are stretching and walking breaks possible? Is there a policy at the hospital to have healthy options available in the cafeteria, on the hospital cart and in other hospital venues? Do vending machines have appropriate size portions of beverages and snacks available? Once an office environmental assessment is completed, the physician and office staff should develop a plan to improve the environment which they can control. They may also want to highlight the changes being made as part of a practice marketing strategy to help raise patient awareness. Physicians can exert significant control over their office environments and should be vocal advocates for healthy change in all work settings (schools, hospitals, worksites, etc.).

Local efforts

Combating obesity can be overwhelming. Physicians report frustration that patients are not adherent to lifestyle change recommendations and admit to little satisfaction in providing weight management services [8]. Efforts to create a supportive community environment can make a significant difference. Adults and children need communities that are conducive to supporting healthy eating and regular physical activity. At times, even when the patient understands and is motivated to implement recommendations, a variety of barriers may keep them from doing so. These factors include the physical and social environments of their communities and organizations, the policies, practices and norms within their social and works settings, and their access to information. Healthcare providers, then, must move outside of the exam room and advocate for social and environmental policies that will promote healthy weight for everyone.

The public health sector has already moved from just providing direct services and has recognized the need to impact policies and environments [9]. Increasingly, the school sector is recognizing that the missions of education and healthcare are merging in the childhood obesity prevention as witnessed by the attention being paid to physical activity and improved child nutrition programs. The environmental and policy changes sought, contribute to behavior change by making it easier for people to engage in the desirable behaviors while making it more difficult to engage in competing and less desirable behaviors. Consider how effective the environmental and social changes addressing tobacco have been over the past 20 years. Policy change generally describes modifications to laws, regulations, formal and informal rules as well as standards of practice. It includes fostering both written and unwritten policies, practices and incentives that provide new or enhanced supports for healthy behaviors and lead to changes in community and societal norms. For example, a policy change related to healthy eating could include a coach encouraging post-game healthy snacks (e.g. orange slices, grapes, raisins, flavored waters). This makes it easier for parents to avoid the child's perceived embarrassment of being the only kid that didn't bring soda and chips.

A faith-based community could have a policy to provide water and healthy food options at all events allowing people with diabetes to participate and still adhere to their dietary prescription. The North Carolina Eat Smart Move More program [10] is one initiative that shares community success stories. See www.eatsmartmovenc.com for additional examples of informal policy changes made at the community level. Policies to support healthy eating and physical activity can also take the form of regulation, many related to school physical activity and food standards, and can be adopted at the local level. Organizations like "Trust for America's Health" (TAH) [11] (www.healthyamericans.org/reports/obesity) argue that current obesity policies are failing in America. Data describing related legislative issues for each state can be found on the TAH website. The National Conference of State Legislatures maintains a list of childhood obesity policy options on its website (www.ncsl.org) [12].

The childhood obesity crisis as a motivator for action

Most experts suggest that the obesity epidemic will be solved at the local level. While the rates of adult obesity have been rising for many years, the current childhood obesity crisis – the increased incidence of type 2 diabetes among youth and other complications of obesity – appear to be motivating leaders across the nation to become involved. Healthcare providers need to be outspoken on children's nutrition needs and habits, obesity, and diabetes. If the talk about a childhood obesity epidemic is to be believed, civic leaders expect primary care providers to validate the concerns and raise awareness of healthful eating and physical activity with civic organizations, business leaders, school leaders, and parents.

Taking action: Join or build coalitions

An important way professional organizations work to affect public policy is through participation in coalitions and other collaborative efforts with related health groups. Such collaborative efforts provide a means through which professional organizations can effectively apply their resources in concert with others and focus them collectively toward a common goal.

The American Academy of Pediatrics (AAP) issued guidelines for the prevention of pediatric overweight and obesity in 2003 [13]. Its major advocacy recommendations include:

1) Help parents, teachers, coaches, and others who influence youth to discuss health habits, not body habitus, as part of their efforts to control overweight and obesity.

2) Enlist policy makers from local, state and national organizations and schools to support a healthful lifestyle for all children, including proper diet and adequate opportunity for regular physical activity.

3) Encourage organizations that are responsible for health care and health care financing to provide coverage for effective obesity prevention and treatment strategies.

4) Encourage public and private sources to direct funding toward research into effective strategies to prevent overweight and obesity and to maximize limited family and community resources to achieve healthful outcomes for youth.

5) Support and advocate for social marketing intended to promote healthful food choices and increased physical activity.

Check professional organizations for their advocacy. For example, the American Academy of Family Physicians (www.aafp.org) [6] has outlined 10 steps for addressing the childhood obesity epidemic at the community level. They are:

1) Students, parents, educators, family physicians, school nurses, school nutritionists, and community leaders should be involved in assessing the schools' eating environment; developing a shared vision and an action plan to achieve it.

2) Adequate funds should be provided by local, state and federal sources to ensure that the total school environment supports the development of healthy eating patterns.

3) Behavior-focused nutrition education should be integrated into the curriculum from pre-K through grade 12 and staff who provide nutrition education should have appropriate training.

4) School meals should meet the USDA (United States Department of Agriculture) nutritional standards as well as provide sufficient choices, including new and newly prepared foods, to meet the taste and cultural preferences of diverse student populations.

5) All students should have designated lunch periods of sufficient length to enjoy healthy foods with friends and these lunch periods will be scheduled as near to the middle of the school day as possible.

6) Schools should provide enough serving areas to ensure student access to school meals with a minimum amount of wait time.

7) Space that is adequate to accommodate all students and pleasant surroundings that reflect the value of the social aspects of eating should be provided.

8) Students, teachers and community volunteers who practice healthy eating should be encouraged to serve as role models in the dining areas.

9) If foods are sold in addition to National School Lunch Program meals, they should be from the five major food groups to foster healthy eating patterns.
10) Decisions regarding the sale of foods in addition to the National School Lunch Program meals should be based on nutrition goals, not on profit-making.

The American Dietetic Association has several position papers outlining strategies to support healthy eating and physical activity [14] (www.eatright .org). This dietetic professional organization also has public policy strategies to reduce the prevalence of obesity and overweight that include:
1) Promote healthy weight for children, emphasizing family and community based interventions that promote healthful eating practices and daily physical activity.
2) Designate obesity a disease by federal agencies and insurers.
3) Support multidisciplinary health initiatives over a substantial period of time, with registered dietetic professionals placed to bring their particular knowledge and skills to bear.
4) Increase funding for basic, translational and outcomes research.
5) Ensure continued, current and adequate monitoring and data collection of food intake, eating behavior and health status.
6) Involve stakeholders to achieve a coordinated effort to address the issue at a national as well as local level.
7) Create and support programs integrating both nutrition and physical activity, and support the individual to be able to make wise lifestyle choices.

Other nationwide organizations, such as Shape Up America, Action for Healthy Kids (AFHK) have state affiliates dedicated to improving the health and educational performance of children through better nutrition and physical activity in school [15] (www.actionforhealthykids.org). In 2005, the Centers for Disease Control and Prevention published a task force report on obesity prevention in schools and worksites [16].

Is there a plan for your community? Find and study the plan

Healthcare providers willing to become advocates should become familiar with action plans that have been developed. In 2001, the U.S. Surgeon General issued a "Call to Action to Prevent and Decrease Overweight and Obesity" [17] (www.surgeongeneral.gov/library). More recently, the Institute of Medicine's action plan, "Preventing Childhood Obesity: Health in the Balance" described population-based strategies [18]. The health departments in many states have also developed plans. To determine if a plan exists in your state to improve policies and environments to support healthy eating and physical activity, check on the local health department's website. Links to state health departments can be found at the United States Department of Health and Human Services' web site [19] (www.dhhs.state.<*state's initials*>.us). The "Nutrition" link will lead to services such as Women, Infant and Children Program (WIC) and other special feeding programs. There might also be a plan for policy and environmental change as well. However, depending on the organization of the state health department, you may need to search for the health promotions branch or section.

Twenty-eight states have been funded by the Centers for Disease Control and Prevention (CDC) DC Division of Nutrition and Physical Activity's National Nutrition, Physical Activity and Obesity Prevention program to develop and implement evidence-based interventions. Twenty-three states were funded for capacity building, and 5 additional states for basic implementation [20] (www.cdc.gov/nccdphp/dnpa). The program's major goals are balancing caloric intake and expenditure; increasing physical activity; improving nutrition through increased consumption of fruits and vegetables; reducing television time; and increasing breastfeeding. Materials from the CDC are available for all states. A resource guide [21] (www.cdc.gov) includes obesity prevention and control (including caloric intake and expenditure), increased physical activity, improved nutrition (including increased breastfeeding and increased consumption of fruits and vegetables), and reduced television time.

Areas where primary care physicians can provide leadership

Several strategies for confronting the childhood obesity epidemic have gained momentum in local communities and four will be described.

BMI report cards

The state of Arkansas made nationwide news when it decided to send Health Report Cards home. In some states, this action was mandated by the state legislature [22] (www.achi.net/current_initiatives/obesity.asp). Some additional states and local communities are following suit. However not all agree that sending report cards is an effective action [23]. Some groups, such as the North Dakota Healthy Weight Council, are preparing position papers to discourage the measurement of children's weight in schools. Physicians can contribute to the debate by evaluating the evidence for potential benefit and harm. If the local decision is made to pursue BMI screening, healthcare providers can work to ensure that the measurements and reporting are done in a sensitive manner and that the collected data are put to positive use. In Arkansas, the mass screening identified the extent of the obesity epidemic among school-age youth. The experience provides a detailed protocol and equipment needed for accurate mass measurement of students [24]. The challenge remains to set goals and monitor outcomes.

Chomitz and colleagues [25] published the first report evaluating risks and benefits associated with using a health report card to inform families about the results of routine BMI screening in schools. The authors concluded that among overweight children, the health report card did increase parental awareness of their child's weight status. But the authors commented that more research is needed to determine the impact of this approach on children's discomfort, self esteem and plans to initiate weight controlling activities. Parent's reactions ranged from disinterest to angry to thankful.

Both the state of Michigan [26] and the Center for Weight and Health at UC Berkeley [27] have published advice on respectful weight screening. Healthcare providers can be involved in training those who will collect the heights and weights to ensure accuracy. They can discuss the need to avoid labeling students, maintaining privacy and confidentiality. Sample letters to parents are available and can be adapted to the situation and physicians can provide leadership for this task and work for understanding that use of the BMI-for-Age is for a screening tool not for diagnosis. Pediatric healthcare providers need to be prepared for parent calls and questions and should seek to build a referral system for further evaluation of children who have no primary care physician. They too can join efforts in determining local programs to address the outcome. Healthcare providers might outline consistent messages that could be included in the report card letter. These messages might be localized but could include strategies such as: increase physical activity to 60 minutes per day, decreasing television and non-productive screen time to less than 2 hours per day, increasing fruit and vegetable intake, decreasing soda and other sweetened beverages, decreasing portion size, eating breakfast, and drinking more low-fat milk and water.

One natural outcome of the screening is the need for treatment services. There is evidence that weight management programs that involve parents can be safe and effective [17,18]. The physician might play a role in planning programs and identifying support from local foundations. The Society for Nutrition Education [30] has outlined guidelines for developing programs that set health, rather than weight, as a goal (www.sne.org/Chi_Obesity.pdf).

In most states, there is limited or no third party reimbursement for weight management services. Physicians need to be active in advocating to insurance companies, state Medicaid officials and others, the need for reimbursement for weight management services for youth at risk for not achieving a healthy weight [18].

School wellness policies

In the 2004 reauthorization of the Child Nutrition and WIC program, a new clause was added that required all school districts with a federally funded school meals program to develop and implement wellness policies that address nutrition and physical activity. This is an important opportunity for the physician advocate. School districts ideally will write policies that meet local needs and reflect community priorities. The National Alliance for Nutrition and Activity has provided model policies that can be adapted [31] (www.SchoolWellnessPolicies.org). Physicians can serve on school health advisory committees or act as consultants in the development and implementation of policies.

Physical activity and physical education in school

Most experts agree that children and youth need 60 minutes of physical activity daily. Many suggest that at least 30 minutes should be during the school day. It is important to distinguish between physical activity and physical education. Does the state have a physical activity policy? How is it implemented at the local level? They can provide leadership for creating and implementing physical activity policies at the local level. Healthcare providers can provide leadership to encourage local groups and foundations to support the creation and maintenance of walking trails and other equipment to support physical activity. Healthcare providers can become members of, or act as consultants to, school health advisory councils and encourage the adoption of active recess (www.choices4health.org) and other policies.

The goal of school physical education programs is to produce an individual who has the knowledge, skill and confidence to enjoy a lifetime of healthful physical activity. Physical education is a curricular area that teaches about physical activity. It is the only curricular subject that develops a child's physical self. States have recommendations for physical education. It is generally about 150 minutes per week for elementary school and at least 225 minutes/week for middle and high school. It is important to note that students who participate in physical education programs do not experience harmful effects on their standardized test scores. Physical activity is a behavior that is part of the solution to childhood obesity.

"No Child Left Behind"

The "No Child Left Behind" (NCLB) legislation [32] (www.ed.gov) has had some unintended consequences. In some communities coaching positions are at risk to keep other "highly qualified teachers." Physical education is decreasing in class time and increasing in class size. This legislation does not list physical education as a "core" subject. Physicians can advocate for physical education using certified physical education teachers and a student–teacher ratio that is consistent with other classrooms; and include adequate facilities. Physicians can also advocate for physical activity with schools offering daily opportunities for structured (during class time) and unstructured (during recess) physical activity. Local boards and superintendents often have the power/authority in this realm and the physician can supply the evidence of efficacy for health. Clinicians interested in more information on programs in this area are referred to the Institute of Medicine's reports on Progress in Preventing Childhood Obesity: Focus on Schools – Brief summary [18] (www.10m-edu/cms/3788/25044/30355, 32913 also .aspx).

Primer for those interested in working on school meal and nutrition education programs

While there are a multitude of factors contributing to the childhood obesity epidemic, many point to the school environment as both a major cause and the easiest setting to fix. It is important to become knowledgeable about the local school food standards and physical activity before criticizing them. While the federally supported child nutrition program provides health promoting foods in age appropriate portions, a number of forces have created a competitive food environment in the schools. Until the late 1970's, child nutrition programs thrived as the "right thing to do for children." But in the 1980's these programs were devastated by major federal budget cuts which shifted the responsibility of feeding school age children to the local communities and charities.

In the 1990's *a la carte* programs were thriving as children developed appetite for the supplemental foods sold and schools developed an appetite for the revenues generated. In the past 30 years there has been a shift in priorities surrounding the Child Nutrition Program. A debate about priorities is needed at the local, state and federal level. Generally, foods sold in competition with the prescribed child nutrition program meal plan are of limited nutritional value and compromise nutrition integrity. Citizens must work to influence the environment in their local schools. Before launching into a crusade to "take all junk foods out of school", it is important to identify the state plan for standards served in schools. In most states, these plans are not mandates but rather guidelines for local districts to follow.

One model plan, which is based on school improvement plan processes, was developed by partnering agencies in North Carolina: "Recommended Standards for All Foods Available in School." It is a blueprint for gradual change that is grade specific, addresses meals, *a la carte*, vending and school events, encourages local policy development, and promotes total school involvement [33] (www.eatsmartmovemorenc.com/tools.htm). In some cases, enforcing already existing federal or state policies, such as the competitive foods rule that says the sale or serving of any food or beverage in competition with the school breakfast or lunch program shall be prohibited on the school campus during the school day until the last child is served lunch for the day, would be a marked improvement. In other schools, optimal food standards meeting the 2005 *Dietary Guidelines for Americans* [34] would be the goal. Barriers to optimal nutrition environment are money, administrative support, lack of value attributed to nutrition as part of the instructional day, limited time and space for meals, student taste preferences, too little nutrition education to influence children's eating habits, and conflicting messages.

In addition to standards, healthcare providers working with local school boards and school superintendents can influence food and beverage contracts to ensure that more healthful choices are available in vending machines outside of the cafeteria. Healthcare providers can also offer suggestions for alternative fund raising events that support health [35] (www.fns.usda.gov/tn/HealthyExecSummary_RevenueInfo.pdf).

There are a plethora of excellent nutrition education curriculums available for use in schools [36] (www.nal.usda.gov). Many of these integrate nutrition into core subjects like reading and math. Unfortunately these curriculums are under utilized. Physicians and other health care providers can and should be advocates for nutrition education in the schools.

Conclusion

To date, consensus has not been reached on the effectiveness of school-based nutrition interventions [37] (Guide to Community Preventive Services: www.thecommunityguide.org/nutrition). Healthcare providers must speak out in support of policies that improve physical activity and healthy eating. They can adopt, in their own practice and environments under their control, healthy eating and physical activity standards and practices. They can work to make their health care facilities serve as model environments for healthy eating and physical activity. They can move outside the exam room and contact public officials to provide evidence for community change to improve opportunities for healthy eating and physical activity for all segments of the population. They can testify in support of legislation. They can contact their legislators, they can lobby, and they can vote. Healthcare providers can respond to news stories, write letters to the editor, and appear on radio and television shows to provide the health care perspective on the need for environmental and policy changes to support healthy eating and physical activity.

References

1 Kleinman LC. Health care in crisis. *JAMA* 1991;265:1991–2.
2 Deen D, Spencer E, Kolasa KM. Nutrition education in family practice residency programs. *Family Medicine* 2003;35(2):105–11.
3 Institute of Medicine. *Preventing Childhood Obesity: Health in the Balance*. National Academy of Sciences. National Academies Press, Washington, DC. 2004.
4 Kolasa KM. "Images" of nutrition in medical education and primary care. *Am J Clin Nutr* 2001;73:1006–9.
5 Dunn C, Deroo L, Rivara FP. The use of brief interventions adapted from motivational interviewing across behavioral domains: a systematic review. *Addiction* 2002;96:1725–42.
6 American Academy Family Physicians. *Healthy Eating in Schools. Policy and Advocacy*. www.aafp.org 2004.
7 American Academy Family Physicians. *AIM Project*. www.aafp.org
8 Soltesz KS, Price JH, Johnson LW, Telljohann SK. Perceptions and practices of family physicians regarding diet and cancer. *Am J Prev Med* 1995;11:197–204.
9 Center for Disease Control. Association of State and Territorial Directors of Health Promotion and Public Health Education. *Policy and Environmental Change: New Directions for Public Health*. Santa Cruz, CA: ToucanEd. www.toucaned.com 2001.
10 Center for Disease Control. *Resource Guide for Nutrition and Physical Activity Interventions to Prevent Obesity and Other Chronic Diseases*. www.cdc.gov 2003.
11 Trust for America's Health. www.healthyamericans.org.
12 The National Conference of State Legislatures. www.ncsl.org
13 Krebs NF, Jacobson MS. American Academy of Pediatrics Committee on Nutrition. Prevention of pediatric overweight and obesity. *Pediatrics* 2003;112(2):424–30. www.aap.org.
14 American Dietetic Association. Policies. www.eatright.org
15 Shape Up America, Action for Healthy Kids. www.actionforhealthykids.org
16 North Carolina Division of Public Health. *North Carolina Blueprint for Changing Policies and Environments in Support of Healthy Eating*. Raleigh, NC 2002. www.EatSmartMoveMoreNC.com.

17 U.S. Department of Health and Human Services. *The Surgeon General's Call to Action to Prevent and Decrease Overweight and Obesity*, 2001. Rockville, MD: US Department of Health and Human Services, Public Health Service, Office of the Surgeon General.

18 Institute of Medicine. *Progress in Preventing Childhood Obesity: Focus on Schools-Brief Summary.* www.iom-edu.

19 United States Department of Health and Human Services' web site. www.dhhs.state. <*state's initials*>.us

20 Division of Nutrition and Physical Activity at the Centers for Disease Control and Prevention www.cdc.gov.

21 Centers for Disease Control and Prevention www.cdc.gov.

22 Arkansas Health Report Cards project www.achi.net.

23 Scheier LM. School health report cards attempt to address the obesity epidemic. *J Am Diet Assoc* 2004 Mar;104:341–4.

24 Gance-Cleveland B, Bushmaiaeer M. Arkansas school nurses' role in statewide assessment of body mass index to screen for overweight children and adolescents. J *School Nursing* 2005;21(2):64–9.

25 Chomitz VR, Collins J, Kim J, Kramer E, McGowan R. Promoting health weight among elementary school children via a Health Report Card approach. *Arch Pediatr Adolesc* 2003;157:765–72.

26 Michigan Department of Education. *The role of Michigan schools in promoting healthy weight. A consensus paper.* Sept 2001. Michigan Department of Education. Lansing, MI.

27 Center for Weight and Health at Berkeley. *Guidelines for Collecting Heights and Weights on Children and Adolescents in School Settings.* www.cnr.berkeley.edu September 2000.

28 Summerbell CD, Ashton V, Campbell KJ, Edmunds L, Kelly S, Waters E. Interventions for treating obesity in children. *Cochrane Database of Systematic Reviews.* Jan 2005. Accession Number 00075320-100000000-01255.

29 Campbell K, Waters E, O'Meara S, Kelly S, Summberbell C. Interventions for preventing obesity in children. *Cochrane Database of Systematic Reviews.* Jan 2005. Accession Number 00075320-100000000-01259.

30 Society for Nutrition Education. Weight Realities Division. *Guidelines for Childhood Obesity Prevention Programs: Promoting Healthy Weight in Children.* www.sne.org and www.healthyweight.net October 2002.

31 National Alliance for Nutrition and Activity. *Model Local School Wellness Policies on Physical Activity and Nutrition.* www.SchoolWellnessPolicies.org March 2005.

32 "No Child Left Behind" legislation (US). www.ed.gov.

33 North Carolina dietary and exercise documents, including school food standards www.eatsmartmovemorenc.com/tools.htm.

34 US Dept. of Health and Human Services, US Dept. of Agriculture. *Dietary Guidelines for Americans.* 2005. www.healthierus.gov. USDA Publication No. Home and Garden Bulletin 232. U.S. Govt. Printing Office, Washington DC.

35 USDA Nutrition Assistance programs www.fns.usda.gov.

36 The National Agricultural Library www.nal.usda.gov.

37 Guide to Community Preventive Services. CDC. www.thecommunityguide.org.

Further reading

Institute of Medicine. Progress in Preventing Childhood Obesity: How do we measure up? National academy of Sciences. National Academies Press. Washington, DC 2006.

Steps to a Healthier US. www.cdc.gov/nccdphp/programs/steps.htm.

Olshansky SJ, Passaro DJ, Hershow RC *et al*. A potential decline in life expectancy in the United States in the 21st century. *N Engl J Med* 2005;352:1138–45.

Price JH, Tellojohann SK. Perceptions and practices of family physicians regarding diet and cancer. *Am J Prev Med* 1995;11:197–204.

Public Health Strategies for Preventing and Controlling Overweight and Obesity in School and Worksite Settings. MMWK2005;54(RRIO:1-12.) www.cdc.gov/mmwr/preview/mmwrhtm/rr5410al.htm.

CHAPTER 17

Cultural considerations

Kim M Gans and Charles B Eaton

Health- and diet-related attitudes and behaviors are primarily determined by cultural, psychosocial, and socioeconomic factors [1]. The cultural milieu that affects a person's diet includes: the rules surrounding the person's upbringing, whether or not the person immigrates to a new society, the degree of acculturation to the new society, and the degree to which traditional foods in the culture of origin are available in the new society [2]. The meanings and uses assigned to foods in a particular culture may be unique to that culture, even though the foods themselves are commonly available and may have different or no special meaning in other cultures [3]. Culture influences many food-related behaviors including food choice, food purchasing, preparation, where and with whom food is eaten, health beliefs related to food, and adherence to dietary recommendations [1,4–6].

Culturally competent health care builds upon the understanding of these cultural influences and facilitates the development of stronger patient–provider relationships with higher levels of trust. This has been shown to be associated with increased use of recommended preventive services in low-income Black/African–American (BA)women. Therefore, understanding the sociocultural context of health for individual patients is very important for effective health care, as culture may influence health knowledge, attitudes, and behaviors, including diet.

The diverse population

The US has become increasingly diverse in the last century, and projections indicate that ethnic minorities will make up one-third of the US population by 2015 and nearly half of the population by 2050. The current US population is 75% white, 12% Black /African-American (BA), 4% Asian and Pacific Islander (API) and 9% other or multiple races [7]. In addition, 12.5% of the population identify as having Hispanic ethnicity. Since 1980, the number of Hispanics in the US has grown five times faster than the rest of the population, making the US the third largest Spanish-speaking country in the world [8]. APIs are the fastest-growing US minority group, having increased by 179% since 1980. In 2000, 1.7 million people in the US identified themselves as South Asians [7].

South Asian cultures include people from India, Pakistan, Bangladesh, and Sri Lanka. The majority of immigrants to the US from South Asia are from India [9].

Cultural issues related to diet

Although distinct populations, the major ethnic minorities in the US have some common cultural beliefs that impact their health behavior. These include strong family values, involvement with complementary and alternative medicine (folk medicine), and strong religious background or spirituality [10–12].

Inclusion of family members in medical decision-making is seen as crucial to many ethnic minority groups [11], but is sometimes overlooked by physicians. Involving the entire family in dietary counseling, especially those who regularly cook the meals, can improve patient compliance. With a child's treatment, it is helpful to involve both parents and sometimes grandparents. Because the family's needs are often considered ahead of the individual's, independence may not be valued, so personal health may be less of a motivator than being a caretaker or role model for the family [4,13–15]. To fully understand difficulties encountered with dietary adherence, primary care providers should explore the role of family support and provide family-level interventions whenever possible.

Although Western cultures rely on science to explain illness and treat disease, other cultures focus more on the spiritual causes of illness with some using home remedies for an illness before visiting a doctor. For example, traditional African-American folk health beliefs describe high blood pressure as "high blood," and remedies may include the ingestion of acid or astringent foods, such as lemon juice, vinegar, sour oranges, or brine from pickles or olives, to "bring the blood down" [12]. Moreover, home remedies such as herbal teas, garlic, and lemon juice may also be used to "bitter" the blood for those with diabetes [12]. Individuals who follow folk beliefs may avoid sharing their beliefs with health care providers. Thus, health care practitioners need to ask questions about the use of specific foods as home remedies. Careful, indirect questions are necessary to find out if your patient believes in such theories. In general, if a belief causes no harm, the provider need not address it; however, harmful practices, such as using high sodium foods to treat hypertension should be addressed [4,6,15,16]. Moreover, providers should encourage patients to use acceptable folk remedies in conjunction with medical treatment when appropriate.

Fatalism can also be an issue in health care. If patients feel powerless, they are less likely to believe that they can assume direct responsibility for their health [13]. Moreover, some ethnic minority groups (especially men) may only seek a health care provider's assistance after a disease has progressed – not for preventive care [1,17].

Creating a positive nutrition counseling relationship

Culture-based food habits are often one of the last traditions people change because they preserve ethnic identity. Therefore, assessing and addressing cultural issues surrounding food and food behaviors may be more likely to enhance permanent dietary change than simply "prescribing a diet" [2,5]. People of all cultural backgrounds can adhere to dietary recommendations; however, the issues and barriers to adherence vary. Clinicians should consider the challenges and barriers that some ethnic minorities and those with limited financial resources face when trying to adhere to a healthy diet and incorporate dietary messages that are culturally sensitive, motivating, and practical [6,18].

Research suggests that minority patients, especially foreign-born immigrants, are less likely than their White counterparts to receive physician advice on prevention and to receive empathy, information, and encouragement to participate in decision making [19–21]. When cultural and linguistic barriers in the clinical encounter negatively affect communication and trust, this leads to patient dissatisfaction, poor adherence, and poorer health outcomes [19,21]. Moreover, when providers fail to take social and cultural factors into account, they may resort to stereotyping, which could lead to biased or discriminatory treatment of patients based on their race/ethnicity, proficiency, or social status [21–23].

Culturally sensitive interviewing

With the huge array of cultures in the US, and the many powerful influences such as acculturation and socioeconomic status leading to intra-group variability, simply learning a set of "facts" about any particular cultural group will not lead to effectiveness in treating individual patients from this group [21]. Cultural competency includes not only possession of knowledge about and respect for different cultural perspectives including traditional dietary practices, but also having skills in cross-cultural communication and being able to use them effectively with patients from different cultural groups [15,16,21,23].

Research suggests that the first thing that a provider should do is to show respect and establish rapport. Place patients at ease by sitting down and maintaining eye contact. Show respect by greeting patients formally using surnames and title (e.g. Mr. and Mrs., unless the patient is a child) for the first meeting, and at all times for the elderly, rather than first names. If you are uncertain about how to pronounce a name, ask. Shake hands at the beginning of each appointment with a firm handshake that is held for several seconds.

Inquire about the patient and his or her family before asking more formal questions. These simple signs of respect will facilitate trust, a key factor in gaining acceptance for new dietary and lifestyle behaviors [6,15,16].

Interview tools have been developed that assist health professionals in obtaining patient information in a culturally unbiased manner [13,15,16,24].

These questions help to elicit information from the patient rather than making assumptions about patients' health beliefs, diet, etc. Use your professional judgment to decide which of the questions to ask. Let patients know that they should inform you if they prefer not to answer any of your questions.
• What do you call this problem you are having? (Use the word(s) the patient uses in place of the words "problem" and "it" in the next questions you ask.)
• What do you think is causing/caused this problem?
• How long have you had this problem(s)?
• Why do you think you have this problem?
• What do you think will help to clear up/treat your problem?
• What results do you hope to receive from treatment?
• How can I help you today?
• Is there anyone else in your family you'd like me to talk to?
• Apart from me, is there anyone else that you think can help you get better?
• What home remedies are common for this sickness? Have you used them?
• Is there anything else you would like me to know about so I can take better care of your health needs?
• Do you have any questions for me?

Before assessing the patient's diet and/or weight, it is helpful to first address the agenda with the patient by expressing the desire to talk about the patient's weight and/or eating habits and why you want to have this discussion [25]. The best approach is to seek the patient's agreement to discuss weight and elicit his/her thoughts about it. For example, *"Could we talk about your weight (eating habits) for a minute? Tell me your thoughts about your weight (eating habits) and health at this time."* If this doesn't elicit a response, follow-up with *"What role do you think your weight (eating habits) plays in your health?"* Tell the patient how risk factors and diet are interrelated. For example, *"I'd like to talk with you about how you are eating, because it can affect your blood cholesterol and your weight."* The terms "obesity" or "excess body fat" can be considered offensive, so instead use words like weight, excess weight or BMI.

Additional questions to understand food habits
• Can the foods you eat help your problem? Or make it worse? How?
• Please describe what you usually eat during the week and on weekends.
• Who does the food shopping and food preparation in your home?
• Do you eat certain foods to keep healthy? To make you strong?
• Do you avoid certain foods? Why?
• Do you balance eating some foods with other foods?
• Are there foods you won't eat? Why?
• How often do you eat traditional foods from your cultural heritage?
• Tell me about your favorite traditional foods so that we may include them in your eating pattern.
• What might make it difficult for you to change your eating habits?

Cross-cultural nutrition counseling

The most effective approach to cross-cultural nutrition counseling is implementing a five-step process of listening, explaining, acknowledging, recommending, and negotiating with the patient. This is called the LEARN approach [13,16,24]. Providing dietary counseling or advice to your patients takes time, but is worth the effort of helping patients to achieve better health as well as improving the doctor-patient relationship (also see Chapter 15).

• **Listen** Use active listening to demonstrate that what your patient has to say is very important to you. Pay attention to the tone and inflection of the speaker's words and the nuances of non-verbal cues as well as listening to the actual words. Be totally attentive to the patient instead of having an internal dialogue and rehearsing rebuttals or questions. Listen to the patient's perception of the problem. Clarify if necessary by saying, "I didn't quite understand that."

• **Explain** To make sure you understand accurately, restate (explain) what you think your patient said. Explain your interpretation of the patient's perception of the problem.

• **Acknowledge** Point out the similarities in what your patient believes and what you feel is appropriate in the cause and/or treatment of the problem. Then talk about the differences. Evaluate the scientific explanation with the patient's explanation to come to an understanding of the problem. For example, *"You told me that you are drinking herbal teas to lower your blood sugar. It is OK to keep doing this, but we also need to talk about important dietary changes you can make to lower your blood sugar."* Do not forego providing comprehensive explanations based on the assumption that patients will not understand them.

• **Recommend** Discuss several options for lifestyle (i.e. dietary) change that are culturally appropriate and practical. Strong, clear, and personalized advice is best. Also, give positive feedback for the healthful behaviors that the patient is already doing, which will help to build confidence.

• **Negotiate** Ask the patient which option(s) they would like to try and where they would like to begin. Negotiate a plan of action. Dietary changes should be gradual so that they can become part of a person's life, and not just a transient "diet." Help the patient set small and achievable goals. Engage participants in an interactive dialogue, encouraging them to discuss individual barriers as well as facilitators to dietary change. Elicit from the patient specific examples of how they can apply the recommendations to their own cultural practices and individual preferences. This collaboration not only empowers the participant, but also further educates the counselor about the culture.

Physicians may provide counseling themselves or provide assistance through the provision of written self-help materials (culturally appropriate and written in the patient's language) and/or referral to other healthcare providers, such as dietitians. Additional assistance is likely to produce better outcomes than advice-only treatment; however, physician advice alone has been shown to be more effective that no intervention at all.

When your patients don't speak English

While ethnicity concordance between patients and physicians has been shown to have little to no effect on physician–patient agreement about recommended changes in patient health behavior, language can be an important barrier [26]. Physicians who have access to trained interpreters report a significantly higher quality of patient–physician communication than physicians who use other methods, such as untrained staff or family members [21]. An ideal interpreter would be older than your patient and of the same gender [13]. Using children to interpret for parents should be a last resort. In general, it is helpful to have bilingual staff or volunteers interpret if a professional interpreter is not available [27]. Tips for working with a foreign language interpreter are shown in Table 17.1.

Health disparities

Though health indicators have improved for most Americans, ethnic minorities experience a disproportionate burden of preventable disease, death, and disability compared with non-minorities. These disparities are caused by

Table 17.1 How to work effectively with a foreign language interpreter.

* Ask patients if they prefer to use an interpreter even if their English seems adequate.
* Schedule enough time: a session with an interpreter will take longer than usual.
* Learn a few words in your patient's language (at least introductory greetings, thank you and good-bye).
* Look at and speak directly to the patient, not the interpreter. Some ethnic groups may show respect by avoiding eye contact with you; however, they will expect you to look directly at them.
* Speak slowly and clearly and in a conversational tone. Raising the volume of your voice will not enhance understanding and may be offensive.
* Speak in short units of speech – not long involved sentences or paragraphs.
* Avoid technical terminology, professional jargon, abstractions, slang, idioms and other expressions that would not be familiar to a non-native English speaker.
* Avoid saying to the interpreter, "Ask him . . ." or "Tell her . . ." Speak in first person.
* Listen to the patient and watch their nonverbal communication.
* Try to convey warmth and acceptance with your body language.
* Repeat important information more than once.
* Check the patient's understanding and accuracy of the translation by asking them to repeat important information in his or her own words, with the interpreter facilitating.
* Realize that the interpreter cannot reveal any information or opinions about the patients.
* Do ask the interpreter to clarify any cultural norms. When possible, reinforce verbal interaction with culturally appropriate materials written in patient's language and/or with visual aids.

Sources: [2,6,13,15,16,24,27].

inequalities in health care as well as a complex interplay of genetic, environmental, socioeconomic, and cultural factors [19].

In general, ethnic minority populations in the US have disproportionately higher rates of diet-related chronic disease, and many chronic disease risk factors [19,21]. Although some evidence suggests that genetic and physiologic differences among people from different cultures may influence illness and disease, health disparities are more likely caused by environmental, behavioral, and socio-political factors [21]. Rates of chronic disease have been shown to increase when the diets of developing countries become more "westernized" [28]. Moreover, migrant studies, which show that some chronic disease rates among migrants are intermediate between that of the country of origin and the adopted country, demonstrate that behavioral factors, such as diet, play a key role in the patterns of disease [29,30]. Among most immigrant groups, number of years of residence in the US is also associated with higher BMI [31,32]. The prevalence of obesity among immigrants living in the US for at least 15 years approaches that of US-born adults [31–33]. This association has been seen in all immigrant subgroups except foreign-born Black/African Americans [31]. This is likely due to adoption of a diet high in fat/calories and low in fruits and vegetables and a physically inactive lifestyle.

Black/African Americans

Disease prevalence

Cardiovascular disease (CVD), which includes coronary heart disease (CHD), stroke, hypertension, and congestive heart failure is the leading killer across most racial and ethnic minority communities in the US [34]. Black / African-Americans have the highest prevalence rates of CVD compared to non-Hispanic Whites (NHW) and Mexican-Americans (MA) [34]. BAs are more likely to have hypertension, CHD (women only), congestive heart failure, and stroke than NHWs and Hispanics/MAs [34,35].

The prevalence of type 2 diabetes has grown to epidemic proportions in the US, and racial and ethnic minority groups are disproportionately affected [36]. The risk of diabetes for Black/African-Americans and MAs is almost twice that for NHWs [34]. BAs have higher rates of diabetes complications, experience greater disability and have death rates attributable to diabetes at a rate 27% higher than Whites [37].

BAs have higher overall cancer mortality compared to other racial/ethnic groups in the US [38]. BA men also have higher incidence rates for all cancers than other groups [38]. In terms of specific cancers, prostate cancer, colorectal cancer and lung cancer have the highest incidence and death rates in BA populations [38]. Although the incidence of breast cancer is lower in BA than in White women, BA women have higher mortality rates than any other racial/ethnic group [38,39].

The prevalence of obesity has increased among all racial and ethnic groups [40]. Overweight and obesity are higher among BA and MA women than in

NHW women [34]. Among BA adults age 18 and older, approximately 70% are overweight or obese [34]. Abdominal (or central) obesity is more common among BA women as in NHW women [35]. BA and Hispanic children are also more likely to be overweight compared with other ethnic groups [34,41].

The prevalence of high blood pressure (HBP) in BA in the US is among the highest in the world. Among BA age 20 and older, 42% of men and 45% of women have HBP [34]. Potential explanations for the higher rates of HBP in BAs include pathophysiologic mechanisms; effect of family history; low socioeconomic status; excess weight; diets with low intake of calcium, potassium, magnesium, and high in fat and salt; and environmental factors such as high levels of chronic stress [42]. Among BA, 11% of men and 18% of women have blood cholesterol levels of 240 mg/dL or higher [34]. Additionally, the prevalence of no leisure-time physical activity is higher in BA compared with NHW [34].

Traditional cuisine of Black/African Americans

BAs are not a homogeneous group, and their dietary habits cannot simply be considered as one culture because their backgrounds, food habits, and traditions are varied. Health beliefs and dietary behaviors of BAs vary according to culture of origin, urban or rural residence, geographic location, social class, and age. However, in general, their dietary habits, food choices, and cooking methods have been distinctively influenced by both custom as well as past slavery and discrimination [3]. Dietary habits of BAs have mostly evolved from family members who lived in the southern US or the Caribbean Islands [5]. Slaves who were brought to the US combined their African cooking methods with British, Spanish, French and Native American techniques with whatever foods were available to produce a distinctive cuisine called "soul food" [4]. Soul food was based on using the parts of the animal not deemed suitable to put on the slave owners' table; for example, pig's feet, salt pork (fat renderings), and chitterlings (pork intestines) and it met the high energy needs of Black slaves performing hard labor [17].

Soul food emphasizes fried, roasted, and boiled food dishes using primarily chicken, pork, pork fat, organ meats, sweet potatoes, corn, and green leafy vegetables [1,4]. Many soul foods have true African roots, such as okra, yams, lentils, chick peas, kidney beans, watermelon, and black-eyed peas [17]. Staples of corn, rice, and beans, with high carbohydrate and fiber content, were important energy sources. For example, the bread and cereal group might include grits, macaroni, corn bread, biscuits, hominy, rice, or hush puppies. Meats, especially chicken, were a source of protein and fat, and dark green leafy vegetables (e.g., collard, turnip, mustard, or kale greens, and spinach) provided essential vitamins and minerals [17]. The liquid from the greens (*pot likker*), which is rich in nutrients, was often served with the greens. Other common foods included sausage, fried chicken and fish, okra, grits, peas, sweet potatoes, tomatoes, and squash. Meats such as pig's feet and chitterlings ("chitlins") are high in saturated fat; however, often it is the cooking method and not the foods themselves that contribute to the health problems [1]. Frying is a very popular cooking method. Meat, pork, and fish are traditionally fried in lard or bacon fat or oil, and vegetables and beans are traditionally cooked with some type of fat, often salt pork, fat back, bacon, or smoked ham hocks.

The current BA food environment has transitioned from a historic experience with a limited food supply to the experience of a great abundance of food available in modern urban settings [43]. Taste, convenience, and health concerns rather than hunger and scarcity are the factors that now drive BA food choices [43]. While soul foods may still be essential to food selection and eating behaviors among some BAs, this may not be true for others. Current issues in the BA diet include the ubiquitous availability of fast foods, snack foods, and convenience foods [43]. Eating at fast-food restaurants is very common among BAs and has been associated with higher fat and lower vegetable intakes in BAs [44].

Recent research has shown that compared with other ethnic groups, BAs had higher intakes of total and saturated fat and sodium and lower intakes of fruits, vegetables, whole grains, and milk [17]. Fewer than 50% of BAs meet the national dietary recommendations for most food groups [45]. BAs are more likely to have high intakes of processed meats, eggs, red meats, and high-fat dairy products than Whites, and less likely to have diets characterized by high intakes of green, leafy vegetables, salad dressings, tomatoes, other vegetables, cruciferous vegetables, and tea [46]. Another study found that BA participants had the highest prevalence of fat-related behaviors compared with NHW and Hispanic participants and were less likely to eat meatless meals, to modify their meals to make them lower in fat, and more likely than NHW participants to fry foods [14]. Lactose intolerance is also more common among BAs, which can result in a lower intake of dairy foods in the diet.

Barriers to eating a healthy diet in BA include: the perception that 'eating healthfully' means giving up cultural heritage and trying to conform to the dominant culture; lack of family and friend support; no sense of urgency; social and cultural symbolism of certain foods; the poor perceived taste of 'healthy' foods, the expense of 'healthy' foods; lack of information on basic nutrition topics such as serving sizes and reading food labels; and fatalism – "everything can cause disease and you have to die of something" [1,4,18,43]. In addition BAs, especially women, may overeat because of their own (or their parent's/grandparents) experiences with food scarcity [47]. Moreover, because BAs are oriented to adjust to environmental stresses, they may be more likely to eat in response to environmental cues (such as seeing food) rather than hunger. When the environment is full of unhealthy choices, this can be problematic [3].

Environmental barriers for low income BAs, as well as other low income ethnic minorities, include lack of supermarkets that carry fresh produce, many fast food establishments and small grocery stores that sell high-fat, energy-dense foods, and high neighborhood crime rates that discourage outdoor activities and limit safe places for physical activity [48]. Another important issue for BAs is the high prevalence of TV watching. BA households watch more TV than

the average American household [49], and one study showed that a significant proportion of BA girls' daily energy intake is consumed while watching
television [49].

The high incidence of diet-related diseases and risk factors among BAs
strongly suggests a need to adopt diets lower in total fat, saturated fat, and
salt and higher in whole grains and fiber. Specific dietary recommendations
are shown in Table 17.2.

Table 17.2 Dietary recommendations for Black Americans.

Eat more traditional high-fiber legumes, such as pinto beans and black-eyed peas, and green leafy
vegetables, such as collard and turnip greens, that are rich in fiber, vitamins and minerals.

Season beans and greens with herbs, onions, garlic, low-sodium chicken broth, and/or smoked
turkey, turkey bacon, or turkey ham rather than pork fat or ham hocks.

Bake, roast, broil, grill, or oven-fry chicken, turkey, or fish instead of frying, and remove skin from
turkey or chicken before cooking or eating.

Cook with canola, olive, or corn oil instead of lard, shortening, or animal fat and limit oil to less than
$^1/_4$ cup.

Choose extra lean ground beef or ground turkey breast instead of regular or lean ground beef.

Make mashed potatoes with low-fat or nonfat milk or buttermilk, and trans free, light margarine
instead of butter and sour cream; top baked potatoes with light or nonfat sour cream.

Make grits and hot cereals with less fat.

Get at least 3 servings of dairy products per day. Use low-fat or non-fat milk, cheese, sour cream,
buttermilk, yogurt, or soy milk instead of whole milk, cheese, sour cream. Use lactose-reduced
products if lactose intolerant.

For snacks, have baked tortilla and potato chips, low-salt pretzels, or air-popped popcorn without
butter instead of regular potato chips, pretzels, salted popcorn with butter.

For desserts, choose graham crackers, dried fruit, fig bars, gelatin desserts, pudding made with
low-fat milk, rice cakes, and use no-calorie sweeteners such as Splenda in baking.

Use low-fat or nonfat salad dressing or mayonnaise or flavored vinegar on salads. Use mustard or
ketchup instead of mayonnaise.

Choose fresh fruit or canned fruit packed in light syrup or juice instead of heavy syrup.

Eat processed meats less often and/or choose lower fat versions of processed meats such as lean
ham, turkey bacon, etc.

Choose water instead of sugar-sweetened sodas and fruit drinks.

To reduce sodium, season with herbs, spices, lemon, vinegar, garlic powder, and salt substitutes
instead of salt, salt pork, garlic salt, celery salt, and seasoning salt and choose lower sodium
processed foods.

Eat high sodium processed foods (smoked, cured, or canned meats; salt pork, ham hocks, pork
feet; cold cuts; salty snacks; canned soups or vegetables; bottled sauces; olives, pickles and
tomato products) less often or buy low sodium varieties.

Eat fast foods less often and make wiser choices at these restaurants such as small hamburgers,
baked or grilled chicken, salads with grilled chicken and light dressing, etc.

Follow guidelines of the DASH eating plan, which has been shown to substantially reduce blood
pressure, particularly among BA [50].

Source: Kim Gans, PhD, RD, Brown University and Lisa Hark, PhD, RD University of Pennsylvania
School of Medicine. 2007. Used with permission.

Note: Health professionals should never make generalizations about food patterns solely on the
basis of race or ethnicity. Although these food recommendations may be appropriate for many BA
patients, physicians need to do an assessment with each individual patient to determine individual
diet habits and counsel accordingly.

Hispanics

Disease prevalence

On average, Hispanics are 1.5 times more likely to have diabetes than NHW of similar age [51]. In the Hispanic population, diabetes rates are highest in MAs and Puerto Ricans. MAs are more than twice as likely to have diabetes as NHWs of similar age [51]. Approximately 24% of MAs, and 26% of Puerto Ricans between the ages of 45–74 years have diabetes [51]. Hispanic populations, particularly MAs also have the highest age-adjusted prevalence of metabolic syndrome (31.9%) compared to NHWs and BAs (23.8% and 21.6%, respectively [34].

Overweight and obesity are higher among MA and BA women than in NHW women. Hispanics also have higher rates of abdominal obesity compared with NHW [30]. Hispanic and BA children are more likely to be overweight compared with other ethnic groups and rates continue to rise [34,41].

Hispanics have lower CVD mortality rates than NHWs and BAs [34,36]. In addition, MAs reveal a slightly lower prevalence of high blood pressure [34,52]. MAs have a higher prevalence of hypertriglyceridemia than other ethnicities [53]. Among MAs, 18% of men and 14% of women have blood cholesterol levels of 240 mg/dL or higher [34]. Notably, Hispanics are less likely to know if they have high cholesterol levels [16].

The frequency of prostate cancer is significantly lower only in MAs, while incidence rates for Puerto Rican and Cuban Americans are comparable to those of NHW men [54]. Hispanic women have lower rates of breast cancer compared to NHW or BA women [38,55], but the incidence of cervical cancer is 2–3 times higher than the rate of NHW women [56]. While rates of stomach cancer have decreased dramatically over the decades among all race and ethnic groups, Hispanics still have risks 30–90% higher than NHW [56]. Rates of liver and gallbladder cancer are also higher in Hispanics compared to non-Hispanics [56].

Traditional cuisine

Hispanics living in the US comprise a heterogeneous population with diverse cultural backgrounds. Certain dietary habits and food preparation techniques are unique to specific countries of origin and even to specific regions within a country [57]. The diets of Hispanics living in the US are influenced by the dietary traditions of individual countries of origin, availability of native foods in the US, and new dietary practices adopted in the US [32,58].

Food plays an important role in the Hispanic culture. Hispanic families are more likely to prepare and serve food at home, as well as to eat with the family. Consumption of fiber through legumes (beans) is higher among Hispanics than other populations, but the types of beans eaten most often differs by subgroup. Hispanics in general are more likely than NHWs to drink whole milk instead of low-fat milk. Hispanics prefer fresh and traditional fruits and vegetables, rather than frozen and canned ones. In many Latin American countries, the midday meal is the largest and snacking is not common; however, this meal pattern may not persist with acculturation. As acculturation occurs, most Hispanics adopt the three-meals-a-day (with the heavier meal in the evening) pattern of the US. It is common for Hispanics to take lunch from home to work.

General nutritional concerns for Hispanic patients include: high fat intake (sometimes in the form of lard); few servings of green or leafy vegetables and milk; a diet high in sugar, including sweetened beverages; and increased incorporation of fast food as acculturation occurs [17,18,27,57,59–61].

Because of the extensive use of frying as a cooking method, the traditional MA diet is often high in fat. The nutrients most likely to be inadequately provided in the MA diet are calcium, iron, vitamin A, folic acid, and vitamin C [62,63]. Tortillas are eaten in the home; bread is usually eaten away from home. Beans may be eaten at all three meals. Rice may be prepared in soup with vegetables and/or meat, or served with vegetables. Rice is usually cooked with lard or oil. One-pot meals of stew or soup, often made with beans and vegetables, are common. Stuffed foods such as enchiladas, burritos, tacos, tamales, and quesadillas are commonly eaten, and they are filled with beans, cheese, meat, poultry, or seafood. Vegetables are usually part of a dish, not served separately. Salsa, which is made primarily from tomatoes, is an important condiment. Milk is not widely consumed among MAs, likely due to lactose intolerance and when it is, it is often whole milk. Cheeses are commonly eaten and can be a major source of saturated fat. Coffee is often served with large amounts of sugar and milk [4,5,17,59,63,64].

MAs have higher total fat and saturated fat intakes than mainland Puerto Ricans and older Cuban Americans, while Puerto Ricans have higher fat intakes than Dominicans, Guatemalans and Colombians [14,59]. The diets of Puerto Ricans, Cuban Americans, and Dominicans are comparable. Rice and beans are staples; however preferred types of beans differ. Rice is usually cooked with lots of oil. Examples of other common foods include meat stew, *morcilla* (blood sausage), other sausages, poultry, beef, pork, spare ribs, and fish, especially *bacalao* (codfish, which is eaten fresh or dried and cured with salt). Tuberous root vegetables (*viandas*) are also staples and include breadfruit, cassava (yuca), taro (dasheen, malanga), potato, yam, plantain, and sweet potato. Lettuce salads with tomato are popular and use of commercial salad dressing, once rare, is increasing in use. Food is seasoned frequently with Sazon, which is mostly monosodium glutamate, cilantro, and sofrito (made from cured ham, onion, green pepper, cilantro, and garlic in oil). *Café con leche*, strong coffee with hot milk and sugar, is a popular beverage [4,5,17,57,63,64]. Gans *et al.* found that compared to NHW and BA, Hispanics in Rhode Island and Massachusetts were more likely to eat fruits and vegetables for snacks and desserts, and less likely to use table fats such as salad dressings, mayonnaise, or spreads [14]. "American" foods, especially convenience and fast foods are also often eaten, especially among Puerto Ricans. Puerto Ricans living on the US mainland have a higher fat intake than immigrants from other Caribbean countries, which is likely due to the fact that they are more acculturated [57,60].

Most studies have shown that the longer Hispanic immigrants live in the US, the more likely they are to increase their consumption of calories, fat, saturated fat, salt, and protein [58,59,61]. Some of the dietary changes with acculturation have been healthy, such as a large decrease in the consumption of lard and *tocino*, and a moderate increase in the consumption of milk. However, acculturation is also associated with the increased use of added fats, a severe decline in the consumption of traditional fruit-based beverages in favor of high-sugar soft drinks, and an increase in sugary cereals, high fat sweets and salty snacks, meats, convenience and fast foods; and decreased consumption of complex carbohydrates (beans, tortillas, pasta, and rice) [58,61,62]. Some studies have shown that fruit and vegetable consumption increases with acculturation [58], while others have shown that its consumption decreases [62].

Barriers to healthy eating include: perceived expense of healthier foods; traditional meals are harder to make because of expense and difficulty finding ingredients; less time for cooking (often both parents work); perceived reluctance of male spouses and children to eat healthier; literacy issues; nutrition misinformation; and a fatalistic viewpoint about health [58]. Hispanics may be more likely to change their eating habits if they receive a diagnosis of a health problem; physician advice to change diet; and/or are concerned for the health of children or spouse [57].

More acculturated Hispanic individuals may need help in selecting a variety of healthful foods including convenience and fast foods, while the less acculturated may need more assistance with modifying traditional dishes for healthier alternatives. It is often harder for people to change traditional food preferences than it is to change food practices such as food-preparation methods, portion sizes, and frequency of consumption. If a favorite traditional food needs to be decreased for health reasons, recommend the 50% rule, patients can enjoy a half portion size of favorite foods or consume them half as frequently [16,57,61]. Table 17.3 provides recommendations for Hispanic patients adapted from many sources [4,5,16,17,27,57,60,61,63,64].

The Food and Drug Administration (FDA) advises that consumers do not eat any unripened raw milk soft cheeses (i.e. queso fresco style cheese) from Mexico, Nicaragua, or Honduras because they are often contaminated with pathogens and can cause serious infectious diseases. These cheeses may be imported or produced in the US. The FDA further recommends that consumers not purchase or consume raw milk soft cheeses from sources such as flea markets, sellers operating door-to-door or out of their trucks or shipped or carried in luggage to and from those countries. This includes cheeses made at home by individuals. This is especially important for high risk groups, such as pregnant women, newborns, older adults, and people with weakened immune systems [65].

Table 17.3 Dietary recommendations for Hispanics.

Encourage Hispanic patients to:

Preserve intake of traditional healthful foods such as rice and beans, root vegetables, corn, fruits, soups, stews, tortillas, salads, etc. Choose flour and corn tortillas instead of fried tortillas (tortillas fritas).

Eat refried beans less often.

Maintain high intake of traditional fruits and vegetables such as avocados, bananas, beans, coconuts, guavas, mangos, papayas, passion fruit, pineapple, *guanabanana*, squash, tomatoes, okra, spinach, kale, onions, yuca, taro, sweet potatoes, cassava, and try new varieties.

Continue the practice of adding vegetables to meats and rice.

Make modifications to traditional foods. For example, add more vegetables to soups or stews; use brown rice instead of white rice; add green leafy and other raw vegetables to salads; and use less fat to prepare rice and beans.

Increase consumption of salads and continue using oil and vinegar or lemon on salads, or make dressings with herbs, garlic, and onions instead of switching to commercial salad dressings.

Continue to use onions, tomatoes, and garlic as condiments in food preparation.

Continue to drink natural fruit juices or water instead of switching to high-sugar sodas and fruit drinks.

Maintain eating bread and potatoes without added fat.

Remove the fat and skin from meat and chicken.

Replace lard and tocino with small amounts of canola or olive oil.

Substitute baking, roasting, grilling or boiling for frying as cooking method.

Decrease red meat intake by increasing the amount of vegetables and decreasing the amount of meat served at meals.

Decrease intake of processed meats such as morcilla, salchicha, linguica, chicharron, chorizo, tripe, salt pork and Spam®.

Sodium Decrease use of salt and Sazon® (a high-sodium commercial product consisting mainly of monosodium glutamate that is used widely by Puerto Ricans and Dominicans). Substitute herbs or sofrito for high sodium seasonings. Decrease intake of bacalao (high in sodium). Continue to stay away from processed foods as much as possible.

Dairy products Switch from whole milk (red top) to 1% or skim milk. Use low-fat milk to make desserts like flan and tembleque. Use lite (skimmed) evaporated milk to make batidos (shakes). Replace whole-milk cheese with part-skim or low-fat cheese like queso cotija anejo. Look for the word "pasteurized" on the cheese label to know that it is safe.

Make small, gradual changes to lower the fat content of favorite foods without sacrificing flavor, and without upsetting the household (e.g., mixing whole with 2% milk).

Snack on low-fat choices, such as baked tortilla chips or fresh vegetables with salsa.

Continue to prepare and eat meals with the family.

Source: Kim Gans, PhD, RD, Brown University and Lisa Hark, PhD, RD, University of Pennsylvania School of Medicine. 2007. Used with permission.

Note: Health professionals should never make generalizations about food patterns solely on the basis of race or ethnicity. Although these food recommendations may be appropriate for many Hispanic patients, physicians need to do an assessment with each individual patient to determine individual diet habits and counsel accordingly.

Asians and Pacific Islanders (South Asians)

Disease prevalence

The API population includes sub-populations at high CVD risk (South Asians) and low CVD risk (Japanese). South Asians have a higher prevalence of and mortality from CHD and stroke than NHW and several-fold higher rates than other ethnic groups in the US [66]. Much of the burden can be attributed to high rates of metabolic syndrome [67]. In addition, elevated homocysteine levels and C-reactive protein have been found to occur in a large percentage of South Asians which may contribute to their increased risk [68,69], and may be related to dietary differences [29,69].

High plasma triglycerides have also been documented in South Asians with higher levels than NHWs and BAs [70]. Total cholesterol (TC) and LDL cholesterol levels in South Asians have been shown to be lower than in NHWs [70], but high density lipoprotein (HDL) levels are also lower than NHWs and BAs, so a majority has high TC/HDL ratios. Atherogenic small dense LDL-cholesterol, and elevated Lp(a) are also prevalent in this population [66,70].

Diabetes is 4.5 times more prevalent in South Asians (19%) compared to Whites (4%) [71]. Insulin resistance and hyperinsulinemia are also more prevalent in South Asian adults and children [71,72]. In addition, South Asians also have a high prevalence of metabolic syndrome [73]. Potential reasons include: increased central obesity and higher visceral fat, genetic factors, and behavioral factors including physical inactivity, diets rich in fat and sugar and high levels of mental stress [74].

South Asians have significantly greater abdominal fat and visceral fat at normal BMIs [72] and a higher percentage of body fat than NHWs [75] classifying them as metabolically obese and prone to diabetes, hypertension, and CHD. Thus, for this group, BMI cut points may not be appropriate and a waist to hip ratio may be a better measurement [76].

Causes of obesity within this population include lower levels of physical activity [33,68,75], which likely decreases with urbanization and acculturation [77].

Since 1980, cancer, rather than heart disease, has been the number one killer of API women [54]. However, overall cancer incidence and mortality rates are lower in API than other ethnic groups [55]. India tends to have lower cancer rates than those in Western countries, but breast and colon cancer rates for immigrants increase with migration from low to high incidence regions [78]. Breast cancer risk varies significantly between South Asians ethnic subgroups, which is partly accounted for by diet and body size [79].

Traditional cuisine

The term "South Asian" refers to all those who trace their origin to the four countries in the Indian subcontinent – India, Pakistan, Bangladesh, and Sri Lanka. These countries have some common dietary patterns and practices; however, there are many differences by subpopulation. For example, in India alone, food practices vary significantly depending on the region. South Asians have considerable intra-group diversity in socioeconomic status, language, and dietary practices based on their region [4,33]. India can be divided into four major regions – North, South, East, and West. Each region has its distinctive languages, dialects, customs and food practices. Northern Indians consume greater amounts of wheat-based products, eggs, dried or pickled fruits, and vegetables, whereas Southerners consume greater amounts of rice, fresh fruits, and vegetables. In the Eastern coastal regions of India, seafood is a common staple [33]. North Indian food is the most popular food in US South Asian restaurants [9].

Religions practiced in these cultures also have a major impact on eating patterns and lifestyle behaviors [9,17]. Hinduism is the predominant religion in India followed by Islam, Buddhism, and many other religions [9]. Pakistan and Bangladesh have a high proportion of Muslims. Most Hindus are lacto-vegetarians. Beef consumption is forbidden in Hinduism. Muslims follow Koranic laws that permit the consumption of meats of certain animals sacrificed in a humane way known as *halal*. If the meat is not obtained according to the Islamic law, it is forbidden, or *haram*. Haram foods also include pork, meat from clawed animals, fish without scales, and alcohol. Crustaceans such as shrimp and lobster are considered undesirable, or *makruh* [17]. Fasting is an important religious practice among South Asians. Hindus follow partial fasting rituals throughout the year, and Muslims observe Ramadan, a month of complete fasting during which neither foods nor fluids are consumed from dawn until sunset. Young children, pregnant and lactating mothers and sick people are exempt [17].

While diets of South Asians differ somewhat by regions and religion, there are some common features. Traditional meals have plenty of whole grains, green vegetables, beans, and lean meats (poultry without skin), and are high in complex carbohydrates, fiber, vitamins, and minerals. However, the overall fat and saturated fat content may be high due to extensive use of milk, butter, and ghee (clarified butter), a source of saturated fat. Rice and wheat are staples, but can be prepared with large amounts of saturated fats such as butter and ghee or "vegetable ghee" (*vanaspati*, a hydrogenated fat containing high amounts of *trans* fatty acids). Rice dishes include *pulao*, and *biryani*, and wheat breads include *puris, parathas,* and *nan*, which are either deep fried or topped with ghee and butter after cooking. A large variety of legumes (or dals), including chickpeas, kidney, black-eyed peas, and lentils, are used in the preparation of curries, in combination with vegetables, meat, and in breads. Legumes fried in hydrogenated fat and oils are also consumed as snacks, usually with mid-afternoon tea [9,17].

Most of the cooking is done on the stovetop using the roasting and frying method [9]. Meat, poultry, fish, and eggs are prepared as curries or kebabs and in combination with grains (*biryani*), legumes, or vegetables. Coconut milk, butter, ghee, and vegetable fats can be used to stir fry and improve texture and flavor. Vegetables are prepared with onions, garlic, spices, oil, butter, cream, or yogurt. Potatoes or legumes are usually cooked with vegetables (for example, spinach with potatoes; zucchini with lentils). Fruits are eaten as desserts, snacks, appetizers with spices and salt (*chat*), or in combination with yogurt as a drink (mango *lassi*). Dairy products such as yogurt cheese (*paneer*), yogurt, and milk are used as ingredients in the preparation of rice dishes, with vegetables, in desserts, or as an accompaniment to the meal. *Chai* (tea) is often drunk with whole milk or half and half [9,17].

There is often a distinct difference in eating between weekdays and weekends. On weekends, there are often social gatherings where traditional "special occasion" (generally high-fat foods) foods are eaten [9]; whereas more restraint may be shown during the week. In general, South Asians eat their own foods for dinner and prefer more convenient foods such as cereals, sandwiches, and pizza for breakfast and lunch. In the larger cities, high-fat, home-style meals are often purchased from Indian and Pakistani restaurants [17]. Acculturation often increases the selection of American or other ethnic foods for main meals or snacks especially by the younger generation [9].

While vegetarianism can be a very healthy lifestyle, many South Asian vegetarian foods, including desserts, are often prepared with butter, ghee, hydrogenated fats (vanaspati), coconut oil, and palm kernel oil, and many are fried. In addition, vegetarians have higher homocysteine levels than omnivores [69], which may be related to vitamin B_{12} deficiency [80].

Traditional South Asian diets are healthful, but as South Asians become more acculturated, they tend to lose some healthful traditional habits while adopting less healthful habits. Dietary changes such as decreasing vegetarianism, changing meal patterns, increasing use of fast and convenience foods, substituting refined grains for unrefined, increasing fat intake; changing frequency of use of traditional foods and the inclusion of other ethnic and American foods as substitutes result in the abandonment of a diet traditionally high in complex carbohydrates and whole grains and low in fat to a diet that is high in saturated fat and animal protein and low in fiber [9,74]. Dietary recommendations for South Asians are shown in Table 17.4 [9,17,74].

Summary

An Institute of Medicine report entitled *Unequal Treatment: Confronting Racial and Ethnic Disparities in Health Care* urges integrating cross-cultural education into the training of all current and future health professionals [19]. Cultural competency not only includes having knowledge about and respect for cultural influences on diet and health, but also having skills in cross-cultural communication and being able to use them effectively with ethnically diverse patients [15,16,21,23]. Primary care providers will be much more effective if they do an assessment with each individual patient to determine individual dietary habits and other health-related cultural issues. Consideration of cultural factors in the medical encounter has a positive impact on patient–provider communication and facilitates shared decision making, which in turn may positively affect adherence and health outcomes, and thus, may help to reduce health disparities.

Table 17.4 Dietary recommendations for South Asians.

Continue the traditional use of unrefined carbohydrates such as whole-grain flour (millet or whole wheat) to make breads such as *chapatis* and *nan*; brown rice to prepare pulao and other rice dishes; and oat and whole-wheat breakfast cereals to prepare savory snacks rather than adopt refined carbohydrates.

Instead of using only rice, select from a variety of grains, such as cracked wheat, oats, and barley. *Roti* and baked *papads* are a better bread choice than *paratha, puri, kachori*, or *nan*, which may be prepared with more fat. *Chapatis* and *nans* are a good choice as long as they are baked and not fried with added ghee or oil.

Continue eating healthful traditional dishes such as: lentil or mulligatawny type soups (avoid creamy soups with coconut); all the vegetable dishes made with garbanzos, lentils, potatoes, spinach, cauliflower, onions and/or tomatoes.

Food preparation Prepare and choose foods that are not fried; for example baked, stir-fried, roasted, grilled, steamed, etc. Tandoori (clay oven) and tikka cooking methods are healthy and low in fat, while bhuna, malai and korma dishes are creamy and high in fat. Prepare dishes with less oil. Shallow frying is better than deep frying and using a non-stick pan usually requires less oil.

Increasing intake of ω-3 fatty acids Mix flax seed powder in curries (eg, *sambar*), dal (lentil soup), vegetable dishes, or chapatis; eat fenugreek leaves *(methi)* as a vegetable; consume fatty fish such as salmon (if religion permits); and use canola oil and walnuts in food preparation.

Decreasing intake of saturated fat, trans fatty acids, and cholesterol Use canola, olive, peanut or sesame oil, or trans free margarine in place of butter, ghee, or *vanaspati* (hydrogenated fat); when any fats are used, use sparingly; substitute almond paste or nonfat yogurt for cream and butter in buttery *makhani* curries; and substitute egg whites for egg yolks in omelets and desserts. Prepare baked goods (pastries, *kulfi, rasmalai,* pies, cakes and cookies) with less fat and/or less saturated fats; choose smaller portions of prepared foods made with these fats in restaurants (fried appetizers, marinated entrees, butter and cream based sauces). Use less coconut.

Using low-fat dairy products Use 1% milk to make desserts, porridge, yogurt, *chenna* (cottage cheese), custards or puddings. Instead of paneer, substitute with tofu or part skim ricotta cheese. Use low-fat or fat-free evaporated milk and unsweetened condensed milk if a recipe calls for regular condensed milk.

Optimizing protein intake Legumes (dried beans and lentils, i.e., *dal*) are naturally low in fat, and high in protein and fiber. Eat *dal*, chicken, and fish cooked in minimal oil instead of fried or creamed. Eat leaner cuts of lamb, goat, pork or beef and in small quantities. Eat fresh or frozen soybeans as savory snacks *(chole, chat, sundal)* and in combination with vegetables such as spinach and zucchini; cook tofu with tomatoes, spinach, onions, or with nonfat yogurt as *raita*.

Increasing intake of fruits and vegetables Choose fruits as snacks, instead of fried legumes such as *bhel;* substitute green leafy vegetables for potatoes with legumes. Recommend against prolonged cooking of vegetables, which can destroy a significant amount of vitamins and minerals. Also cook vegetables with minimal oil instead of creamed or fried vegetables. While using potato, green plantain or other starchy vegetables, cut down on the amount of rice eaten. Select a green vegetable more often than starchy ones. Salads are good with any meal. Simple lemon or vinegar dressings may be freely used.

Decreasing intake of salt Use herbs such as cilantro and mint; cook with spices such as cumin, black pepper, cardamom, saffron, poppy seeds, basil leaves, cumin seeds, garlic, turmeric, and cinnamon that enhance food flavors. Continue traditional practice of serving salt separately on the plate for optional use. Condiments like *raita*, and most *chutney*, like mint and tamarind, are low in sodium, but the pickles and some other *chutney* may contain a lot of sodium.

(Continued)

Table 17.4 Dietary recommendations for South Asians *(Continued)*.

Optimizing intake of calcium and vitamin D Consume non-fat milk, non-fat yogurt, and non-fat milk powder in combination with fruit as shakes and dessert. Try using soy milk with fresh fruit to make smoothies. Use lower fat milks in the preparation of *chai* and desserts.

Minimizing sugar and caloric sweeteners Continue the practice of serving water with meals and limit sugary soft drinks; use non-calorie sweeteners in the preparation of sweets and desserts, and/or reduce the portion sizes. Use $1/4$ the amount of sugar suggested in the recipe and add the rest with non-calorie sweetener if you cannot make the entire dish with non-calorie sweetener. Squeeze the syrup out from sweets that are immersed in sugar syrup.

Physical activity If women are uncomfortable exercising in public for religious or cultural reasons, suggest using videos to exercise at home or join women-only facilities such as Curves®.

Source: Kim Gans, PhD, RD, Brown University and Lisa Hark, PhD, RD, University of Pennsylvania School of Medicine. 2007. Used with permission.

Note: Health professionals should never make generalizations about food patterns solely on the basis of race or ethnicity. Although these food recommendations may be appropriate for many South Asian patients, physicians need to do an assessment with each individual patient to determine individual diet habits and counsel accordingly.

References

1 James DC. Factors influencing food choices, dietary intake, and nutrition-related attitudes among African Americans: application of a culturally sensitive model. *Ethn Health* 2004;9(4):349–67.

2 Curry KR, Jaffe A (eds). *Nutrition Counseling and Communication Skills*, WB Saunders Company, Philadelphia, PA, 1998.

3 Airhihenbuwa CO, Kumanyika S, Agurs TD, Lowe A, Saunders D, Morssink CB. Cultural aspects of African American eating patterns. *Ethn Health* 1996;1(3):245–60.

4 Kittler PG, Sucher KP. *Food and Culture in American: A Nutrition Handbook*. 2nd edition. Belmont, CA: West/Wadsworth Publishing; 2001.

5 Burrowes JD. Incorporating ethnic and cultural food preferences in the renal diet. *Adv Ren Replace Ther* 2004;11(1):97–104.

6 Graves, DE, Suitor, CW. *Celebrating Diversity: Approaching Families Through Their Food*. National Center for Education in Maternal and Child Health: Arlington, VA. 1998.

7 US Census 2000. Your Gateway to the Census 2000. Available at www.census.gov.

8 US Census Bureau, The Hispanic population in the United States: March 2002. Current Population Reports. 2003. Report P20-545. Available at: www.census.gov/prod/2003pubs/p20-545.pdf.

9 Patel TG, *The Subcommittee of the Public Health Committee of AAPI (eds); Indian Foods: AAPI's Guide To Nutrition, Health and Diabetes*. Allied Publishers, Chennai, India, 2002.

10 Ramirez AG. Consumer–provider communication research with special populations. *Patient Education and Counseling* 2003;50(1):51–4.

11 Napoles-Springer AM, Santoyo J, Houston K, Perez-Stable E, Steware AL. Patients' perceptions of cultural factors affecting the quality their medical encounters. *Health Expectations* 2005;8:4–17.

12 Blue AV. The Provision of Culturally Competent Health Care. Medical University of South Carolina. www.musc.edu/fm_ruralclerkship/culture.html

13 Boyle M. *Community Nutrition in Action. 3rd edition*. Belmont, Calif: Wadsworth Publishing; 2003.

14 Gans KM, Burkholder GJ, Risica PM, Lasater TM. Baseline fat-related dietary behaviors of white, Hispanic, and black participants in a cholesterol screening and education project in New England. *J Am Diet Assoc* 2003;103:699–706.

15 Salimbene A. What Language Does Your Patient Hurt In? A Practical Guide to the Culturally Competent Health Care. Diversity Resources, 2005.

16 Batty PA, Kurko MJ (eds). Spanish for the Nutrition Professional. American Dietetic Association, 2005.

17 Sarieddine H, Hark LA, Hamdan W, Maldonado GA, Karmally W: Chapter 15 *Multicultural Nutrition Strategies. In Cardiovascular Nutrition, Disease Management and Prevention*, Editors: Carson J, Burke F, Hark LA, American Dietetic Association, 2004.

18 Horowitz CR, Tuzzio L, Rojas M, Monteith SA, Sisk JE. How do urban African Americans and Latinos view the influence of diet on hypertension? *J Health Care Poor Underserved* 2004;15(4):631–44.

19 Smedley BD, Stith AY, Nelson AR (Eds). Institute of Medicine Committee on Understanding and Eliminating Racial and Ethnic Disparities in Health Care. Unequal Treatment: Confronting Racial and Ethnic Disparities in Health Care. National Academies Press. Washington, DC, 2003.

20 Honda K. Factors underlying variation in receipt of physician advice on diet and exercise: applications of the behavioral model of health care utilization. *Am J Health Promot* 2004;18:370–7.

21 Betancourt JR, Green JR, Carrillo JE, Ananeh-Firempong O. Defining Cultural Competence: A practical framework for addressing racial/ethnic disparities in health and health care. *Public Health Rep* 2003;118(4):293–302.

22 Betancourt JR, Carrillo JE, Green AR. Hypertension in multicultural and minority populations: linking communication to compliance. *Curr Hypertens Rep* 1999;1(6):482–8.

23 Brach C, Fraser I. Can cultural competency reduce racial and ethnic health disparities? A review and conceptual model. *Med Care Res Rev* 2000;57 Suppl 1:181–217.

24 Magnus M. What's your IQ on cross-cultural nutrition counseling? *The Diabetes Educator* 1996;96:57–62.

25 Sciamanna, C, Gans, KM, Goldstein M. Counseling patients to change diet behavior. *Medicine and Health/Rhode Island* 2000;83(11):354–8.

26 Clark T, Sleath B, Rubin RH. Influence of ethnicity and language concordance on physician-patient agreement about recommended changes in patient health behavior. *Patient Educ Couns* 2004;53(1):87–93.

27 Clutter A. Understanding the Hispanic culture. Ohio State University fact sheet. HYG-5237-00. Available at http://ohioline.osu.edu/hyg-fact/5000/5237.html.

28 Popkin BM. The nutrition transition: an overview of world patterns of change. *Nutr Rev* 2004;62(7 Pt2):S140–3.

29 Chambers JC, Kooner JS. Diabetes, insulin resistance and vascular disease among Indian Asians and Europeans. *Semin Vasc Med* 2002;2(2):199–214.

30 Kuller LH. Ethnic differences in atherosclerosis, cardiovascular disease and lipid metabolism. *Curr Opin Lipidol* 2004;15(2):109–13.

31 Goel MS, McCarthy EP, Phillipa RS, Wee CC. Obesity among US immigrant subgroups by duration of residence. *JAMA* 2004;292(23):2860–7.

32 Ayala GX, Elder JP, Campbell NR *et al*. Correlates of body mass index and waist-to-hip ratio among Mexican women in the United States: implications for intervention development. *Womens Health Issues* 2004;14(5):155–64.

33 Jonnalagadda SS, Diwan S. Regional variations in dietary intake and body mass index of first generation Asian-Indian immigrants in the United States. *J Am Diet Assoc* 2002;102(9):1286–9.

34 American Heart Association. *Heart Disease and Stroke Statistics – 2005 Update*. Dallas, Texas: American Heart Association; 2004. www.americanheart.org.

35 Mensah GA, Mokdad AH, Ford ES, Greenland KJ, Croft JB. State of Disparities in Cardiovascular Health in the United States. *Circulation* 2005;111:1233–41.

36 US Department of Health and Human Services. Eliminating Minority Health Disparities, 2004. http://raceandhealth.hhs.gov.

37 National Institute for Diabetes and Digestive and Kidney Disease. Diabetes in African Americans. Available at: http://diabetes.niddk.nih.gov/dm/pubs/africanamerican.

38 American Cancer Society. Cancer Facts and Figures 2005. Available at www.cancer.org.

39 National Cancer Institute. Cancer Health Disparities: Fact Sheet. Available at www.cancer.gov.

40 Flegal KM, Carroll MD, Ogden CL, Johnson CL. Prevalence and trends in obesity among US adults, 1999–2000. *JAMA* 2002;288:1723–7.

41 Hedley AA, Ogden CL, Johnson CL, Carroll MD, Curtin LR, Flegal KM. Prevalence of overweight and obesity among US children, adolescents, and adults, 1999–2002. *JAMA* 2004;291(23):2847–50.

42 Jamerson KA. The disproportionate impact of hypertensive cardiovascular disease in African Americans: getting to the heart of the issue. *J Clin Hypertens* 2004;6(4 Suppl 1):4–10.

43 Hargreaves MK, Schlundt DG, Buchowski MS. Contextual factors influencing the eating behaviors of african american women: A focus group investigation. *Ethnicity & Health* 2002;7(3):133–47.

44 Satia JA, Galanko JA, Siega-Riz AM. Eating at fast-food restaurants is associated with dietary intake, demographic, psychosocial and behavioral factors among African Americans in North Carolina. *Public Health Nutr* 2004;7(8):1089–96.

45 Basiotis PP, Lino M, Anand RS. Report card on the diet quality of African Americans. *Nutr Insights* 1998;11:61–3. Available at www.cnpp.usda.gov.

46 Kerver JM, Yang EJ, Bianchi L, Song WO. Dietary patterns associated with risk factors for cardiovascular disease in healthy US adults. *Am J Clin Nutr* 2003;78(6):1103–10.

47 Wilson DB, Musham C, McLellan MS. From mothers to daughters: transgenerational food and diet communication in an underserved group. *J Cult Divers* 2004;11(1):12–17.

48 Fitzgibbon ML, Stolley MR. Environmental changes may be needed for prevention of overweight in minority children. *Pediatr Ann* 2004;33(1):45–9.

49 Matheson DM, Wang Y, Klesges LM, Beech BM, Kraemer HC, Robinson TN. African–American girls' dietary intake while watching television. *Obes Res* 2004;12 Suppl:32S–37S.

50 Sacks FM, Svetkey LP, Vollmer WM *et al*. Effects on blood pressure of reduced dietary sodium and the dietary approaches to stop hypertension (DASH) Diet. *N Engl J Med* 2001;344:3–10.

51 American Diabetes Association. National Diabetes Fact Sheet. General information and national estimates on diabetes in the United States, 2002. www.diabetes.org.

52 Hertz RP, Unger AN, Ferrario CM. Diabetes, hypertension, and dyslipidemia in Mexican Americans and non-Hispanic Whites. *Am J Prev Med* 2006;30(2):103–10.

53 Ford ES, Giles WH, Dietz WH. Prevalence of the metabolic syndrome among US adults. *JAMA* 2002;286:356–9.

54 Intercultural Cancer Council. Hispanics/Latinos & Cancer. Available at: http://iccnetwork.org/cancerfacts/ICC-CFS4.pdf.

55 National Cancer Institute. Cancer Health Disparities: Fact Sheet. Available at www.cancer. gov/newscenter/healthdisparities.

56 Intercultural Cancer Council. Asian Americans & Cancer. Available at: http:// iccnetwork.org/cancerfacts/cfs3.htm.

57 Gans KM, Lovell HJ, Fortunet R, McMahon C, Crton-Lopez S, Lasater TM. Implications of qualitative research for nutrition education geared to selected Hispanic audiences. *J Nutr Educ* 1999;31:331–8.

58 Romero-Gwynn E, Gwynn D, Grivetti L *et al.* Dietary acculturation among Latinos of Mexican descent. *Nutr Today* 1993;28:6–12.

59 Artinian NT, Schim SM, Vander Wal JS, Nies MA. Eating Patterns and Cardiovascular Disease Risk in a Detroit Mexican American Population. *Public Health Nursing* 2004;21(5):425–34.

60 Gans KM, Burkholder DI, Upegui MA, Risica PM, Lasater TM, Fortunet R. Comparison of baseline fat-related eating behaviors of Puerto Rican, Dominican, Colombian, and Guatemalan participants who joined a cholesterol education project. *J Nutr Educ Behav* 2002;34:202–10.

61 Neuhouser ML, Thompson B, Coronado GD, Solomon CC. Higher fat intake and lower fruit and vegetables intakes are associated with greater acculturation among Mexicans living in Washington State. *J Am Diet Assoc* 2004;104(1):51–7.

62 Warrix M. Cultural diversity: eat ing in America: Mexican-American. Ohio State University extension fact sheet. HYG-52255-95. Available at http://ohioline.osu.edu/hyg-fact/5000/5255.html.

63 Sanjur D. Hispanic Foodways, Nutrition and Health, Allyn & Bacon, Needham, MA, 1995.

64 Syracuse CJ. Cultural diversity: eating in America: Puerto Rican. Ohio State University extension fact sheet. HYG=5257-95. Available at: http://ohioline.osu.edu/hyg-fact/5000/5257.html.

65 Food and Drug Administration. FDA Issues Health Advisory About Certain Soft Cheese Made From Raw Milk, March 14, 2005, www.fda.gov/bbs/topics/news/2005/NEW01165.html.

66 Enas EA, Mehta J. Malignant coronary artery disease in young Asian Indians: thoughts on pathogenesis, prevention, and therapy. *Clin Cardiol* 1995a;18:131–5.

67 Brady LM, Williams CM, Lovegrove JA. Dietary PUFA and the metabolic syndrome in Indian Asians living in the UK. *Proc Nutr Soc* 2004;63(1):115–25.

68 Vikram NK, Misra A, Dwivedi M *et al.* Correlations of C-reactive protein levels with anthropometric profile, percentage of body fat and lipids in healthy adolescents and young adults in urban North India. *Atherosclerosis* 2003;168:305–13.

69 Carmel R, Mallidi PV, Vinarskiy S, Brar S, Frouhar Z. Hyperhomocysteinemia and cobalamin deficiency in young Asian Indians in the US (New York). *Am J Hematol* 2002;70(2):107–14.

70 Enas EA, Davidson MA, Garg A, Nair VM, Yusuf S. Coronary heart disease and its risk factors in first-generation immigrant Asian Indians to the United States of America. *Indian Heart J* 1996;48(4):343–53.

71 McKeigue PM, Shah B, Marmot MG. Relation of central obesity and insulin resistance with high diabetes prevalence and cardiovascular risk in South Asians. *Lancet* 1991;337:382–6.

72 Raji A, Seely EW, Arky RA, Simonson DC. Body fat distribution and insulin resistance in healthy Asian Indians and Caucasians. *J Clin Endocrinol Metab* 2001;86:5366–71.

73 Tillin T, Forouhi N, Johnston DG, McKeigue PM, Chaturvedi N, Godsland IF. Metabolic syndrome and coronary heart disease in South Asians, African-Caribbeans and White Europeans: a UK population-based cross-sectional study. *Diabetologia* 2005;48(4):649–56.

74 Mohan V. Why are Indians more prone to diabetes? *J Assoc Physicians India* 2004;52:468–74.

75 Kamath SK, Hussain EA, Amin D *et al.* Cardiovascular disease risk factors in 2 distinct ethnic groups: Indian and Pakistani compared with American premenopausal women. *Am J Clin Nutr* 1999;69(4):621–31.

76 Deurenberg-Yap M, Chew SK, Deurenberg P. Elvated body fat percentage and cardio-vascular risks at low body mass index levels among Singaporean Chinese, Malays and Indians. *Obes Rev* 2002;3(3):209–15.

77 Dhawan J, Bray CL. Asian Indians, coronary artery disease, and physical exercise. *Heart* 1997;78(6):550–4.

78 Smith-Blesch K, Davis F, Kamath SK. A comparison of breast and colon cancer incidence rates among Native Asian Indians, US immigrant Asian Indians, and Whites. *J Am Diet Assoc* 1999;99:1275–7.

79 McCormack VA, Mangtani P, Bhakta D, McMichael AJ, dos Santos Silva I. Heterogeneity of breast cancer risk within the South Asian female population in England: a population-based case-control study of first-generation migrants. *Br J Cancer* 2004;90(1):160–6.

80 Gupta AK, Damji A, Uppaluri A. Vitamin B12 deficiency. Prevalence among South Asians at a Toronto clinic. *Can Fam Physician* 2004;50:743–7.

Further reading

Gans KM, Kumanyika SK, Lovell HJ *et al.* The development of Sistertalk: a cable TV–delivered weight control program for Black women. *Prev Med* 2003;37:654–67.

Appendices

Developed by Susan Zogheib and Lisa Hark

*Appendices A–P used *www.nutritiondata.com*

Appendix A Food sources of vitamin A.

Food, Standard Amount	Serving Size	Vitamin A (μg RE)
Margarine	1 Tbsp	
Liver (beef, veal, goose, and turkey)	3 oz	13,000–19,000
Liver (chicken, lamb)	3 oz	6000–10,000
Various ready-to-eat cereals, with added Vitamin A	1 oz	180–376
Instant cooked cereals, fortified	1 packet	285–376
Beets	1 cup	3.4
Apricots, dried	$1/2$ cup	80
Broccoli, fresh, cooked	1 cup	120.2
Herring, Atlantic	3 oz	219
Cantaloupe, raw	$1/4$ medium melon	233
Chinese cabbage, cooked	1 cup	360
Red sweet pepper, cooked	1 cup	371
Peppers, chili	1 cup	405
Mustard greens, cooked	1 cup	442
Milk, (all types) with added vitamin A	1 cup	478
Winter squash, cooked	1 cup	535
Turnip greens, cooked from frozen	1 cup	549
Collards, cooked from frozen	1 cup	771
Kale, cooked from frozen	1 cup	885
Spinach, cooked from frozen	1 cup	943
Mixed vegetables, canned	1 cup	949
Pumpkin, canned	$1/2$ cup	953
Carrots, raw	1 cup	1026
Sweet potato with peel, baked	1 medium	1096
Mango, raw	1 cup	1262
Carrot juice	$3/4$ cup	1692
Tomatoes and vegetable juice	1 cup	3770
Fish oil, cod liver	1 Tbsp	4051

Source: www.nutritiondata.com

The Complete Guide to Nutrition in Primary Care by Darwin Deen, MD and Lisa Hark, PhD, RD.
Blackwell Publishing 2007.

Appendix B Food sources of vitamin D.

Food, Standard Amount	Serving Size	Vitamin D (IU)
Herring, Atlantic	3 oz	1384
Fish oil, cod liver	1 Tbsp	1350
Fish, sardines, salmon, codfish	3 oz	649–71.4
Catfish	3 oz	425
Oysters	3 oz	268.8
Egg, yolk, raw, fresh	1 large	260
Milk (all types)	1 cup	299–97.6
Milk, whole	1 cup	100
Margarine	1 Tbsp	60
Cereals ready-to-eat	1 cup	126–88
Butter, salted	1 Tbsp	7.8
Cheddar Cheese	1.5 oz	5.1

Source: www.nutritiondata.com

The Complete Guide to Nutrition in Primary Care by Darwin Deen, MD and Lisa Hark, PhD, RD. Blackwell Publishing 2007.

Appendix C Food sources of vitamin E.

Food, Standard Amount	Serving Size	Alpha Tocopherol (mg)
Fortified ready-to-eat cereals	1 cup	33.8–13.5
Sunflower seeds, dry roasted	1 oz	7.4
Almonds	1 oz	7.3
Sunflower oil	1 Tbsp	5.6
Tomato sauce	1 cup	5.0
Safflower oil	1 Tbsp	4.6
Spinach, frozen, cooked	1 cup	3.7
Swiss chard, cooked	1 cup	3.3
Mixed nuts, dry roasted	1 oz	3.1
Turnip greens, frozen, cooked	1 cup	2.7
Pine nuts	1 oz	2.6
Peanut butter	2 Tbsp	2.5
Canola oil	1 Tbsp	2.4
Wheat germ, toasted, plain	2 Tbsp	2.3
Peanuts	1 oz	2.2
Avocado, raw	$1/2$ avocado	2.1
Carrot juice, canned	$3/4$ cup	2.1
Corn oil and olive oil	1 Tbsp	1.9
Mustard greens, frozen, cooked	1 cup	1.7
Sardine, Atlantic, in oil, drained	3 oz	1.7
Radicchio	1 cup	0.9
Herring, Atlantic,	3 oz	0.9
Margarine	1 Tbsp	0.8
Salad dressing (Italian)	1 Tbsp	0.7

Source: www.nutritiondata.com

The Complete Guide to Nutrition in Primary Care by Darwin Deen, MD and Lisa Hark, PhD, RD. Blackwell Publishing 2007.

Appendix D Food sources of vitamin K.

Food, Standard Amount	Serving Size	Phyloquinone per serving (μg)
Kale, frozen, cooked	1 cup	1062
Collard greens, frozen, cooked	1 cup	1060
Spinach, frozen, cooked	1 cup	889
Turnip greens, frozen, cooked	1 cup	529
Mustard greens, frozen, cooked	1 cup	419
Parsley, raw	$^1/_4$ cup	246
Brussels sprouts, fresh	1 cup	218
Broccoli, fresh	1 cup	110
Asparagus, fresh	1 cup	91
Okra, frozen, cooked	1 cup	88
Cabbage, fresh	1 cup	67.6
Green peas, frozen, cooked	1 cup	38.4
Cauliflower	1 cup	17.2
Celery, raw	1 medium stalk	17
Carrot, raw	1 cup	16.1
Grapes, red/green, seedless, raw	1 $^1/_2$ cup	12
Plums, raw	2 medium	11
Pear, raw	1 medium	8.1
Tomato juice, bottled	8 fluid oz	5.6
Tomato, red, raw	1 medium	4.4
Avocado, raw	1/5 medium	4.3
Apricot, raw	$^1/_2$ cup	2.5

Source: www.nutritiondata.com

The Complete Guide to Nutrition in Primary Care by Darwin Deen, MD and Lisa Hark, PhD, RD. Blackwell Publishing 2007.

Appendix E Food sources of vitamin C.

Food, Standard Amount	Serving Size	Vitamin C (mg)
Guava, raw	$1/2$ cup	188
Peppers (all types), raw	1 cup	155
Peppers (all types) cooked	1 cup	150
Broccoli, cooked	1 cup	101.2
Strawberries, raw	1 cup	100
Brussels sprouts, cooked	1 cup	96.8
Kohlrabi, cooked	1 cup	90
Broccoli, raw	1 cup	81.2
Peas, Snowpeas, Sugar snap peas, cooked	1 cup	76.6
Kiwi fruit	1 medium	70
Orange, raw	1 medium	70
Orange juice	$3/4$ cup	61–93
Peas, edible-podded, raw [Snowpeas, Sugar snap peas]	1 cup	58.8
Tangerines, (mandarin oranges), raw	1 cup	52.1
Green pepper, sweet, cooked	$1/2$ cup	51
Grapefruit juice	$3/4$ cup	50–70
Vegetable juice cocktail	$3/4$ cup	50
Cantaloupe	$1/4$ medium	47
Papaya, raw	$1/4$ medium	47
Tomato juice	$3/4$ cup	33
Raspberries, raw	1 cup	32.2
Melons, honeydew, raw	1 cup	31.9
Sweet potato, cooked	1 medium	22.3

Source: www.nutritiondata.com

The Complete Guide to Nutrition in Primary Care by Darwin Deen, MD and Lisa Hark, PhD, RD. Blackwell Publishing 2007.

Appendix F Food sources of folate.

Food, Standard Amount	Serving Size	Folate (μg)
Ready-to-eat cereals	1 cup	1010
Chicken liver	3 oz	495
Beef liver	3 oz	243.6
Spinach, frozen, cooked	1 cup	230
Lentils, cooked	$^1/_2$ cup	180
Tomato	1 medium	75–97
Mustard and turnip greens, frozen, cooked	1 cup	170
Seaweed, kelp, raw	1 cup	144
Chickpeas, canned	$^1/_2$ cup	140
Okra, frozen, cooked	1 cup	134
Collard greens, frozen, cooked	1 cup	129
Asparagus, fresh, cooked	1 cup	121.2
Peas, green, boiled	1 cup	94.4
Brussels sprouts, raw	1 cup	93.6
Broccoli, fresh, cooked	1 cup	84.2
Lettuce, romaine	1 cup	63.9
Orange juice	6 oz	55.8
Cauliflower	1 cup	54.6
Potato, baked with skin	1 medium	40
Egg, boiled	1 large	24

Source: www.nutritiondata.com

The Complete Guide to Nutrition in Primary Care by Darwin Deen, MD and Lisa Hark, PhD, RD. Blackwell Publishing 2007.

Appendix G Food sources of calcium (dairy).

Food, Standard Amount	Serving Size	Calcium (mg)
Lactose-Free Calcium Fortified Milk	1 cup	500
Plain yogurt, non-fat	8 oz	452
Romano cheese	1.5 oz	452
Plain yogurt, low-fat	8 oz	415
Soy Milk, calcium fortified	1 cup	368
Fruit yogurt, low-fat	8 oz	345
Swiss cheese	1.5 oz	336
Ricotta cheese, part skim	1/2 cup	335
Pasteurized process Swiss cheese	1.5 oz	324
Provolone cheese	1.5 oz	321
Egg, yolk, raw, fresh	1 large	313
Mozzarella cheese, part-skim	1.5 oz	311
Cheddar cheese	1.5 oz	307
Fat-free (skim) milk	1 cup	306
Muenster cheese	1.5 oz	305
1% low-fat milk	1 cup	290
Low-fat chocolate milk (1%)	1 cup	288
2% reduced fat milk	1 cup	285
Reduced fat chocolate milk (2%)	1 cup	285
Buttermilk, low-fat	1 cup	284
Chocolate milk	1 cup	280
Whole milk	1 cup	276
Yogurt, plain, whole milk	8 oz	275
Ricotta cheese, whole milk	1/2 cup	255
Pasteurized process American cheese food	1.5 oz	232
Blue cheese	1.5 oz	225
Mozzarella cheese, whole milk	1.5 oz	215
Feta cheese	1.5 oz	210

Source: www.nutritiondata.com

The Complete Guide to Nutrition in Primary Care by Darwin Deen, MD and Lisa Hark, PhD, RD. Blackwell Publishing 2007.

Appendix H Food sources of calcium (non-dairy).

Food, Standard Amount	Serving Size	Calcium (mg)
Soy beverage, calcium fortified	1 cup	368
Collard greens, frozen, cooked	1 cup	357
Sardines, Atlantic, in oil, drained	3 oz	325
Tofu, firm, prepared with nigari	$^1/_2$ cup	253
Spinach, frozen, cooked	1 cup	245
Turnip greens, frozen, cooked	1 cup	197
Pink salmon, canned, with bone	3 oz	181
Okra, frozen, cooked	1 cup	176
Molasses, blackstrap	1 Tbsp	172
Beet greens, fresh, cooked	1 cup	164
Pak-choi, Chinese cabbage, cooked from fresh	1 cup	158
Soybeans, green, cooked	$^1/_2$ cup	130
Ocean perch, Atlantic, cooked	3 oz	116
White beans, canned	$^1/_2$ cup	96
Kale, frozen, cooked	1 cup	93.6
Clams, canned	3 oz	78
Nuts, almonds, oil roasted	1 oz	74.5
Rainbow trout, farmed, cooked	3 oz	73
Oatmeal, plain and flavored, instant, fortified	1 packet prepared	99–110

Source: www.nutritiondata.com

The Complete Guide to Nutrition in Primary Care by Darwin Deen, MD and Lisa Hark, PhD, RD. Blackwell Publishing 2007.

Appendix I Food sources of sodium.

Food, Standard Amount	Serving Size	Sodium (mg)
Salt (sodium chloride)	1 tsp	2325
Pickle relish, sweet	1 cup	1987
Soup, canned (all types)	1 cup	850–2500
Tomato sauce	1 cup	1284
Soy sauce made from soy (tamari)	1 Tbsp	1006
Sauerkraut, canned	1 cup	939
Chicken Pot pie, frozen entree	1 pie	841
Potato chips, regular and baked	1 bag (1 oz)	837
Pretzels, hard, plain, salted	10 twists	814
Cheese American	1.5 oz	670
Tomato juice, canned, with salt added	1 cup	654
Vegetable juice cocktail, canned	1 cup	653
Pickles, kosher dill	1 medium	569
Beef frankfurter, hot dog	1 frank	461
Olives, canned or bottled, green	1 oz	440
Scrapple, pork	2 oz	369
Gravy, canned	$1/4$ cup	352
Canned tuna	3 oz	320
Canned vegetables	1 cup	243
Lunch meats (turkey, ham, salami, pastrami)	3 slices	250–500
Barbeque Sauce	1 Tbsp	212
Noodles, Chinese, chow mein	1 cup	198
Cheese Pizza	1 slice	194
Beef sausage, fresh, cooked	1 oz	184
Salad dressings	1 Tbsp	147
Peanuts, oil-roasted, with salt	1 oz	121
Frozen Dinner	1 dinner	360–768

Source: www.nutritiondata.com

The Complete Guide to Nutrition in Primary Care by Darwin Deen, MD and Lisa Hark, PhD, RD. Blackwell Publishing 2007.

Appendix J Food sources of potassium.

Food, Standard Amount	Serving Size	Potassium (mg)
Beet greens, cooked	1 cup	1309
Spinach, cooked	1 cup	839
Tomato sauce	1 cup	810
Sweet potato, baked	1 medium	694
Potato, baked, flesh	1 medium	610
White beans, canned	$^1/_2$ cup	595
Yogurt, plain, non-fat	8 oz	579
Tomato puree	$^1/_2$ cup	549
Clams, canned	3 oz	534
Yogurt, plain, low-fat	8 oz	531
Prune juice	$^3/_4$ cup	530
Carrot juice	$^3/_4$ cup	517
Apricots, dried	$^1/_2$ cup	514
Blackstrap molasses	1 Tbsp.	498
Halibut, cooked	3 oz	490
Soybeans, green, cooked	$^1/_2$ cup	485
Tuna, yellow fin, cooked	3 oz	484
Lima beans, cooked	$^1/_2$ cup	484
Artichokes, (globe or French), raw	1 artichoke	474
Winter squash, cooked	1 cup	449
Soybeans, mature, cooked	$^1/_2$ cup	443
Rockfish, Pacific, cooked	3 oz	442
Cod, Pacific, cooked	3 oz	439
Bananas	1 medium	422
Tomato juice	$^3/_4$ cup	417
Peaches, fresh	1 medium	398
Prunes, stewed	$^1/_2$ cup	398
Milk, non-fat	1 cup	382
Pork chop, center loin, cooked	3 oz	382
Rainbow trout, farmed, cooked	3 oz	375
Pork loin, center rib (roasts), lean, roasted	3 oz	371
Buttermilk, cultured, low-fat	1 cup	370
Cantaloupe	$^1/_4$ medium	368
1%–2% milk	1 cup	366
Honeydew melon	1/8 medium	365
Lentils, cooked	$^1/_2$ cup	365
Plantains, cooked	$^1/_2$ cup slices	358
Kidney beans, cooked	$^1/_2$ cup	358
Orange juice	$^3/_4$ cup	355
Split peas, cooked	$^1/_2$ cup	355
Yogurt, plain, whole milk	8 oz container	352

Source: www.nutritiondata.com

The Complete Guide to Nutrition in Primary Care by Darwin Deen, MD and Lisa Hark, PhD, RD. Blackwell Publishing 2007.

Appendix K Food sources of magnesium.

Food, Standard Amount	Serving Size	Magnesium (mg)
Beet greens, cooked	1 cup	97.9
Okra, cooked from frozen	1 cup	93.8
Halibut, cooked	3 oz	91
Quinoa, dry	1/4 cup	89
Almonds	1 oz	78
Soybeans, mature, cooked	1/2 cup	74
Nuts, (various types)	1 oz	70–107
White beans	1/2 cup	67
Pollock, walleye, cooked	3 oz	62
Black beans, cooked	1/2 cup	60
Oat bran, raw	1/4 cup	55
Soybeans, green, cooked	1/2 cup	54
Tuna, yellow fin, cooked	3 oz	54
Lima beans, baby, cooked from frozen	1/2 cup	50
Navy beans, cooked	1/2 cup	48
Tofu, firm, prepared with nigari	1/2 cup	47
Soy beverage	1 cup	47
Cowpeas, cooked	1/2 cup	46
Hazelnuts	1 oz	46
Great northern beans, cooked	1/2 cup	44
Oat bran, cooked	1/2 cup	44
Buckwheat groats, roasted, cooked	1/2 cup	43
Brown rice, cooked	1/2 cup	42
Haddock, cooked	3 oz	42
Spinach, frozen, cooked	1 cup	157
Pumpkin and squash seed kernels, roasted	1 oz	151
Bran ready-to-eat cereal (100%)	1 oz	103

Source: www.nutritiondata.com

The Complete Guide to Nutrition in Primary Care by Darwin Deen, MD and Lisa Hark, PhD, RD.
Blackwell Publishing 2007.

Appendix L Food sources of iron.

Food, Standard Amount	Serving Size	Iron (mg)
Spinach, frozen, cooked	1 cup	6.4
Liver (various types) cooked	3 oz	5.0–9.9
Fortified instant cooked cereals (various)	1 packet	5.0–8.1
Soybeans, mature, cooked	¹/₂ cup	4.4
Pumpkin and squash seed kernels, roasted	1 oz	4.2
White beans, canned	¹/₂ cup	3.9
Blackstrap molasses	1 Tbsp	3.5
Lentils, cooked	¹/₂ cup	3.3
Fortified ready-to-eat cereals (various)	1 cup	19–28
Clams, canned, drained	3 oz	23.8
Clams, canned	3 oz	23.8
Kidney beans, cooked	¹/₂ cup	2.6
Sardines, canned in oil, drained	3 oz	2.5
Chickpeas, cooked	¹/₂ cup	2.4
Duck, meat only, roasted	3 oz	2.3
Prune juice	³/₄ cup	2.3
Shrimp, canned	3 oz	2.3
Cowpeas, cooked	¹/₂ cup	2.2
Ground beef, 15% fat, cooked	3 oz	2.2
Tomato puree	¹/₂ cup	2.2
Lima beans, cooked	¹/₂ cup	2.2
Soybeans, green, cooked	¹/₂ cup	2.2
Navy beans, cooked	¹/₂ cup	2.1
Refried beans	¹/₂ cup	2.1
Tomato paste	¹/₄ cup	2.0
Oysters, eastern, wild, cooked	3 oz	10.2
Beef, lean ground, raw	3 oz	1.5
Beef, sirloin steak or filet mignon, raw	3 oz	1.2
Lamb, shoulder, arm, raw	3 oz	1.1

Source: www.nutritiondata.com

The Complete Guide to Nutrition in Primary Care by Darwin Deen, MD and Lisa Hark, PhD, RD. Blackwell Publishing 2007.

Appendix M Food sources of omega-3 fatty acids.

Food, Standard Amount	Serving Size	Omega-3 FA (g)
Flaxseed oil	1 Tbsp	6.7
Salmon, Atlantic, wild, cooked	3.0 oz	2.198
Flaxseeds	1 Tbsp	2.63
Walnuts	1 oz	2.5
Soybeans, cooked	$1/2$ cup	2.1
Canola oil	1 Tbsp	1.4
Walnut oil	1 Tbsp	1.3
Sardine	3.0 oz	1.2
Tuna, white, canned in water	3.0 oz	0.81
Wheat germ oil	1 Tbsp	0.86

Source: www.nutritiondata.com

The Complete Guide to Nutrition in Primary Care by Darwin Deen, MD and Lisa Hark, PhD, RD. Blackwell Publishing 2007.

Appendix N Food sources of oxalic acid.

Food, Standard Amount	Serving Size	Oxalic acid (mg)
Spinach, frozen	1 cup	1230
Beans in tomato sauce	1 cup	1148
Beetroot, pickled	1 cup	1135
Chard, Swish, boiled	1 cup	1129
Spinach, boiled	1 cup	420
Okra, boiled	1 cup	234
Chard, Swiss, raw	1 cup	232
Tea, Indian, 6 minute infusion	1 cup	185
Potato, sweet, boiled, mashed	1 cup	184
Peanuts, roasted	2 oz	137
Cocoa, dry powder	$^1/_4$ cup	134
Berries, green goose	1 cup	132
Crackers, soybean	2 oz	118
Pecans	2 oz	111
Leeks, raw, boiled	1 cup	110
Grits, white corn, cooked	1 cup	99
Collards, raw, boiled	1 cup	95
Chocolate, plain	2 oz	66
Raspberries, black	1 cup	65
Parsley, raw	1 cup	64
Grapes, concord	1 cup	40
Squash, summer	1 cup	40
Berries, black	1 cup	26
Celery	1 cup	24
Berries, blue	1 cup	22
Wheat germ	1 Tbsp	19
Raspberries, red	1 cup	18
Eggplant, boiled	1 cup	17
Dandelion greens, raw	1 cup	14
Pepper, green	1 cup	12
Escarole, raw	1 cup	9

Source: www.nutritiondata.com

The Complete Guide to Nutrition in Primary Care by Darwin Deen, MD and Lisa Hark, PhD, RD. Blackwell Publishing 2007.

Appendix O Food sources of dietary fiber.

Food, Standard Amount	Serving Size	Dietary Fiber (g)
Cereal, All-Bran	1 cup	25.8
Wheat bran	1 cup	24.6
Cereal, Fiber One	1 cup	23.8
White beans, great-northern, canned	1 cup	14.4
Kidney beans, red, cooked	1 cup	13.8
Navy beans, cooked	1 cup	13.0
Black beans, cooked	1 cup	12.2
Pinto beans, cooked	1 cup	11.8
Lentils, cooked	1 cup	10.4
White beans, great northern beans, cooked	1 cup	10.0
Lima beans, canned	1 cup	8.6
Chickpeas, cooked	1 cup	8.6
Peas, cooked	1 cup	8.6
Peas, green, cooked	1 cup	8.6
Okra, frozen, cooked	1 cup	8.2
Brussels sprouts, cooked	1 cup	7.6
Split peas, cooked	1 cup	6.2
Pear, fresh with skin	1 small	6.0
Cracker, Matzo	6 crackers	6.0
Bread, pumpernickel	2 slices	5.4
Spaghetti, whole-wheat, cooked	1 cup	5.4
Figs, dried	3 pieces	4.6
Carrots, cooked	1 cup	4.0
Applesauce, canned, unsweetened	1 cup	4.0
Prunes, dried, stewed	6 pieces	3.4
Raspberries, fresh	1 cup	3.3
Spinach, cooked	1 cup	3.2
Orange, fresh without skin	1 small	3.0
Carrots, canned	1 cup	3.0
Apple, fresh with skin	1 small	2.8

Source: www.nutritiondata.com

The Complete Guide to Nutrition in Primary Care by Darwin Deen, MD and Lisa Hark, PhD, RD. Blackwell Publishing 2007.

Appendix P Food sources of purine.

Food, Standard Amount	Purine (mg/100 g)
Sweetbreads	825
Anchovies	363
Brains	363
Sardines	295
Scallops	295
Liver, calf/beef	233
Mackerel	233
Kidney, beef	200
Game meats	200
Herring	200
Asparagus	50–150
Bread and cereals, whole grain	50–150
Cauliflower	50–150
Fish, fresh and saltwater	50–150
Legumes, beans/lentils/peas	50–150
Meat-beef/lamb/pork/veal	50–150
Mushrooms	50–150
Oatmeal	50–150
Peas, green	50–150
Poultry, chicken/duck/turkey	50–150
Shellfish, crab/lobster/oysters	50–150
Spinach	50–150
Wheat germ and bran	50–150

Source: www.nutritiondata.com

The Complete Guide to Nutrition in Primary Care by Darwin Deen, MD and Lisa Hark, PhD, RD. Blackwell Publishing 2007.

Appendix Q Therapeutic lifestyle changes (TLC) diet (low-fat, low-saturated fat diet).

Food Items to Choose More Often	Food Items to Choose Less Often
Breads and Cereals	
≥6 servings per day, adjusted to caloric needs	Many bakery products, including doughnuts, biscuits, butter...croissants, Danish, pies, cookies
Breads, cereals, especially whole grain; pasta; rice; potatoes; dry beans and peas; low fat crackers and cookies	Many grain-based snacks, including chips, cheese puffs, snack mix, regular crackers, buttered popcorn
Vegetables and Fruits	
4–5 servings vegetables/day fresh, frozen, or canned, without added fat, sauce, or salt	Vegetables fried or prepared with butter, cheese, or cream sauce
3–4 servings fruits per day fresh, frozen, canned, dried	Fruits fried or served with butter or cream
Dairy Foods	
3 servings/day fat-free, 1% low-fat milk, buttermilk, low-fat yogurt, 1% low-fat cottage cheese; fat-free, low-fat cheeses	Whole milk, 2% milk, whole-milk yogurt, ice cream, cream, full-fat cheese
Eggs	
≤2 egg yolks per week	>3 egg yolks, whole eggs
Egg whites or egg substitute	
Meat, Fish & Poultry	
≤6 oz per day	Higher fat meat cuts: ribs, t-bone steak, regular hamburger, bacon, sausage; cold cuts: salami, bologna, hot dogs; organ meats: liver, brains, sweetbreads; poultry with skin; fried meat; fried poultry; fried fish
Lean cuts loin, leg, round; extra lean hamburger; cold cuts made with lean meat or soy protein; skinless poultry; fish, shellfish without butter	
Fats and Oils	
Amount adjusted to caloric level: Unsaturated oils; soft tub or liquid margarines and vegetable oil spreads, salad dressings, seeds, nuts, nut butters	Butter, shortening, stick margarine, coconut and palm oil, trans fats, partially hydrogenated vegetable oils

Source: National Heart, Lung, and Blood Institute *Third Report of the National Cholesterol Education Program Expert Panel on Detection, Evaluation, and Treatment of High Blood Cholesterol in Adults (Adult Treatment Panel III). Executive Summary.* Bethesda, MD: National Institutes of Health; 2001. NIH publication 01-3670.

The Complete Guide to Nutrition in Primary Care by Darwin Deen, MD and Lisa Hark, PhD, RD. Blackwell Publishing 2007.

Appendix R DASH diet this DASH eating plan is based on 2,000 calories daily. The number of servings may vary from those listed depending on caloric needs.

Food Group	Daily Servings	Serving Sizes
Grains & grain products	7–8	1 slice bread 1 cup dry cereal* $1/2$ cup cooked rice, pasta or cereal
Vegetables	4–5	1 cup raw leafy vegetables $1/2$ cup cooked vegetables 6 oz low-sodium vegetable juice
Fruits	4–5	6 oz 100% fruit juice 1 medium fruit $1/4$ cup dried fruit $1/2$ cup fresh, frozen or canned fruit
Low-fat or fat free dairy foods	3	8 oz 1% low-fat or fat-free milk 1 cup low-fat yogurt 1 $1/2$ oz low-fat cheese
Meats, poultry, and fish	2 or less	3 oz cooked meats, poultry, or fish
Nuts, seeds, and dry beans	4–5/week	1/3 cup or 1 $1/2$ oz nuts 2 Tbsp or $1/2$ oz seeds $1/2$ cup cooked dry beans
Fats and oils	2–3	1 Tbsp soft tub "light" margarine 1 Tbsp low-fat mayonnaise 2 Tbsp "light" salad dressing 1 tsp vegetable oil
Sweets	5/week	1 Tbsp sugar 1 Tbsp jelly or jam $1/2$ oz jelly beans 8 oz lemonade

*Serving sizes may vary between $1/2$–1 $1/4$ cups.
Source: Appel LJ, Brands MW, Daniels SR, Karanja N, Elmer PJ, Sacks FM. Dietary approaches to prevent and treat hypertension. A Scientific Statement from the American Heart Association. *Hypertension*. 2006;47:296–308.

The Complete Guide to Nutrition in Primary Care by Darwin Deen, MD and Lisa Hark, PhD, RD. Blackwell Publishing 2007.

Review questions

Chapter 1: Nutrition and the primary care clinician

1) *Healthy People 2010* nutrition objectives state that 75% of primary care clinician office visits should include nutrition counseling for which of the following conditions?
(a) Hyperlipidemia
(b) Diabetes
(c) Hypertension
(d) All of the above

2) According to the *US Dietary Guidelines*, adult patients should be advised to consume how many cups of fruits and vegetables per day?
(a) 3 cups fruit and 1 cup vegetables per day
(b) 1 cup fruit and 1 cup vegetables per day
(c) 1 ½ cups fruit and 1 ½ cups vegetables per day
(d) 2 cups fruit and 2 ½ cups vegetables per day

3) According to data from NHANES III, what percentage of Americans do not get the recommended amount of fruits and vegetables in their diet?
(a) 25%
(b) 50%
(c) 75%
(d) 100%

4) According to the 2005 *US Dietary Guidelines*, children 9 years of age and older should be advised to consume how many servings of low-fat dairy foods per day?
(a) 1 serving of a low-fat dairy food per day
(b) 2 servings of low-fat dairy foods per day
(c) 3 servings of low-fat dairy foods per day
(d) None of the above

5) TK is a 16-year-old female who is brought to her doctor by her parents for a sports physical. Her BMI is 17 and she has missed her period several times this year. She is very active, running almost every day. Which of the following statements is the most appropriate next step in the management of this patient?
(a) Ask the patient to cut back on her physical activity
(b) Refer the patient to a behavioral therapist
(c) Give the patient a prescription for a multivitamin
(d) Tell the parents she is fine and schedule a 1-year follow-up appointment

6) FD is a 59-year-old female who requests help from her primary care clinician to lose weight. She has many questions about nutrition and is referred to the registered dietitian working in the office. What is the most appropriate next step for the physician in the management of this patient?
(a) Schedule the patient for a 1-year follow-up appointment
(b) Give the patient a prescription for a weight loss medication
(c) Suggest the patient consider a low carbohydrate diet
(d) Support the dietitian's plan and provide on-going guidance

7) According to a report from the Pew Research Center, 90% of Americans recognize that as a nation, we are obese. What percentage of respondents felt that this was a potential problem for them?
(a) 30%
(b) 40%
(c) 50%
(d) 60%

8) PS is a 10-year-old boy who comes to his doctor for an annual check-up. His parents express concern that he's overweight and watches too much TV. The child's weight and height are documented and BMI is calculated, indicating that PS is in fact overweight (90th %ile). The child's TV and video game use is assessed and he is watching 4 hours of screen time per day during the week

and 6 hours on weekend days. What is the most appropriate next step in the management of this patient?
(a) Limit screen time to less than 2 hours per day including weekends
(b) Tell the parents he is fine and schedule a 1- year follow-up appointment
(c) Tell the child he is not allowed to watch any TV
(d) Prescribe a weight loss diet

9) Some studies indicate that primary care clinicians lack the inclination to provide dietary advice to their patients because they face several barriers. Which of the following barriers were cited in these studies for lack of nutrition counseling by primary care clinicians? (May be more than one correct answer)
(a) Lack of nutrition knowledge
(b) Lack of available office space
(c) Lack of time
(d) Lack of confidence in teaching nutrition

10) RP is a 65-year-old-female who is hospitalized to rule out a myocardial infarction and is visited by her primary care clinician during rounds. Which of the following best describes the role of the primary care clinician with regard to RP's medical nutrition therapy in this setting?
(a) Counsel the patient on a low-sodium diet
(b) Confirm that the patient is receiving a low-sodium diet and has an appetite
(c) Perform a thorough nutrition assessment
(d) Identify nutrition-related risks while the patient is hospitalized

11) KL is a 45-year-old male who comes to see his primary care clinician for a physical. He has not seen a doctor in several years. He reports that he has gained approximately 20 pounds over the past 2 years because he has a sedentary job and has limited free time to devote to exercise. What is the most appropriate next step in the management of this patient with regard to his lack of physical activity?
(a) Recommend KL incorporate exercise into his everyday life
(b) Recommend KL join a gym
(c) Recommend KL play softball at night
(d) Write a prescription stating 60 minutes of physical activity every day

Chapter 2: Changing the office culture to make it work

1) Which of the following statements are TRUE regarding coding for nutrition counseling visits? (May be more than one correct answer)
(a) Nutrition counseling visits can never be billed
(b) Nutrition counseling visits are billable when provided by a physician
(c) Nutrition counseling visits are billable when provided by a registered dietitian
(d) Nutrition counseling visits are billable only for certain diagnoses

2) TV is a 57-year-old male with a sedentary lifestyle whose brief diet history reveals excessive saturated fat intake. He is informed of the health risks associated with his diet and is advised to make some changes. He indicates a willingness to change his diet and begin exercising immediately. According to our proposed model, what is the most appropriate next step in the management of this patient?
(a) Schedule a follow-up appointment in 6 months
(b) Initiate a counseling session immediately, since he is interested
(c) Refer him to a registered dietitian for a more thorough investigation of his dietary intake
(d) Request that he make a follow-up appointment with you in 2 weeks to discuss these issues

3) The AFFECTS questionnaire addresses which of the following lifestyle risks?
(a) Tobacco use
(b) Drug use
(c) Alcohol use
(d) Sugar containing beverages

4) Body mass index is the relationship of body weight to which of the following variables?
(a) Age
(b) Waist circumference
(c) Height
(d) Gender

5) Including nutrition assessment and counseling services is highly recommended as a routine part of patient care. The rationale for providing nutrition services is related to which of the following potential outcomes?
(a) Reducing disease risk and attenuate severity
(b) Reducing primary care office setting costs
(c) Insurance companies require a formal nutrition assessment as part of the annual health maintenance visit
(d) Patient compliance with prescription medications improves

6) Which of the following has been identified as a barrier to providing screening or intervention for behavior change in the primary care office setting?
(a) Physicians doubt their effectiveness
(b) The sensitive nature of discussing lifestyle choices
(c) Limited time and poor reimbursement
(d) All of the above

7) FD is a 56-year-old female with hyperlipidemia who you feel would benefit from a consultation with a registered dietitian. When making a referral, what information should be included to make the visit reimburseable?
(a) Patient's diagnosis and ICD-9 codes for the disease
(b) Patient's social security number
(c) Patient's demographic information
(d) All of the above

8) To improve practice efficiency, certain tasks may be performed by non-clinician providers and office staff members. Which of the following tasks can be performed by non-clinician providers and office staff members?
(a) Distribution of education materials
(b) Measurement of height, weight and calculation of body mass index
(c) Providing copies of laboratory results
(d) All of the above

9) Dietary counseling issues vary by patient age, disease state and food preferences. Column A lists food preferences and disease states. Match those listed in Column A with the appropriate dietary recommendation in Column B.

Column A	Column B
Vegetarian	a. Limit sodium
Congestive Heart Failure	b. Increase protein, B_{12}, iron, calcium
Malabsorption	c. Increase vitamins A, D, E, K, reduce fat

10) When submitting claims for processing with the expectation of reimbursement, codes from what types of code sets should be provided? (May be more than one correct answer)
(a) Procedural codes (CPT-codes)
(b) Diagnostic codes (ICD-9 codes)
(c) Clinical laboratory codes
(d) All of the above

11) Medicare reimburses for Medical Nutrition Therapy (nutrition counseling) for which of the following diseases or conditions? (May be more than one correct answer)
(a) Obesity
(b) Hyperlipidemia
(c) Diabetes mellitus
(d) Chronic renal disease

Chapter 3: Methods of weight control

1) JJ is a 55-year-old female who has been frustrated for some time because she has not been able to lose weight. She comes to see you for a yearly physical and requests a drug to help treat her obesity. Assuming JJ meets the criteria for prescribing an obesity medication such as Meridia (Sibutramine), approximately how much weight should you tell her she can expect to lose on this medication?
(a) 1 to 3% of her body weight
(b) 5 to 10% of her body weight
(c) 12 to 15% of her body weight
(d) 20 to 22% of her body weight

2) MJ is a 35-year-old man who comes to his primary care clinician requesting a referral for surgery so he can have a gastric bypass procedure to treat his obesity. Which of the following must be true for him to be considered for this surgery? (May be more than one correct answer)
(a) BMI ≥ 40
(b) BMI ≥ 35 for those with weight related co-morbidities
(c) Unable to participate in regular physical activity
(d) None of the above

3) Medications for weight loss that affect norepinephrine such as Meridia (Sibutramine) and the generic phentermine, include guidelines for regular monitoring of which of the following parameters? (May be more than one correct answer)
(a) Depression
(b) Blood pressure
(c) Ferritin
(d) Hemoglobin

4) What are the two medications for weight loss that are approved for long-term use?
(a) Tenuate and Adipex
(b) Phentermine and Bontril
(c) Didrex and Phentermine
(d) Orlistat and Sibutramine

5) A version of Orlistat (Xenical) has been approved for over-the-counter use. Xenical will remain a prescription drug. Which of the following will be the over-the-counter dosage for Orlistat?
(a) 60 mg
(b) 120 mg
(c) 30 mg
(d) 25 mg

6) Obesity is associated with a greater than 50% increase in the risk of premature death from all causes compared to normal weight individuals. A modest weight loss has clearly been shown to have significant improvements in the health profile. Which of the following percent reductions in body weight is the minimum needed to achieve a reduction in risk?
(a) <5% weight loss
(b) 5–10% weight loss
(c) 10–15% weight loss
(d) 15–20% weight loss

7) Rimonabant is a new weight loss drug currently pending FDA approval for long-term use. Rimonabant blocks the CB1 receptor of the endocannabinoid system. In addition to weight loss, which of the following best describes the benefits associated with Rimonabant therapy compared to control groups?
(a) Increased HDL-C, increased LDL-C particle size, decreased waist circumference
(b) Increased HDL-C, decreased triglycerides, reduced insulin resistance
(c) Decreased HDL-C, decreased LDL-C particle size, increased waist circumference
(d) Decreased HDL-C, increased triglycerides, increased insulin resistance

8) Which of the following best describes the mechanism by which Orlistat (Xenical) causes patients to experience weight loss?
(a) Appetite suppressant
(b) Reduced absorption of carbohydrate calories
(c) Increases metabolic rate
(d) Reduced absorption of fat calories

9) AM is a 54-year-old post-menopausal woman who wants to lose weight. She is 5′6″ (168 cm) and weighs 190 pounds (86.4 kg). What is her BMI?
(a) $BMI = 19 \, kg/m^2$
(b) $BMI = 24 \, kg/m^2$
(c) $BMI = 31 \, kg/m^2$
(d) $BMI = 36 \, kg/m^2$

10) Over the past decade overweight and obesity has increased dramatically in both adults and children in the U.S. Which of the following hypotheses offers the best explanation for the increased prevalence in overweight and obesity?
(a) Change in the gene pool
(b) Decrease in sedentary behavior
(c) Increase in calorie intake
(d) All of the above

11) KM is a 60-year old post-menopausal woman who wants to lose weight. She is 5'6" (168 cm) and weighs 230 pounds (104.5 kg). Her body mass index (BMI) is calculated to be 37 kg/m². According to KM's BMI, in which of the following classifications does she present?
(a) Class I obesity
(b) Class II obesity
(c) Class III obesity
(d) Morbid obesity

12) Which of the following best describes the clinical findings of the recent study comparing the Atkins diet with a conventional high-carbohydrate, low-fat diet?
(a) After one year there was no statistically significant difference in weight loss between the two diet groups
(b) HDL cholesterol levels dropped as a result of weight loss in both diet plans
(c) Triglyceride levels increased in participants following the Atkins diet plan
(d) The participants following the Atkins diet achieved a greater statistically significant weight loss at one year compared to those following the conventional diet

13) The Dean Ornish diet plan is an example of which of the following diet categories?
(a) High-carbohydrate, low-fat
(b) Low-carbohydrate, high-fat
(c) Moderate carbohydrate and fat
(d) High protein, low carbohydrate

14) According to many authors of popular weight loss diet books, which of the following statements best characterizes the "perfect diet"?
(a) The perfect diet is one that is nutritionally balanced in protein (~20%), fat (~30%) and carbohydrate (~50%)
(b) The perfect diet is one that can be incorporated into the dieter's lifestyle successfully
(c) The perfect diet allows 1 day of "cheating" on special treats
(d) All of the above

15) Which of the following guidelines can help a health care provider evaluate a weight loss diet approach?
(a) Whether the dietary approach will compromise the patient's health
(b) Whether the dietary approach fosters the patient's adherence for the long-term
(c) Whether or not the dietary approach was successful in reducing weight by 5% to 10%
(d) All of the above

Chapter 4: Growing up healthy

1) JK is a 13-year-old boy who comes to see his primary care clinician because he needs a physical before going to overnight camp. JK is 5'10" and weighs 190 pounds. He is at the 90th percentile for BMI. According to his BMI percentile, what is this patient's diagnosis as it relates to his body weight?
(a) The child is obese
(b) The child is overweight
(c) The child is at a normal BMI
(d) Unable to assess with only one value

2) Why does the American Academy of Pediatrics recommend delaying the introduction of solid foods until infants are at least 6 months of age?
(a) They may stimulate the development of food allergies
(b) They may increase the amount of iron in the infant's diet
(c) They may lead to overeating in childhood
(d) They may interfere with quantity of breast milk or formula consumed

3) Which of the following recommendations should be given to parents regarding fluoride to avoid the development of dental caries in children?
(a) Begin fluoride supplements if living in an area without fluoridated water
(b) Begin fluoride supplements for infants exclusively breastfed after 6 months
(c) Begin brushing with fluoridated toothpaste when teeth erupt
(d) All of the above

4) Adolescent girls who develop amenorrhea secondary to low levels of estrogen are at increased risk for which of the following conditions?
(a) Liver disease
(b) Cystic fibrosis
(c) Osteoporosis
(d) Arthritis

5) CJ is an 11-month-old baby girl who is seen by her primary care clinician for a well visit. She is described by her mother as an irritable child. On physical examination you notice that the child is pale. You obtain a complete blood count (CBC) which shows that the child's hemoglobin is 5 g/dL (normal 10.5–13.5 g/dL). Mean corpuscular volume (MCV) is 62 fL (normal 70–84 fL). The child is diagnosed with iron deficiency anemia. Which of the following explanations is the most likely cause of iron deficiency in this child?
(a) The child began drinking apple juice at 6 months
(b) The child began drinking cow's milk at 7 months
(c) The child began eating rice cereal at 5 months
(d) The child began eating fruits and vegetables at 6 months

6) BJ is an 11-year-old girl who comes to see her primary care clinician for a physical before school starts. She has gained 8 pounds since last year and is now considered overweight. When asked about her favorite activities, she states that she loves to watch TV and play on the computer. According to the American Academy of Pediatrics, what is the maximum total number of hours per day that children should spend watching TV, and/or playing computer and video games?
(a) Less than 2 hours per day
(b) Less than 3 hours per day
(c) Less than 4 hours per day
(d) Less than 5 hours per day

7) MK is a 5-month-old baby who is brought to her doctor because of a 3-day history of runny nose and dry erythematous rash on her trunk. According to her mom she started eating solid foods 2 weeks ago, which included rice cereal mixed with formula, eggs and pureed fruits. You believe her symptoms may be the result of an allergic reaction. Which of the following foods would be the most likely cause of these symptoms?
(a) Eggs
(b) Cereal
(c) Formula
(d) Pureed fruits

8) RM is a 2-year-old child who is brought to her primary care physician for a well-child visit. She is at the 45th percentile of weight-for-age and height-for-age and has been growing steadily and normally at this percentile since birth. Her parents express concern that she is a picky eater and that she is not eating enough. Which of the following is the most appropriate response to say to the parents?
(a) Have the parents document everything the child eats and drinks and return in one week
(b) Assure the parents that the child is growing normally and avoid forcing her to eat
(c) Give the child a high-calorie, high-protein food plan
(d) Recommend that the child eat snacks between meals and at bedtime

9) Why is malnutrition especially important to detect, treat, and prevent in children under 3 years old? (Early malnutrition defined as occurring prior to 3 years of age).
(a) Early malnutrition can have a lifelong impact on a child's hemoglobin levels
(b) Early malnutrition can have a lifelong impact on a child's immune function
(c) Early malnutrition can have an impact on brain growth
(d) Early malnutrition can have an impact on fertility

10) MM is a 15-year-old teenager who is brought to see her primary care clinician for a check-up. She is very active with sports and plays all year long. Her parents state that she doesn't seem to eat much, just moves food around on her plate when they eat together. She is 5'2" and weighs 85 pounds (BMI = 15.5). She has lost 15 pounds since her last visit one year ago. She has missed her period for 7 months and currently has amenorrhea. What is the most appropriate next step in the management of this patient?
(a) Refer the patient to a gynecologist
(b) Ask the patient if she uses laxatives after eating
(c) Give the patient a prescription for birth control pills
(d) Refer the patient to a psychiatrist or psychologist specializing in eating disorders

11) Mrs. Jones brings Jane, her 15-year-old daughter, to see her primary care clinician. Jane's grandmother, who has severe osteoporosis, fell last week and broke her hip. Mrs. Jones and Jane are in the midst of a fight because Jane refuses to drink milk. Mrs. Jones wants Jane to drink milk to prevent her daughter from developing osteoporosis later in life. Which of the following statements is correct?
(a) Dairy foods are not recommended for adolescents because so many of them are lactose intolerant
(b) Dairy foods are not recommended because they are a significant source of saturated fat, which promotes atherosclerosis and diabetes
(c) Dairy foods are an efficient source of calcium that promote proper bone mineralization and are required by children and adolescents
(d) Dairy foods are not important for adolescents because bone mineralization ends before puberty starts

12) Joan Smith gives birth to triplets: Jennifer, Tiffany, and Fred. At six months of age the children are seen by their primary care clinician. Mr. Smith asks about changing the children from formula to regular cow's milk (whole milk) when they are six months old. Which of the following is the best response?
(a) The introduction of cow's milk before one year of age may induce a low-grade loss of blood from the GI tract
(b) Although cow's milk is relatively low in iron, the iron is very bioavailable, and milk can be introduced before one year of age
(c) The high renal solute load of cow's milk helps stimulate the development of an infant's kidneys
(d) Cow's milk is high in the vitamins and minerals that infants need at six months of age

13) Mrs. Y and her husband bring their 14-month-old twins to their primary care clinician for a well baby visit. Mr. and Mrs. Y are both from Bangledesh and are both following a low-fat diet because of hyperlipidemia. Their 6-year-old daughter is also following a low-fat diet. Mrs. Y wants to know if it is appropriate to begin skim milk and other fat-free foods for the twins at 18 months-of-age? Which of the following would be the best response?
(a) The children's cholesterol levels should be measured due to their father's history of heart disease; if levels come back high then they can be placed on a low-fat diet
(b) The children should be placed on a low-fat diet immediately
(c) Children should not be placed on low-fat diets until two years of age
(d) None of the above

Chapter 5: Feeding the mother-to-be

1) AB is a 24-year-old woman who comes to the OB/GYN clinic because she has missed her period. A pregnancy test is performed and she is found to be 8 weeks gestation. AB is 5'7" and her pre-pregnancy weight was 135 lbs. According to the National Academy of Sciences, what is the total amount of weight AB should gain during her pregnancy? (Pre-pregnancy BMI = 21.2)
(a) 5–10 lbs
(b) 15–25 lbs
(c) 25–35 lbs
(d) 35–45 lbs

2) Pregnancy is an anabolic state resulting in an increased need for energy. How many additional calories from the diet are required on a daily basis during the second trimester of pregnancy?
(a) No additional calories are required during the second trimester
(b) An additional 100 kcal/day are required during the second trimester
(c) An additional 340 kcal/day are required during the second trimester
(d) An additional 452 kcal/day are required during the second trimester

3) Pregnant women are now routinely prescribed prenatal vitamins during pregnancy to prevent the development of neural tube defects in their fetus. At what point during gestation does the neural tube close.
(a) 18th to 30th day
(b) 35th to 60th day
(c) 3 months to 4 months
(d) By 6 months

4) RS is a pregnant woman who likes to drink one glass of wine when she goes out to dinner on the weekends. Which of the following statements is most correct concerning alcohol intake during pregnancy?

(a) Alcohol during pregnancy always causes fetal alcohol syndrome and birth defects
(b) Alcohol during the first trimester of pregnancy is safe in moderation
(c) Alcohol during the third trimester of pregnancy is safe in moderation
(d) Alcohol is not recommended for pregnant women

5) According to the Dietary Reference Intake (DRI), how many additional calories from the diet are required on a daily basis when a woman is lactating during the first 6 months?
(a) No additional calories are required from the diet during lactation
(b) An additional 100 kcal/day are required during the first 6 months
(c) An additional 300 kcal/day are required during the first 6 months
(d) An additional 500 kcal/day are required during the first 6 months

6) LH, a 32-year-old woman planning her second pregnancy, has already delivered an infant with a neural tube defect (spina bifida) and asks if there is anything she can do to prevent a recurrence. Which vitamin supplement has been shown to decrease the incidence of neural tube defects in newborns when given to pregnant women who have previously delivered a child with such a defect?
(a) Vitamin B_{12}
(b) Folic acid
(c) Thiamin
(d) All of the above

7) CB begins to successfully breast-feed her new baby after speaking to a lactation consultant in the hospital. Which of the following statements regarding maternal milk production is correct?
(a) Breast-milk production is dependent on maternal nutritional status
(b) Breast-milk production is independent of the weight of the infant
(c) Breast-milk production is determined by the frequency of nursing
(d) Breast-milk production is unaffected by smoking as none of the circulating components of cigarette smoke pass into breast milk

8) CB asks what vitamins, if any, are lacking in breast milk. Excluding vitamin K, which is routinely given to all infants, which of the following vitamins are typically present in low levels in breast milk, depending on the mother's diet and genetic makeup?
(a) Vitamin A
(b) Vitamin D
(c) Folate
(d) Vitamin B_6

9) NM, a 15-year-old girl, comes to the OB/GYN clinic for her first prenatal visit. She reports having begun menstruation at age 13. NM is 5'7", and her pre-pregnancy weight was 115 pounds (BMI = 18). Based on NM's pre-pregnancy weight status, how much weight should she gain during her pregnancy?
(a) 15–20 pounds
(b) 20–25 pounds
(c) 25–30 pounds
(d) 30–45 pounds

10) Megavitamin therapy is a common practice for many patients, however, some may not recognize the potential for toxicity. Of the following vitamins, which of the following is associated with teratogenic effects (birth defects in the developing embryo) if taken during pregnancy in doses exceeding the Dietary Reference Intake Tolerable Upper Limit?
(a) Vitamin C
(b) Vitamin A
(c) Vitamin B_{12}
(d) Folate

11) Iron controls the production of red blood cells in both the mother and her developing fetus. During which trimester of pregnancy are iron requirements the highest?
(a) 1st trimester
(b) 2nd trimester
(c) 3rd trimester
(d) Iron requirements do not change during pregnancy

12) Gestational diabetes mellitus is commonly seen in approximately 4% of pregnant women. In reviewing a patient's history, which of the following is considered a risk factor for gestational diabetes?
(a) Individuals of African-American descent
(b) Under-nutrition
(c) Maternal age
(d) First degree relative with cardiovascular disease

Chapter 6: Staying healthy in later life

1) Metabolic changes that are associated with aging include which of the following descriptions?
(a) Lean body mass increases, body fat decreases
(b) Lean body mass decreases, body fat increases
(c) Lean body mass increases, body fat increases
(d) Lean body mass decreases, body fat decreases

2) Appetite stimulants are appropriately used in which of the following cases?
(a) Patients lose weight due to dysphagia
(b) Patients lose weight due to depression

(c) Patients lose weight due to a lack of appetite or interest in food
(d) Patients are nearing death due to a terminal illness

3) Calcium requirements increase as people grow older in order to compensate for the decreased production of $1,25(OH)_2D$ by the kidney and for the accelerated bone mineral losses. According to the Dietary References Intake (DRI) for males and females age 51 years and older, how much calcium is required on a daily basis?
(a) 800 mg/day
(b) 1000 mg/day
(c) 1200 mg/day
(d) 2000 mg/day

4) The absorption and bioavailability of vitamins and minerals may decline as a normal consequence of aging. Which of the following age-related physiological changes can cause these nutritional problems?
(a) Reduced gastric acid secretion
(b) Reduced T-cell function
(c) Reduced glomerular filtration rate
(d) Reduced bone density

5) Constipation is very common in older adults due to decreased GI motility, inadequate fiber and fluid intake and use of certain medications. Which of the following foods contains the most amount of fiber and can be recommended to treat constipation?
(a) Gatorade
(b) Pasta
(c) Oatmeal
(d) Yogurt

6) Monitoring nutritional status, identifying risk factors, and intervening to promote adequate nutrition is most important in which of the following patients?
(a) All patients over the age of 55 due to changes in macronutrient and micronutrient needs
(b) All patients with unintentional weight loss
(c) All patients on a therapeutic diet for a chronic condition
(d) All patients with constipation

7) Older adults are frequently prescribed multiple medications to be taken on a daily basis. How can medications affect the nutritional status of older adults?
(a) Alter food intake by decreasing appetite, taste, and smell
(b) Decrease absorption and function of nutrients
(c) Cause gastrointestinal disturbances such as nausea or constipation
(d) All of the above

8) Which of the following body mass index (BMI) cut-offs should be used as the criteria in older adults to prompt further evaluation of nutritional status?
(a) BMI < 25
(b) BMI < 22
(c) BMI < 20
(d) BMI < 18

9) Decreased ability to taste food may be caused by which of the following in older adults?
(a) Age-related changes in odor perception
(b) Adverse effects of medication
(c) Alzheimer's Disease
(d) All of the above

10) FD is a 72-year-old male with Parkinson's Disease who has lost 30 pounds over a one year period due to a significant decline in appetite and interest in eating. He is 6'1" and now weighs 150 pounds (BMI = 20, Albumin = 2.0 mg/dL). He is admitted to the hospital for a medical work-up and treatment of malnutrition and the Nutrition Support Service is consulted. After a 3-day calorie count revealed poor oral intake despite adding nutritional supplements and snacks to his diet, enteral nutrition support is recommended. Which of the following statements best describes the scientific rationale for choosing enteral and not parenteral nutrition support for this patient?
(a) Enteral nutrition supplies more calories than parenteral nutrition
(b) The patient's gastrointestinal tract is functional
(c) Malnutrition will be reversed sooner when enteral nutrition is provided
(d) The patient's albumin is under 2.5 mg/dL

11) RD is an 88-year-old male who is admitted to the rehabilitation center following a stroke 2 weeks ago. Physical examination shows dry skin and dry mucous membranes. He has had minimal urine output since admission. He is 5'8" and weighs 151 pounds (BMI = 23) and his weight has remained stable over the past 2 weeks. His kidney function is adequate for his age. He is presently receiving 6 cans of Ensure over 24-hours via a continuous feeding tube at a rate of 60 cc per hour. Which of the following interventions should be recommended at this time?
(a) Add an additional can of Ensure (240 ml)
(b) Decrease the tube feeding rate to 40 cc per hour
(c) Flush the tube with 100 cc of water every 4 hours
(d) Change to bolus feedings rather than continuous

12) Nutritional frailty is defined as which of the following in older adults?
(a) Albumin <2.5 mg/dL
(b) BMI <18
(c) Sarcopenia and rapid, unintentional weight loss
(d) Complaints of food tasting bland

13) Feeding tubes are appropriate in which of the following situations?
(a) To meet nutritional needs during an acute but reversible illness that compromises oral intake
(b) For a patient whose chronic illness compromises oral nutrition and who is able to understand and accept the benefits and risks associated with prolonged use of a feeding tube
(c) To supplement oral intake when the patient has an intact GI tract but has trouble consistently consuming adequate nutrients
(d) All of the above

Chapter 7: Dyslipidemia, hypertension and metabolic syndrome

1) Which of the following risk factors for metabolic syndrome has different criteria among various ethnic groups?
(a) Hypertension
(b) Fasting plasma glucose levels
(c) Waist circumference
(d) HDL levels

2) Omega-3 fatty acids (eicosapentanoic acid and docosahexenoic acid) are effective at reducing which of the following serum levels if they are abnormally elevated?
(a) Triglycerides
(b) LDL-cholesterol
(c) Lp(a)
(d) All of the above

3) JK is a 45-year-old male who comes to see his primary care clinician for a routine physical examination. He is 5'8", weighs 210 pounds (BMI) = 32). His waist circumference is 41 inches and his most recent lab work showed an abnormal glucose of 109 mg/dL and triglycerides of 282 mg/dL. He reports that he has been traveling lately and that his diet has been poor. He is recommended to make some changes to his diet over the next 3 months and have repeat lab work done at that time. Which of the following dietary interventions will most likely improve JK's abnormal laboratory findings?
(a) Reduction in saturated fat intake
(b) Reduction in simple carbohydrate intake
(c) Reduction in trans fat intake
(d) Increase in monounsaturated fat intake

4) The metabolic syndrome, which is targeted by the National Cholesterol Education Program ATP III guidelines for intensive lifestyle change, includes low HDL cholesterol and waist circumference defined in women as which of the following?
(a) HDL < 50 mg/dL and waist circumferance >35 inches
(b) HDL < 40 mg/dL and waist circumferance >40 inches
(c) HDL < 35 mg/dL and waist circumferance >40 inches
(d) HDL < 35 mg/dL and waist circumferance >35 inches

5) Which of the following dietary approaches was just as effective as low dose statin therapy reducing LDL cholesterol levels?
(a) Dietary Approaches to Stop Hypertension (DASH)
(b) Diabetes Prevention Program
(c) Portfolio Diet Study
(d) Lyon Diet Heart Study

6) Which of the following characterizes atherogenic dyslipidemia often seen in patients with metabolic syndrome?
(a) Reduced levels of HDL-cholesterol
(b) Increased levels of apolipoprotein B
(c) Increased small LDL-cholesterol particles
(d) All of the above

7) The 2005 *U.S. Dietary Guidelines* advises eating as little trans fat as possible. Which of the following statements is true regarding trans fats?
(a) Trans fats are saturated fats found in animal product
(b) Trans fats raise both LDL and HDL cholesterol levels
(c) Trans fats raise LDL cholesterol and lower HDL cholesterol levels
(d) Trans fats are polyunsaturated fats found in liquid vegetable oils

8) The National High Blood Pressure Education Program estimates that a reduction in systolic blood pressure by which of the following mm Hg is thought to save more than 70,000 lives in the US each year?
(a) 0.5 mm Hg
(b) 2 mm Hg
(c) 4 mm Hg
(d) 7 mm Hg

9) Which of the following daily combined number of fruit and vegetable servings were included in the Dietary Approaches to Stop Hypertension (DASH) trial?
(a) 2 to 4 servings of fruits and vegetables per day
(b) 3 to 6 servings of fruits and vegetables per day
(c) 6 to 7 servings of fruits and vegetables per day
(d) 8 to 10 servings of fruits and vegetables per day

10) Which of the following statements is correct regarding the relationship between an individual's alcohol consumption, blood pressure (BP), and lifestyle?
(a) The relationship between alcohol and BP is dependent on both the amount and type of alcohol consumed
(b) The relationship between alcohol and BP is dependent on the amount of alcohol consumed, not the type of alcohol
(c) The relationship between alcohol and BP is dependent on the effects of obesity and sodium intake
(d) There is no relationship between alcohol and BP

11) Which of the following recommendations is included as part of ATP III's Therapeutic Lifestyle Changes?
(a) Balancing calorie intake with expenditure to maintain a healthy weight
(b) Substituting unsaturated fat for saturated and trans fat
(c) Supplementing the diet with 2 gm plant stanol/sterol esters daily
(d) All of the above

12) Low density lipoprotein (LDL) cholesterol has been identified by ATP III as the most atherogenic lipoprotein, making it the primary target for cholesterol lowering therapy. Nutritional analysis of your patient's food record provides the following calorie distribution:
    54% of calories from carbohydrate
    30% of calories from fat (6% saturated, 14% monounsaturated, 10% polyunsaturated)
    16% of calories from protein
    250 mg cholesterol
    14 gm dietary fiber (4 gm soluble fiber)

Which of the following dietary interventions will most likely lower the patient's elevated LDL cholesterol levels?
(a) Further reduction in dietary cholesterol intake
(b) Increase in dietary fat intake
(c) Increase in dietary fiber and soluble fiber intake
(d) Increase in dietary protein intake

13) Which of the following fats is highest in trans fatty acids?
(a) Stick margarine
(b) Olive oil
(c) Butter
(d) Sunflower oil

Chapter 8: Diabetes, pre-diabetes, and hypoglycemia

1) Which of the following outcomes should be used to evaluate the effectiveness of medical nutrition therapy on glycemia in patients with diabetes?
(a) Outcomes from medical nutrition therapy should be evaluated within one month after initiation
(b) Outcomes from medical nutrition therapy should be evaluated at 6 months after initiation
(c) The expected outcome from medical nutrition therapy is a 1% to 2% decrease in A1C
(d) Medical nutrition therapy for diabetes has an immediate effect on lipids

2) Which of the following statements best summarizes the initial priority of medical nutrition therapy in patients with type 1 diabetes?
(a) Focus on developing a meal plan emphasizing weight reduction
(b) Focus on developing an insulin regimen that integrates physiological insulin therapy into the patient's lifestyle after the meal plan is developed
(c) Focus on getting the patient to eat 3 meals and 3 snacks at consistent times each day
(d) Focus on getting the patient to include regular physical activity

3) Which of the following statements best summarizes the initial priority of medical nutrition therapy in patients with type 2 diabetes?
(a) Focus on achieving an ideal body weight
(b) Focus on eliminating sugars and starches made from white flour
(c) Focus on utilizing nutrition interventions that will improve metabolic outcomes, such as glucose, lipids, and blood pressure
(d) Focus on abstaining from drinking alcohol

4) Which of the following statements is correct regarding carbohydrate intake in patients with diabetes?
(a) The total amount of carbohydrate ingested is more important than the source or the type
(b) Any increase in fiber will improve glycemia
(c) Implementing a low glycemic index diet will improve glucose and lipid levels
(d) Sugars cause a rapid increase in blood glucose concentrations

5) Using the carbohydrate counting method for meal panning, which of the following grams of carbohydrate equals one carbohydrate serving?
(a) 5 grams of carbohydrate
(b) 10 grams of carbohydrate
(c) 15 grams of carbohydrate
(d) 20 grams of carbohydrate

6) According to the NCEP Adult Treatment Panel III guidelines and the American Diabetes Association, what is the target LDL cholesterol goal for all adults with diabetes?
(a) <190 mg/dL
(b) <160 mg/dL
(c) <130 mg/dL
(d) <100 mg/dL

7) There is general consensus on which of the following dietary guidelines for healthy eating?
(a) Carbohydrates should be restricted
(b) Protein intake should be increased
(c) Saturated and *trans* fat intake should be lowered
(d) Only monounsaturated fats should be used to replace saturated fats

8) Which of the following recommendations regarding alcohol consumption in persons with type 1 diabetes is most appropriate?
(a) Alcohol should be consumed without food to avoid excess calories
(b) Alcohol should be consumed with food to prevent hypoglycemia
(c) Avoid sweet wines because they raise blood glucose
(d) Alcoholic beverages should not be consumed for good glycemic control

9) Two major studies showed a 58% reduction in the onset of diabetes in a population of people with pre-diabetes. What percentage weight loss was necessary to achieve this risk reduction?
(a) 7%
(b) 15%
(c) 25%
(d) 58%

10) Which of the following must be reduced for successful weight loss?
(a) Carbohydrate
(b) Protein
(c) Fat
(d) Calories

11) Which of the following strategies may help patients with hypoglycemia of non-diabetic origin avoid symptoms?
(a) Eat a high protein, high fat diet
(b) Eat small meals, with snacks interspersed between meals
(c) Avoid all foods containing carbohydrate
(d) Exercise before eating a meal

12) Which of the following actions by a health professional is likely to be beneficial for behavior change in individuals in the pre-contemplation Stage of Change?
(a) Specific guidelines on actions to implement are recommended
(b) Highlight the relationship between the individual's risk for potential disease outcome and the individual's behavioural change
(c) Engaging family members in supporting behavior change is essential
(d) Help the patient set realistic goals for two behavior changes

Chapter 9: Gastrointestinal disorders

1) JT is a 54-year-old male with chronic liver disease and ascites. He is not currently experiencing encephalopathy. What dietary recommendation is most appropriate for JT at this time?
(a) Low-sodium diet
(b) Low-sodium, low-protein diet
(c) High-protein diet
(d) Low-fat diet

2) Medical nutrition therapy for patients with peptic ulcer disease should include which of the following recommendations? (May be more than one correct answer)
(a) Avoid alcohol
(b) Limit caffeine
(c) Avoid dairy foods
(d) Eat small, frequent meals

3) Patients with a variety of GI disorders may benefit from ingesting more soluble fiber. Which of the following foods would be considered the best source of soluble fiber?
(a) Carrots
(b) Oatmeal
(c) Wheat bran
(d) Watermelon

4) Recent research has focused on the health benefits of probiotics in gastrointestinal health. What dietary recommendation can be given to patients with inflammatory bowel disease or irritable bowel syndrome to increase their intake of probiotics?
(a) Increase intake of fresh fruits and vegetables
(b) Take a soluble fiber supplement
(c) Consume yogurt with live, active cultures (i.e., lactobacillus)
(d) Drink soy milk fortified with vitamins and minerals

5) Individuals with celiac disease are advised to avoid all foods containing rye, wheat, and barley because they are especially sensitive to which of the following proteins?
(a) Albumin
(b) Gluten
(c) Gliadin
(d) Casein

6) Which of the following populations have a high prevalence of lactose intolerance (more than 50% may experience lactose intolerance)? (May be more than one correct answer)
(a) Latinos
(b) African American
(c) Native American
(d) Asians

7) RT is a 45-year-old female with chronic diarrhea. A comprehensive GI workup has failed to determine a cause of her diarrhea. She has no abnormalities in her blood work and her weight has been stable. Her biggest complaint is

the impact on her quality of life. What adjustments to her diet may help to decrease her diarrhea?
(a) Eliminate fruits and vegetables
(b) Increase intake of fish and poultry
(c) Choose foods high in soluble fiber or take a soluble fiber supplement
(d) Include fruit juices or Gatorade in her diet to replace electrolyte losses

8) FC is a 28-year-old obese female diagnosed with gallstones. Her body BMI is 37. Her primary care clinician recommends that she try to lose weight to help control her gallstone formation. What would be the maximum amount of weight that she should lose each week to prevent additional gallstones?
(a) 1/2 to 1 pound per week
(b) 1 to 2 pounds per week
(c) 3 to 4 pounds per week
(d) 5 pounds per week

9) Pl is a 24-year-old male who was diagnosed with Crohn's disease several years ago. He has lost a significant amount of weight and complains of poor appetite most of the time. Which of the following factors could contribute to anorexia in patients with Crohn's disease and therefore lead to weight loss? (May be more than one correct answer)
(a) Elevated levels of tumor necrosis factor-alpha
(b) Elevated levels of cytokines
(c) Reduced levels of lactase enzyme
(d) Taste changes secondary to medications

10) DM is a 30-year-old female with ulcerative colitis who has been prescribed Sulfasalazine. Which of the following vitamins should be prescribed to patients who are being treated with Sulfasalazine?
(a) Folate
(b) Vitamin A
(c) Vitamin C
(d) Thiamin

11) MT is a 42-year-old male experiencing the following symptoms: abdominal pain, altered bowel motility, and bloating. The physician suspects irritable bowel syndrome (IBS). Which other etiologies of such symptoms should be ruled out prior to diagnosing IBS? (May be more than one correct answer)
(a) Lactose malabsorption
(b) Inflammatory bowel disease
(c) Colon polyps
(d) Fructose malabsorption

12) PR is a 50-year-old female with chronic pancreatitis who is hospitalized for surgical evaluation. Assuming that PR takes pancreatic enzymes and can tolerate food, what diet should be prescribed for her at this time?
(a) Low-sodium diet
(b) Low-protein diet
(c) Low-fat diet
(d) Low-fiber diet

Chapter 10: Everything else

1) Dietary protein is restricted for individuals with chronic kidney disease (CKD) prior to initiating dialysis for which of the following reasons?
(a) To preserve lean body mass
(b) To prevent weight loss
(c) To minimize the symptoms of uremia
(d) All of the above

2) The goal of medical nutrition therapy for patients with nephrolithiasis (kidney stones) is to eliminate the diet related risk factors for stone formation. Which of the following recommendations is most critical for patients with a history of kidney stones?
(a) Increase fluid intake
(b) Increase protein intake
(c) Decrease calcium intake
(d) Decrease magnesium intake

3) Medical nutrition therapy for patients with calcium oxalate stones includes which of the following recommendations?
(a) Low calcium diet (< 500 mg/d)
(b) Low sodium diet (< 1500 mg/d)
(c) Low oxalate diet ($< 40\text{-}50$ g/d)
(d) Low fiber diet (< 8g/d)

4) MR is a 30-year-old male who is HIV positive but has not progressed to acquired immunodeficiency syndrome (AIDS). His primary care clinician has stressed to him the importance of maintaining optimal nutrition status. Which of the following should be included by the clinician as part of early nutritional counseling? (May be more than one correct answer)
(a) Establish appropriate calorie intake
(b) Assess BMI, waist and hip circumference, waist-to-hip ratio
(c) Recommend mega-doses of vitamin and mineral supplements
(d) Assess lipids, albumin, and glucose levels

5) TY is a 45-year-old alcoholic who presents to the Emergency Room with pain in his stomach. Laboratory tests reveal he has iron deficiency anemia. What other clinical manifestations of this type of anemia may be encountered during TY's physical exam? (May be more than one correct answer)
(a) Tachycardia
(b) Peripheral neuropathy
(c) Arthralgia
(d) Pallor

6) MA is a 24-year-old female experiencing a urinary tract infection (UTI). Which of the following is the most likely pathogen leading to her UTI?
(a) Staphylococcus
(b) Escherichia coli (E. coli)
(c) Proteus mirabilis
(d) Group B strep

7) MA's grandmother (in the above question) insists she drink cranberry juice to lower her incidence of UTIs. MA thinks this is an old wives' tale, but decides to ask her primary care clinician. To MA's surprise her clinician agrees with her grandmother. By what mechanism can cranberry juice exert a bacteriostatic effect?
(a) Acidifying of urine to destroy pathogen
(b) Reducing ability of pathogen to bind to uroepithelial cells
(c) Inducing dehydration by increasing urine output
(d) Restoring normal urogenital flora with lactobacillus

8) Patients may experience migraine headaches following exposure to certain dietary-related triggers. Match the dietary trigger in Column A with its chemical ingredient in Column B.

Column A	Column B
Diet Soda	(a) Nitrites
Chocolate	(b) Tyramine
Wine, beer	(c) Phenylethylamine
Hot dogs	(d) Aspartame

9) Many commercial foods are higher in sodium than consumers would expect. Which of the following foods contains a high sodium content (> 400 mg/serving)? (May be more than one correct answer)
(a) Tomato juice
(b) Ham
(c) Grilled chicken
(d) Soy sauce

10) LT is a 33-year-old Asian female who is experiencing recurrent migraines. Her history reveals a headache following the consumption of fried rice and pan-fried pork dumplings for lunch. Which of the following additives may be the chemical trigger for LT's migraines?
(a) Phenolic amine
(b) Histamine
(c) Monosodium glutamate
(d) Nitric Oxide

11) SM is a 23-year-old female with a history of dysfunctional uterine bleeding, who is admitted to the Emergency Department. Her laboratory tests reveals iron-deficiency anemia with a hemoglobin of 8.6 g/dL. Which of the following is the optimal daily dose of elemental iron that she should be prescribed at this time?
(a) 60 mg, 3 times daily
(b) 60 mg, 2 times daily
(c) 45 mg, 3 times daily
(d) 45 mg, 2 times daily

12) The glomerular filtration rate (GFR) is used to determine whether protein restriction should be initiated in patients with chronic kidney disease (CKD). At what GFR level should a CKD patient be prescribed a low-protein diet? (Select the best answer.)
(a) GFR < 60 ml/min.
(b) GFR < 30 ml/min.
(c) GFR < 20 ml/min.
(d) GFR < 15 ml/min.

13) PF is a 50-year-old male with human immunodeficiency virus (HIV). He has been treated with highly active antiretroviral therapy (HAART) for several years. His lipid levels are significantly elevated. He complains that his legs are skinny and he looks like he has a beer gut. Which of the following HAART complications has PF developed?
(a) Opportunistic infections
(b) Lypodystrophy
(c) Polyphagia and obesity
(d) Hypoglycemia and hypertension

Chapter 11: Vitamins

1) The National Academy of Sciences Institute of Medicine has updated the Recommended Dietary Allowance (RDA) for certain vitamins and minerals to focus more on the prevention of disease rather than the reversal of deficiency states. Which of the following is the updated term used that includes current

vitamin and mineral requirements, tolerable upper limit, and adequate intake established by the Institute of Medicine?
(a) Dietary Reference Intake (DRI)
(b) Recommended Dietary Intake (RDI)
(c) International Reference Unit (IRU)
(d) Reference Daily Allowance (RDA)

2) DH is a 56-year-old male who has had ulcerative colitis for the past 30 years. Ten years ago he was treated with a resection of his terminal ileum. He has not taken any vitamin supplements following this procedure. He presents to his primary care clinician complaining of numbness and tingling in his hands and feet. Which of the following vitamin deficiency should be suspected?
(a) Vitamin C
(b) Vitamin D
(c) Vitamin B_{12}
(d) Vitamin K

3) BT is an 18-year-old teenager who comes to his primary care clinician complaining of headaches and hair loss. He has started taking large doses of vitamins because a friend told him this would improve his acne. Mega doses of which of the following vitamins could contribute to headaches and hair loss (above the tolerable upper limit recommendation)?
(a) Vitamin A
(b) Vitamin B_{12}
(c) Vitamin E
(d) Vitamin B_6

4) GL is a 56-year-old female with atrial fibrillation who has recently been prescribed Coumadin by her cardiologist. Her primary care clinician notes that her prothrombin time (PT) seems to fluctuate and asks her to keep a food record. Which of the following foods should be monitored based on her medical history?
(a) Green leafy vegetables
(b) Breads and cereals
(c) Dairy foods
(d) Meats and poultry

5) Recent evidence has shown that individuals who eat a diet rich in phytochemicals may have a lower incidence of which of the following conditions?
(a) Cancer
(b) Bone disease
(c) Ear infections
(d) Alopecia

6) Phytochemicals are naturally occurring compounds which have antioxidant properties. They are found primarily in plant foods, as well as in red wine. Drinking small amounts of red wine on a daily basis has been shown to have cardiovascular benefits. Which of the following phytochemicals are found in red wine?
(a) Sopinins
(b) Terpines
(c) Polyphenols
(d) Resveratrol

7) PL is a 25-year-old female who takes birth control pills and vitamin supplements. Due to the potential drug-nutrient interaction, which of the following vitamin supplements should be limited?
(a) Vitamin A
(b) Vitamin C
(c) Vitamin D
(d) Folate

8) An elderly couple comes to see their primary care clinician for a check-up. They are in good health and take large doses of vitamin supplements. The wife reports that her husband has been bruising easily and that after a shaving cut, he could not get the bleeding to stop. After reviewing their list of supplements, you advise him to discontinue which of the following supplements?
(a) Beta-carotene (10,000 IU daily)
(b) Alpha-tocopheral (1000 mg daily)
(c) Ascorbic acid (500 mg daily)
(d) Sublingual vitamin B_{12} (1 mg daily)

9) Older adults frequently experience achlorhydria, which is a normal process associated with aging. Which of the following nutrient groups may not be adequately absorbed in older adults secondary to achlorhydria?
(a) Fiber
(b) Carbohydrates and protein
(c) Calcium and iron
(d) Fat-soluble vitamins

10) What is the current Recommended Daily Allowance (RDA) for folate in non-pregnant women according to the Dietary Reference Intake (DRI)?
(a) 100 micrograms/day
(b) 400 micrograms/day
(c) 600 micrograms/day
(d) 1000 micrograms/day

11) CK is an 18-year-old teenage boy who has been taking Monocycline (antibiotic) for acne for the past 5 years. Based on this history, what vitamin deficiency is CK at risk of developing?
(a) Vitamin B_{12}
(b) Vitamin C
(c) Vitamin K
(d) Vitamin A

12) Vitamin C intake enhances the absorption of which of the following minerals?
(a) Fluoride
(b) Iron
(c) Sodium
(d) Calcium

13) MT is a 35-year-old homeless man who presents to the Emergency Department with magenta tongue, soreness of the lips and mouth, and cheilosis. Which of the following vitamin deficiencies should be suspected in this patient?
(a) Vitamin C deficiency
(b) Iron deficiency
(c) Niacin deficiency
(d) Folate deficiency

Chapter 12: Minerals

1) Which of the following statements best describes why calcium requirements increase as people grow older?
(a) To compensate for the decreased production of $1,25(OH)_2D$ by the kidney
(b) Bone mineral losses have declined
(c) Lactase enzyme activity has declined
(d) All of the above

2) JR is a 16-year-old adolescent boy who runs cross-country and plays basketball. He skips lunch and has a snack before track in the afternoon. He drinks predominantly soda, sports drinks, and juices and his mother is concerned that he is not getting enough calcium. According to the DRIs, how much dietary and/or supplemental calcium is required on a daily basis for a teenager?
(a) 500 mg/day
(b) 800 mg/day
(c) 1000 mg/day
(d) 1300 mg/day

3) The DASH diet research has demonstrated that lifestyle changes can be effective in reducing blood pressure. During the routine medical history, what dietary factors should be elicited to prescribe DASH-related interventions?
(a) Sodium, fruits, vegetables and saturated fat intake
(b) Sodium, vegetables, and fiber intake
(c) Sodium, fruits, vegetables, dairy and saturated fat intake
(d) Sodium, dairy, fruits, and vegetable intake

4) Which of the following diseases may result in zinc deficiency?
(a) Kidney stones
(b) Multiple sclerosis
(c) Hyperlipidemia
(d) Crohn's disease

5) Match the mineral in Column A with the food source in Column B. Answers in Column B can only be used once.

Column A	Column B
Iron	(a) Whole grains
Sodium	(b) Potatoes
Potassium	(c) Luncheon meats
Magnesium	(d) Dried apricots

6) Which of the following minerals functions as an antioxidant by working with enzymes that protect cells from the damaging effects of free radicals?
(a) Zinc
(b) Selenium
(c) Potassium
(d) Chromium

7) MN is a 48-year-old male with hypertension. He is interested in managing his blood pressure with non-pharmacological treatment, such as diet and exercise. Diets high in which of the following minerals have been shown to reduce blood pressure? (May be more than one correct answer)
(a) Fluoride
(b) Potassium
(c) Calcium
(d) Zinc

8) OK is a 68-year old man with congestive heart failure who is being treated with an ACE inhibitor. His most recent blood work shows a serum potassium level of 4.8 MEq/dL and he is diagnosed with hyperkalemia. He is told to decrease his dietary potassium intake. In addition to bananas, which of the following foods are high in potassium and should be limited?

(a) Orange juice
(b) White bread
(c) Turkey
(d) Green beans

9) In the United States, the average daily sodium intake is approximately how many milligrams?
(a) 2400 mg
(b) 4500 mg
(c) 5500 mg
(d) 6000 mg

10) MT is a 31-year-old female who was diagnosed with inflammatory bowel disease and reports occasional blood in her stools. She complains of fatigue, and feeling cold, and she chews on ice. Which of the following mineral deficiencies should be suspected in this patient?
(a) Magnesium
(b) Phosphorus
(c) Iron
(d) Calcium

11) SR is a 65-year-old female who has been taking antacids with calcium carbonate for several years to prevent osteoporosis. Which of the following minerals binds with antacids and may lead to a deficiency of this mineral?
(a) Magnesium
(b) Phosphorous
(c) Potassium
(d) Zinc

Chapter 13: Dietary and nutritional supplements

1) Which of the following dietary supplements can have anti-inflammatory properties?
(a) Vitamin C
(b) Omega-3-fatty acids
(c) Zinc
(d) Vitamin B6

2) Which of the following dietary recommendations should be provided to all patients receiving Warfarin therapy for anticoagulation?
(a) Maintain daily consistency in vitamin K intake
(b) Maintain daily consistency in vitamin C intake
(c) Eat a diet low in vitamin A
(d) Eat a diet low in vitamin D

3) Patients who suffer from migraine headaches may benefit from taking which of the following supplements? (May be more than one correct answer)
(a) Vitamin B_{12}
(b) Vitamin A
(c) Magnesium
(d) Folate

4) RS is a 25-year-old female who avoids eating dairy foods because she is lactose intolerant. She has tried lactose-free products but her symptoms do not improve. Patients who avoid eating dairy foods would benefit most from taking which of the following two supplements?
(a) Vitamin E and folate
(b) Vitamin C and iron
(c) Vitamin A and riboflavin
(d) Vitamin D and calcium

5) Folate supplementation is used in the treatment of which of the following conditions?
(a) Fibromyalgia
(b) Hyperhomocysteinemia
(c) Hypertriglyceridemia
(d) Coagulopathy

6) DD is a 55-year-old female who is scheduled for an elective cholecystectomy. Which of the following supplements should be discontinued 2 weeks prior to surgery?
(a) Vitamin C
(b) Iron
(c) Calcium
(d) Vitamin E

7) RS is a 79-year-old female with Parkinson's disease who was started on L-Dopa by her neurologist. You know that she is taking multiple dietary supplements. Which of the following would you advise that she discontinue because it interferes with the effectiveness of L-Dopa?
(a) Vitamin B_{12}
(b) Coenzyme Q10
(c) Calcium
(d) Vitamin B_6

8) PJ is a 54-year-old male who has recently been diagnosed with calcium oxalate stones. Which of the following supplements should not be prescribed for patients with calcium oxalate kidney stones because it has been shown to cause hyperoxaluria (increased urinary oxalate) and may contribute to more stones?
(a) Beta-carotene
(b) Calcium

(c) Vitamin C
(d) Zinc

9) TR is a 40-year-old female who has experienced constipation for many years. Which of the following dietary supplements can be prescribed to help reduce her constipation?
(a) Glucoseamine sulfate
(b) Probiotics
(c) Vitamin A
(d) Iron

10) MR is a 73-year-old male who has been taking thiazide diuretics for hypertension for the past 15 years. He regularly takes a potassium supplement. Which of the following minerals should also be prescribed to MR because its excretion also increases in patients taking thiazide diuretics?
(a) Phosphorus
(b) Iron
(c) Zinc
(d) Calcium

11) WS is a 55-year-old female who is complaining of intermittent flushing, itching, and heartburn for several months. Mega-dosing of which of the following vitamins may result in these symptoms?
(a) Niacin
(b) Riboflavin
(c) Vitamin B_{12}
(d) Vitamin E

12) Mineral oil is no longer prescribed to children as a laxative because it interferes with the absorption of certain nutrients. Which of the following group of nutrients is most affected by mineral oil?
(a) Electrolyte absorption
(b) Water-soluble vitamin absorption
(c) Fat-soluble vitamin absorption
(d) Mineral absorption

13) Metformin is commonly prescribed to patients with diabetes. Which of the following vitamin supplements should not be taken at the same time as Metformin because of a potential drug-nutrient interaction which may result in decreased vitamin absorption?
(a) Vitamin B_6
(b) Thiamin
(c) Riboflavin
(d) Vitamin B_{12}

Chapter 14: Considering the alternatives

1) The Specific Carbohydrate Diet (SCD) is a low disaccharide diet in which almost all foods containing disaccharides and polysaccharides are eliminated. This therapeutic diet can be extremely helpful to patients with which of the following conditions?
(a) Diverticulitis
(b) Crohn's disease
(c) Ulcerative colitis
(d) All of the above

2) Which of the following foods are allowed on The Specific Carbohydrate Diet?
(a) Honey
(b) Cornflakes
(c) White rice
(d) Wheat bread

3) Elimination diets may be prescribed to children with which of the following conditions?
(a) Failure-to-thrive
(b) Excema
(c) Scoliosis
(d) Constipation

4) The anti-inflammatory diet is commonly prescribed to patients with which of the following conditions?
(a) Allergic disorders
(b) Rheumatoid arthritis
(c) Metabolic syndrome
(d) All of the above

5) An anti-inflammatory diet is characterized by modifying which of the following:
(a) Antioxidants and anti-inflammatory spices
(b) Fat, sugar, antioxidants, allergenic foods, and anti-inflammatory spices
(c) Fat, sugar, antioxidants, and allergenic foods
(d) None of the above

6) Which of the following fatty acids are involved in the metabolic pathway of linoleic acid to arachadonic acid?
(a) Eicosatraenoic acid
(b) Alpha-linolenic acid
(c) Gamma-linolenic acid
(d) Steridonic acid

7) According to current research, daily supplementation of which of the following antioxidants may reduce the likelihood of asthma exacerbations?
(a) Vitamin A
(b) Vitamin C
(c) Vitamin E
(d) All of the above

8) Match the diet in Column A with its appropriate principle in Column B.

Column A	Column B
Anti-Inflammatory Diet	(a) Prescribed for food sensitivities
Specific Carbohydrate Diet	(b) Indicated in Maldigestion/Malabsorption
Elimination Diet	(c) Increases foods high in antioxidants

9) Asthma is the most common chronic disease of childhood. In clinical practice, which of the following diets has been shown to be most beneficial in the treatment of asthma in children and adults?
(a) Elimination Diet
(b) Specific Carbohydrate Diet
(c) Anti-Inflammatory Diet
(d) None of the above

10) Including dietary antioxidants on a regular basis may help reduce systemic inflammation. Which of the following foods and/or beverages are an excellent source of antioxidants?
(a) Ginger
(b) Green tea
(c) Dark green leafy and cruciferous vegetables
(d) All of the above

11) Which of the following statements is true concerning the purpose of the anti-inflammatory diet?
(a) To decrease omega-3 fatty acids and increase omega-6 fatty acids, saturated fats and trans fatty acids
(b) To increase omega-3 fatty acids and decrease omega-6 fatty acids, saturated fats and trans fatty acids
(c) To increase omega-3 fatty acids and increase omega-6 fatty acids, saturated fat and trans fatty acids
(d) To decrease omega-3 fatty acids and decrease omega-6 fatty acids, saturated fats and trans fatty acids

12) Which of the following dietary regimens is most likely to increase postprandial insulin levels and promote inflammation?
(a) Low carbohydrate, low fiber diets
(b) High carbohydrate, high fiber diets
(c) High carbohydrate, low fiber diets
(d) Low carbohydrate, high fiber diets

13) Which of the following vegetable oils contains the highest amount of omega-3 fatty acids per serving?
(a) Canola oil
(b) Safflower oil
(c) Flax seed oil
(d) Sunflower oil

Chapter 15: It's all about changing behaviors

1) RP is a 50-year-old male who comes to see his primary care clinician for a blood pressure check. He is 5'10" and weighs 190 pounds (BMI = 27). His blood pressure is 140/90. He works at a sedentary job and does not exercise on a regular basis. When he is asked to begin a walking program or join a gym to reduce his blood pressure, he states that he knows he "should" exercise but he is too busy and does not believe he can find time. Which of the following stages of change does RP exhibit in the Prochaska Model, based on his responses to the suggestion about increasing his exercise?
(a) Precontemplation
(b) Contemplation
(c) Preparation
(d) Action

2) FM is a 48-year-old female who makes an appointment with her primary care clinician for help with weight loss. She has tried lots of different diets in the past but is currently not doing anything about her weight. Which of the following stages of change does FM exhibit in the Prochaska Model, based on her request to lose weight at this time?
(a) Precontemplation
(b) Contemplation
(c) Action
(d) Relapse

3) Which of the following behavioral qualities in a practitioner has been shown to facilitate positive behavior changes in patients?
(a) Empathy
(b) Warmth
(c) Genuineness
(d) All of the above

4) Which of the following statements best defines motivational interviewing?
(a) A group approach which can be used to provide support to help patients make changes
(b) A client-centered directive approach which helps patients explore and resolve ambivalence

(c) A Socratic approach in which the counselor asks patients to make choices about changes
(d) A counselor-centered approach which applies stages of change to help patients make changes

5) AD is a 37-year-old male who has followed a low-fat diet for the past five years after his father's cardiac bypass surgery. AD states that he just went on a cruise for his honeymoon and has been having difficulty getting back on his low-fat dietary regimen. Which of the following stages of change does AD fall into at this time?
(a) Precontemplation
(b) Contemplation
(c) Action
(d) Relapse

6) The National Cancer Institute's 5 A's Model for behavior change includes which of the following components?
(a) Ask, Abdicate, Answer, Agree, Abstract
(b) Answer, Attend, Allow, Acquaint, Acquire
(c) Assess, Advise, Agree, Assist, and Arrange
(d) Allow, Attain, Affiliate, Alter, Amend

7) Which of the following health care provider behaviors has been shown to be the most effective counseling technique across all behavior change models?
(a) Asking probing questions
(b) Interrupting to clarify statements
(c) Taking notes during the interview
(d) Active listening

8) Current evidence suggests that behavior change is most effective when it is?
(a) Initiated by a consultant
(b) Reinforced by patient education materials
(c) Reinforced by the primary care clinician
(d) Discussed primarily by the registered dietitian

9) According to the American Heart Association's physical activity recommendations, how many days per week should an individual engage in at least 30 minutes of exercise?
(a) One day a week
(b) Two days a week
(c) Three days a week
(d) Most days of the week

10) GR is a 53-year-old male who is being treated by his primary care clinician for diabetes and hypertension. As part of his treatment, he is referred to the local hospital to attend a Diabetes Education Program for one week. He is then scheduled for follow-up in the primary care office and asked about what changes he has made. Which step in the 5 A's Model does this referral process represent?
(a) Advise
(b) Arrange
(c) Assist
(d) Assess

11) JJ is a 32-year-old female who is seeing her primary care clinician for the first time. JJ exercises 5 days a week and has been doing so for the past month to improve her health and lose weight. Which of the following stages of change does JJ exhibit in the Prochaska Model, based on her current exercise behavior?
(a) Contemplation
(b) Preparation
(c) Action
(d) Relapse

12) Which of the following questions represents the starting point for promoting behavior changes using the Choices and Change Model?
(a) How important do you feel that it is to make this change at this time?
(b) How confident do you feel that you can make this change at this time?
(c) How will it make you feel if you are able to make this change at this time?
(d) All of the above

Chapter 16: Community counts

1) Which statement best exemplifies the traditional role of the primary care clinician in promoting desired lifestyle changes for individuals?
(a) Advocates for physical activity and nutrition at school board meetings
(b) Negotiates with insurers for third party payment for nutrition and weight loss counseling and treatment
(c) Provides face to face counseling about nutrition and physical activity in the office/clinic setting
(d) Talks with legislators about needed regulations to help prevent obesity

2) Which of the following are evidence-based approaches to raising awareness of obesity? (May be more than one correct answer)
(a) Annual monitoring of patients' weight and BMI
(b) Measuring adults' waist circumference
(c) Plotting BMI on growth charts for children
(d) Telling the patient to reduce calorie intake

3) Which of the following are examples of environmental changes that primary care clinicians might consider in the work environment to improve awareness of healthy eating and physical activity?
(a) Providing a private location for women to breastfeed
(b) Hanging BMI charts in each exam room
(c) Having water available in the waiting room or office
(d) All of the above

4) Which of the following statements is an example of a policy change that would encourage healthy eating and physical activity?
(a) Providing non-candy treats such as stickers to pediatric patients
(b) Providing office staff with a 10 minute break twice a day in addition to their lunch
(c) Allowing sales representatives to bring food and beverages into the office for the physician and staff
(d) All of the above

5) Which of the following statements best identifies what schools should consider when sending BMI report cards home?
(a) Schools should expect that all parents will welcome the information
(b) Schools should explore the risks, benefits and costs of doing so in their environment
(c) Schools should make better use of tax dollars since all parents are aware of their children's weight
(d) Schools should use passive consent from children and their parents when implementing these BMI report cards

6) Which of the following statements is correct regarding teaching physical education in schools?
(a) If taught in schools, it guarantees each child gets 150 minutes/week of physical activity
(b) If negatively taught it affects test scores in math and science
(c) Is a curricular area that provides important skills
(d) Is only needed for elementary school children

7) Which of the following statements is correct regarding the Child Nutrition Program?
(a) Has control over the food and beverages available on school grounds
(b) Has standards that if followed provide healthy meals at affordable prices to students
(c) Is adequately funded to serve healthy meals to all children in public schools
(d) Serves similar portions of food to all students

8) The American Dietetic Association and the Centers for Disease Control and Prevention concluded that physical activity is an important tool to decrease childhood obesity. How much daily physical activity is required as a partial solution to this epidemic?
(a) 30 minutes/day
(b) 45 minutes/day
(c) 60 minutes/day
(d) 90 minutes/day

9) The socio-ecological model represents the positive and negative influences on the eating and physical activity behaviors of an individual. Which of the following are the main focuses of this model?
(a) Individual, Community, Physician and Public Policy
(b) Individual, Family, Organizations, Community and Public Policy
(c) Individual, Family, Community and Public Policy
(d) Individual, Family, Community, and Physician

10) Which of the following has resulted from the "No Child Left Behind" legislation that President Bush signed in 2002 with regard to physical education?
(a) Physical education is now listed as a "core" subject
(b) Physical education class time is increasing
(c) Physical education class size is decreasing
(d) Coaching positions are at risk in some communities

11) Arkansas is the first state to implement Health Report Cards. Results have concluded which of the following?
(a) The obesity epidemic among school-age youth is not significant in Arkansas
(b) Among overweight children, the health report card increased parental awareness of their child's weight status
(c) All states agree that sending health report cards is an effective action plan
(d) None of the above

12) Which of the following statements is correct about the healthcare environment?
(a) The skilled clinician is required to audit the office to see if change is warranted
(b) The healthcare environment is required to support healthy behaviors
(c) The motivated patient is required to make lifestyle changes for good health and well being
(d) All of the above

13) One natural outcome of childhood obesity screening is the need for treatment services. Which of the following statements is correct regarding developing programs to treat the childhood obesity epidemic?
(a) Most states have adequate 3rd party reimbursement for weight management programs
(b) Weight programs should set health, rather than weight goals
(c) Weight management programs that involve parents are not used properly
(d) All of the above

Chapter 17: Cultural considerations

1) Which of the following statements is correct regarding ethnic minorities in the US?
(a) Ethnic minorities will make up one-third of the US population by the year 2015
(b) Ethnic minorities will make up one-fourth of the US population by the year 2015
(c) Ethnic minorities will make up one-half of the US population by the year 2015
(d) None of the above

2) Which of the following common cultural beliefs of the major US ethnic minorities may impact health behavior?
(a) Strong family values
(b) Involvement with folk medicine
(c) Strong religiosity or spirituality
(d) All of the above

3) Which of the following statements is correct?
(a) Culturally based food habits are often one of the first traditions people change
(b) Inclusion of family members in medical decision-making is not important for most ethnic minority groups
(c) Stereotyping based on race/ethnicity can lead to biased or discriminatory treatment of patients
(d) Ethnic minority patients are more likely than white patients to receive physician advice on prevention

4) To become culturally competent one must achieve which of the following skills or behaviors? (May be more than one correct answer)
(a) Knowledge about different cultural perspectives
(b) Learning a set of "facts" about cultural competency
(c) Respect for different cultural perspectives
(d) Proficiency in cross cultural communication

5) An effective approach to cross-cultural nutrition counseling is implementing a five-step process called the LEARN approach. What does the acronym LEARN stand for?
(a) Listen, Explain, Acknowledge, Recommend, Negotiate
(b) Listen, Encourage, Assess, Recognize, Negotiate
(c) Listen, Encourage, Advise, Respond, Negotiate
(d) Listen, Endorse, Assist, Reply, Negotiate

6) Which of the following statements is correct?
(a) Ethnic minorities in the US experience a disproportionate burden of preventable disease, death, and disability compared with non-minorities.
(b) Health disparities are more likely caused by environmental, behavioral, and sociopolitical factors than genetic factors.
(c) Among most immigrant groups, number of years of residence in the US is associated with increased body mass index (BMI).
(d) All of the above

7) Which of the following risk factors for cardiovascular disease (CVD) are found to be significantly higher in the Black-American population compared to whites?
(a) Low density lipoprotein levels
(b) Cigarette smoking
(c) Hypertension
(d) Hypertriglyceridemia

8) Which of the statements below may help explain why Black-Americans are at greater risk for CVD than whites?
(a) Black-Americans have higher rates of cigarette smoking than whites
(b) Black-Americans have higher rates of obesity than whites
(c) Black-Americans have higher cholesterol levels than whites
(d) All of the above

9) Asian Indian immigrants to the U.S. include individuals from which of the following countries?
(a) India, both North and South
(b) India, Nepal and Malaysia
(c) Pakistan and Afghanistan
(d) India, Pakistan and Bangladesh

10) Which of the following nutrition messages should Black-American patients focus on?
(a) Increase carbohydrate intake
(b) Reduce sodium and saturated fat intake
(c) Increase intake of dairy products
(d) Increase protein intake

11) Which of the following traditional or emerging risk factors for coronary heart disease (CHD) are found to be significantly higher in the Asian Indian population compared to European Americans?
(a) Lipoprotein (a)
(b) Low density lipoprotein (LDL) cholesterol
(c) Cigarette smoking
(d) Family history of premature CHD disease

12) Which statement below may help to explain why Asian Indians living in the U.S. are at greater risk for CVD compared to their Caucasian counterparts?
(a) Asian Indians have higher LDL cholesterol levels compared to Caucasians
(b) Asian Indians have a greater body mass index compared to Caucasians
(c) Asian Indians are 4.5 times more likely than Caucasians to have diabetes
(d) All of the above

13) Which of the following CVD risk factors is found to be significantly higher in the Hispanic population compared to other ethnic groups?
(a) Hypertriglyceridemia
(b) Cigarette smoking
(c) Lipoprotein(a)
(d) All of the above

14) Which of the following health problems is significantly higher in the Hispanic population compared to Non-Hispanic whites?
(a) Cardiovascular disease
(b) Diabetes
(c) Hypercholesterolemia
(d) Breast cancer

15) Which of the following dietary behaviors is most likely to occur when Hispanics become acculturated in the U.S.?
(a) Increased intake of fat
(b) Increased intake of complex carbohydrates
(c) Increased intake of protein
(d) Increased intake of dairy foods

Review answers

Chapter 1: Nutrition and the primary care clinician

1) d
2) d
3) c
4) c
5) b
6) d
7) b
8) a
9) a,c,d
10) b
11) a

Chapter 2: Changing office culture to make it work

1) b,c
2) d
3) a,c,d
4) c
5) a
6) d
7) a
8) d
9) b,a,c
10) a,b
11) c,d

Chapter 3: Methods of weight control

1) b
2) a,b
3) b
4) d
5) a
6) b
7) b
8) d
9) c
10) c
11) b
12) a
13) a
14) b
15) d

Chapter 4: Growing up healthy

1) b
2) a
3) d
4) c
5) b
6) a
7) a
8) b
9) c
10) d
11) c
12) a
13) c

Chapter 5: Feeding the mother-to-be

1) c
2) c
3) a
4) d
5) d
6) b
7) c
8) b
9) d
10) b
11) c
12) a

Chapter 6: Staying healthy in later life

1) b
2) c
3) c
4) a
5) c
6) b
7) d
8) b
9) d
10) b
11) c
12) c
13) d

Chapter 7: Dyslipidemia, hypertension and metabolic syndrome

1) c
2) a
3) b
4) a
5) c
6) d
7) c
8) b
9) d
10) b
11) d
12) c
13) a

Chapter 8: Pre-diabetes, diabetes and hyperglycemia

1) c
2) b
3) c
4) a
5) c
6) d
7) c
8) b
9) a
10) d
11) b
12) b

Chapter 9: Gastrointestinal disorders

1) a
2) a,b,d
3) b
4) c
5) b
6) a,b,c,d
7) c
8) b
9) a,b,d
10) a
11) a,b,d
12) c

Chapter 10: Everything else

1) c
2) a
3) c
4) a,b,d
5) a,d
6) b
7) b
8) d,c,b,a
9) a,b,d
10) c
11) a
12) a
13) b

Chapter 11: Vitamins

1) a
2) c
3) a
4) a
5) a
6) d
7) a
8) b
9) c
10) b
11) c
12) b
13) c

Chapter 12: Minerals

1) a
2) d
3) c
4) d
5) d,c,b,a
6) b
7) b,c
8) a
9) b
10) c
11) b

Chapter 13: Dietary and nutritional supplements

1) b
2) a
3) c
4) d
5) b
6) d
7) d
8) c
9) b
10) c
11) a
12) c
13) a,d

Chapter 14: Considering the alternatives

1) d
2) a
3) b
4) d
5) b
6) c
7) b
8) c,b,a
9) a
10) d
11) b
12) c
13) c

Chapter 15: It's all about changing behaviors

1) a
2) b
3) d
4) b
5) d
6) c
7) d
8) c
9) d
10) b
11) c
12) d

Chapter 16: Community counts

1) c
2) a,b,c
3) d
4) a
5) b
6) c
7) b
8) c
9) b
10) d
11) b
12) d
13) b

Chapter 17: Cultural considerations

1) a
2) d
3) c
4) a,c,d
5) a
6) d
7) c
8) b
9) d
10) b
11) a
12) c
13) a
14) b
15) a

Index

abdominal pain, and IBS, 191
acid reflux. *See* gastroesophageal reflux disease
acquired immunodeficiency virus (AIDS)
  food safety issues, 216
  nutritional risk stratification, 213–214
  symptom nutritional guidelines, 214–218
active listening technique, 319
acupuncture, 293
adolescents
  and diabetes, 166
  physical activity requirements, 78
  and pregnancy, 96–97
  and vegetarianism, 81
Adult Treatment Panel III (ATP III), 135, 136, 138, 148
AFFECTS Questionnaire, 18
African Americans
  and cardiovascular disease, 347–348
  and childhood obesity, 60, 61
  and diabetes, 347
  dietary recommendations for, 350
  disease prevalence, 347–348
  folk remedies, 342
  and gestational diabetes mellitus, 98
  and lactose deficiency, 180
  traditional cuisine of, 348–350
alcohol. *See also* fetal alcohol syndrome; maternal alcoholism; National Institute of Alcohol Abuse and Alcoholism
  and cirrhosis, 194
  and diabetes, 165
  and hypertension, 145–146
  and magnesium excretion, 252
  and migraine headaches, 204
allergies
  elimination diet, 296–297
  and infants, 72–73
  testing for, 294

American Academy of Family Physicians (AAFP), 106, 329, 332
American Academy of Pediatrics (AAP), 62, 101, 106, 332
American Diabetes Association (ADA), 98, 147, 163, 171
American Dietetic Association, 24, 101, 106
American Heart Association, 140
American Medical Association (Council on Scientific Affairs), 92
Americans in Motion program, 329
anemia. *See* dilutional anemia; iron deficiency anemia; megaloblastic anemia; nutritional anemia; pernicious anemia
anorexia nervosa, 80–81, 124, 194
anthropometrics/vital signs assessments, 32
antihypertensive therapy, 144–145
anti-inflammatory diet, 301–304
  antioxidant aspect of, 304
  carbohydrate modifications, 303–304
  fat aspect of, 301–303
  food sensitivities/elimination trial, 304–305
  herbs/spices, 304
appointment system, of primary care clinicians, 16–17
arachidonic acid, 302
ascites, and cirrhosis, 195
ascorbic acid. *See* Vitamin C
Ashkenazi Jews, and lactose deficiency, 180
Asians
  disease prevalence, 354–355
  and lactose deficiency, 180
  traditional cuisine, 355–357
assessment
  of biochemical data, 35
  models for, 16
  of patient readiness, 4
  transtheoretical dietary model, 313, 314

ANSWER SHEET/ENROLLMENT FORM FOR DIETITIANS AND DIETETIC TECHNICIANS

Continuing Professional Education: Level 3

The Complete Guide to Nutrition in Primary Care
Edited by Darwin Deen, MD and Lisa Hark, PhD, RD

This self-study learning activity is pre-approved for **42 credits** by the American Dietetic Association, Commission on Dietetic Registration. Credits are awarded for the completion of the entire book, you can not received credits for individual chapters. There are no additional charges for credits. Follow the instructions below.

1. Read *The Complete Guide to Nutrition in Primary Care*, and complete the test questions in the back of the book after completing each chapter.
    Write the correct answers on the dietitian answer sheet.

2. Grade yourself using the answers in *The Complete Guide to Nutrition in Primary Care*. Successful completion of this independent learning activity requires that you attain at least 80% correct (>172 correct). If you do not attain this score, retest yourself again and indicate the corrected score on the form. Please note, credits are awarded for completion of the entire book only.

3. If you are on the ADA Professional Development Portfolio, you do not need to submit any forms to ADA. Following the directions in #4. If your state requires licensure, the Certificate of Completion is at the back of the book. YOU DO NOT SEND ANY FORMS TO THE PROVIDER.

4. Visit ADA Professional Development Portfolio (www.cdrnet.org).
    Log in and enter the following information into your activity log:
    Activity Title: *The Complete Guide to Nutrition in Primary Care*
    Activity Type: Conventional: Self-Study Print
    Activity Topic: CL0000: Clinical Nutrition
    Learning Need: 5000: Medical Nutrition Therapy CPE Level: 3
    42 CPE Credit Units from September 1, 2007 to August 31, 2010

THERE ARE NO ADDITIONAL CHARGES FROM ADA. MORE THAN ONE DIETITIAN MAY READ THE BOOK AND COPY THIS FORM AND THE ANSWER SHEET. THIS INDEPENDENT LEARNING ACTIVITY IS VALID UNTIL AUGUST 31, 2010.

Name _____ Credentials _____
ADA Registration # _____ Date completed _____
Address _____
_____
City _____ State _____ Zip _____
Email _____

Provider questions contact Dr. Lisa Hark, (215) 349-5795 or email to lhark@mail.med.upenn.edu. For more information, contact our web site at www.lisahark.com.

Pre-approved by the: American Dietetic Association,
Commission on Dietetic Registration

Continuing Professional Education
Certificate of Completion for Dietitians and Dietetic Technicians

Title of Program: The Complete Guide to Nutrition in Primary Care
Edited by Darwin Deen, MD and Lisa Hark, PhD, RD

Program Provider's Name: Lisa Hark, PhD, RD
Activity Type: 720: Conventional: Self-Study Print
Activity Topic: CL0000: Clinical Nutrition
Learning Need: 5000: Medical Nutrition Therapy CPE Level: 3
Approved for 42 CPE Credit Units from September 1, 2007 to August 31, 2010

ATTENDEE COPY

Participant Name
Registration Number
Date Completed

Pre-approved by the: American Dietetic Association,
Commission on Dietetic Registration

Continuing Professional Education
Certificate of Completion for Dietitians and Dietetic Technicians

Title of Program: The Complete Guide to Nutrition in Primary Care
Edited by Darwin Deen, MD and Lisa Hark, PhD, RD

Program Provider's Name: Lisa Hark, PhD, RD
Activity Type: 720: Conventional: Self-Study Print
Activity Topic: CL0000: Clinical Nutrition
Learning Need: 5000: Medical Nutrition Therapy CPE Level: 3
Approved for 42 CPE Credit Units from September 1, 2007 to August 31, 2010

STATE LICENSURE COPY

Participant Name
Registration Number
Date Completed

ANSWER SHEET FOR REGISTERED DIETITIANS and DTRs

The Complete Guide to Nutrition in Primary Care

Fill in the correct answers and grade yourself when finished. Expiration date: August 31, 2010. DO NOT SEND ANY FORMS TO ADA OR THE PROVIDER.
Complete the other side. No additional self-reporting form is needed.
Visit the ADA Professional Development Portfolio (www.cdrnet.org).
Log in and enter the following information into your activity log:
Activity Title: *The Complete Guide to Nutrition in Primary Care*
Activity Type: Conventional: Self-Study Print
Activity Topic: CL0000: Clinical Nutrition
Learning Need: 5000: Medical Nutrition Therapy CPE Level 3
Approved for: 42 CPE Credit Units from September 1, 2007 to August 31, 2010
More than one dietitian may read the book and copy these forms. There are no fees.
Credits are awarded for completion of the entire book only, not for individual chapters.

Chapter 1	Chapter 2	Chapter 3	Chapter 4
1)	1)	1)	1)
2)	2)	2)	2)
3)	3)	3)	3)
4)	4)	4)	4)
5)	5)	5)	5)
6)	6)	6)	6)
7)	7)	7)	7)
8)	8)	8)	8)
9)	9)	9)	9)
10)	10)	10)	10)
11)	11)	11)	11)
		12)	12)
		13)	13)
		14)	
		15)	

Chapter 5	Chapter 6	Chapter 7	Chapter 8
1)	1)	1)	1)
2)	2)	2)	2)
3)	3)	3)	3)
4)	4)	4)	4)
5)	5)	5)	5)
6)	6)	6)	6)
7)	7)	7)	7)
8)	8)	8)	8)
9)	9)	9)	9)
10)	10)	10)	10)
11)	11)	11)	11)
12)	12)	12)	12)
	13)	13)	

Chapter 9	Chapter 10	Chapter 11	Chapter 12
1)	1)	1)	1)
2)	2)	2)	2)
3)	3)	3)	3)
4)	4)	4)	4)
5)	5)	5)	5)
6)	6)	6)	6)
7)	7)	7)	7)
8)	8)	8)	8)
9)	9)	9)	9)
10)	10)	10)	10)
11)	11)	11)	11)
12)	12)	12)	
	13)	13)	

Chapter 13	Chapter 14	Chapter 15	Chapter 16
1)	1)	1)	1)
2)	2)	2)	2)
3)	3)	3)	3)
4)	4)	4)	4)
5)	5)	5)	5)
6)	6)	6)	6)
7)	7)	7)	7)
8)	8)	8)	8)
9)	9)	9)	9)
10)	10)	10)	10)
11)	11)	11)	11)
12)	12)	12)	12)
13)	13)		13)

Chapter 17
1)
2)
3)
4)
5)
6)
7)
8)
9)
10)
11)
12)
13)
14)
15)

Correct _____ /215 _____

Answers to these questions are located in *The Complete Guide to Nutrition in Primary Care*. Completion of this independent learning activity requires that you attain at least 80% correct (>172 correct). If not, retest yourself and indicate the corrected score on the form. You do not need to send this form to anyone once you have logged this activity with CDR. Questions, please call Lisa Hark, PhD, RD at 215-349-5795, lhark@mail.med.upenn.edu